Anesthesia of the Upper Limb

Fernando Alemanno
Mario Bosco · Aldo Barbati
Editors

Anesthesia of the Upper Limb

A State of the Art Guide

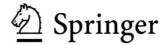

Editors
Fernando Alemanno
Institute of Anesthesiology
Resuscitation and Pain Therapy
University of Verona
Verona
Italy

Aldo Barbati
Pain Therapy Service
Padre Pio Hospital
Mondragone, CE
Italy

Mario Bosco
Department of Anesthesiology
and Critical Care Medicine
Catholic University of the Sacred Heart
Rome
Italy

ISBN 978-88-470-5417-2   ISBN 978-88-470-5418-9   (eBook)
DOI 10.1007/978-88-470-5418-9
Springer Milan Heidelberg New York Dordrecht London

Library of Congress Control Number: 2013939040

The contents of this book are based on: L'Anestesia dell'arto superiore. F. Alemanno, M. Bosco, A.Barbati (eds)
© Verduci Editore 2011 Translated from the Italian by Anthony Steele MA (Oxon), former Senior Lecturer in Medical English. Faculty of Medicine and Surgery, University of Verona.

© Springer-Verlag Italia 2014
This work is subject to copyright. All rights are reserved by the Publisher, whether the whole or part of the material is concerned, specifically the rights of translation, reprinting, reuse of illustrations, recitation, broadcasting, reproduction on microfilms or in any other physical way, and transmission or information storage and retrieval, electronic adaptation, computer software, or by similar or dissimilar methodology now known or hereafter developed. Exempted from this legal reservation are brief excerpts in connection with reviews or scholarly analysis or material supplied specifically for the purpose of being entered and executed on a computer system, for exclusive use by the purchaser of the work. Duplication of this publication or parts thereof is permitted only under the provisions of the Copyright Law of the Publisher's location, in its current version, and permission for use must always be obtained from Springer. Permissions for use may be obtained through RightsLink at the Copyright Clearance Center. Violations are liable to prosecution under the respective Copyright Law.
The use of general descriptive names, registered names, trademarks, service marks, etc. in this publication does not imply, even in the absence of a specific statement, that such names are exempt from the relevant protective laws and regulations and therefore free for general use.
While the advice and information in this book are believed to be true and accurate at the date of publication, neither the authors nor the editors nor the publisher can accept any legal responsibility for any errors or omissions that may be made. The publisher makes no warranty, express or implied, with respect to the material contained herein.

Printed on acid-free paper

Springer is part of Springer Science+Business Media (www.springer.com)

It would be easier for me to list the defects and flaws of this book rather than its merits and positive qualities. Before putting pen to paper I knew that I would inevitably have come to this conclusion, but I wrote the book all the same because I enjoyed writing it, and because I hope someone will enjoy reading it…..

Indro Montanelli,
The History of the Greeks
Rizzoli Editore, Milan 1959

This book is dedicated to the memory of Andrea Casati who we shall always remember as the worthiest young representative of Italian anesthesiology at the turn of the millennium.

Fernando Alemanno
Mario Bosco
Aldo Barbati

About the Editors

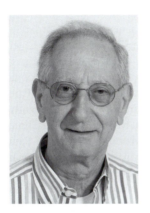

Fernando Alemanno born in Scorzé (Venice). Graduated in Medicine and Surgery at the University of Ferrara. Postgraduate specialization in Anesthesia and Resuscitation at Padua University. Hospital career as Assistant, Padua University General Hospital Anesthesia and Resuscitation Service; Jointly Responsible Head Deputy, Treviso Regional Hospital; Head of Department, Bolzano Regional Hospital. Contract Professor, Institute of Anesthesiology, University of Verona, where he continues to deliver lectures and hold conferences every year. Professor Alemanno has been a speaker at numerous national and international congresses and ECM accredited courses. He has published 36 scientific papers in national and international journals and chapters of books regarding anesthesiology, intensive care, and pain therapy. He is the author of an original brachial plexus block technique. He is a member of the scientific societies SIAARTI and ESRA.

fernando@alemannobpb.it
www.alemannobpb.it

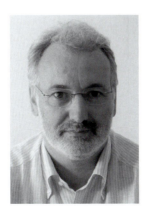

Mario Bosco born in Palermo. Graduated in Medicine and Surgery at the Catholic University of the Sacred Heart, Rome. Postgraduate specialization in Anesthesiology and Resuscitation at the same university. His current post is Head of a 'Simple Structure' with functions of coordination and acting Director of the Operative Unit of Anesthesiology and Resuscitation of the Columbus Integrated Complex, Catholic University of the Sacred Heart, Rome, where he also works as a Researcher and Lecturer in the Postgraduate School of Anesthesiology and Resuscitation. He is the author of more than 100 scientific publications in national and international journals, chapters of texts, and monographic studies. He has been a speaker at numerous congresses, meetings, and accredited ECM updating courses. He has also organized congresses, seminars, and ECM accredited updating courses on regional anesthesia, anesthesia in odontostomatology, intravenous anesthesia, and pain therapy. He is the author of an original technique for performing parasacral sciatic nerve blocks. He is a member of the scientific societies SIAARTI, ESRA (board member, treasurer), AINOS (board member), ESA and World-SIVA (founder member).

mbosco@rm.unicatt.it

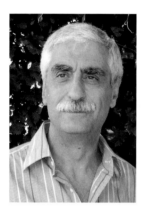

Aldo Barbati born in Avella (AV). Graduated in Medicine and Surgery with postgraduate specialization in Anesthesia and Resuscitation at the Federic II University of Naples. Hospital career: Assistant and later chef of the Pain Unit at the Orthopedic Department of the A. Cardarelli Hospital, Naples. Medical Director and Chief Anesthetist at the Casa di Cura Santa Maria di Castellanza (VA) and then for the 'Policlinico di Monza' Group. Medical Director of the Pain Unit at the Cava de' Tirreni Hospital. Currently he works as a Consultant for the Padre Pio Clinic in Mondragone (CE) where he is Head of Pain Therapy. His publications mainly relate to topics in the field of regional anesthesia and pain therapy, with more than 90 scientific papers published in national and international journals. He has also written books and manuals as well as chapters in Italian and overseas books on invitation. He has been President of FADO (Forum of Anesthesia and Pain in Orthopedics and Traumatology) and board member of the Italian Chapter of ESRA. He is currently a board member of SIARED.

aldobarbati@hotmail.com

Foreword

In the year commemorating the unity of Italy I am pleased to present this book which in some ways epitomizes that unity over the past 150 years. The book is the fruit of the work of three authors who have shared the by no means easy task of writing a monographic study on brachial plexus anesthesia, a topic already expertly addressed in the past by both Italian and non-Italian authors. Perhaps, by some curious geographical coincidence, the authors divided the task between them and addressed the subject matter in three sections: the topographically higher, supraclavicular techniques were addressed by Fernando Alemanno, resident in Alto Adige (northern Italy); the intermediate, infraclavicular, and axillary techniques were addressed by Mario Bosco, resident in Rome (central Italy), while the topographically lower techniques, the truncular anesthesia techniques, were addressed by Aldo Barbati of Naples (southern Italy).

An important aspect of this work is also the collaboration of many other specialists who have devoted years of work and study to the brachial plexus block techniques and more besides, despite each of them continuing to practice general anesthesia, intensive care and pain therapy, regarding the perfection of these techniques not as time taken away from the study of the others, but as the possibility of integrating them overall with a view to optimizing the results.

A great deal of importance has been attributed to the iconography. The advent of ultrasound as applied to regional anesthesia that has occurred over the past decade has made it possible to extend the study of anatomy from the purely dissective realm, as pertaining strictly to the anatomical theater, burdened with all manner of logistic and legislative difficulties, to the virtual '*in corpore viri*' realm of the ultrasound image in which the scholar can compare the real, individual anatomy and all its variants, with his or her memories of classical anatomy learnt in books and atlases and above all in the anatomical theater. We should, in fact, stress that the fluorescent screen of the ultrasound appliance fails to show the minimal details that can be noted in the dissecting room, and therefore ultrasound anatomy cannot do without a sound knowledge of normal human anatomy.

I would like to emphasize once again that the three authors have succeeded in demonstrating that the solving of problems not only in terms of content, but also in terms of organization, including not least those in the publishing sphere, can only come about as a result of a profitable effort of collaboration and integration on the part of the many centers of excellence present in Italy. We are always hearing the media talking about the 'brain drain' and the success Italians are achieving abroad and would never have been able to achieve in Italy. In my opinion, this is only partly true; the real reason for the success lies in the basic scientific preparation of our scholars and their culture. With these two qualities, combined with a good measure of determination and tenacity, characteristic of Italians when they want to achieve their goals, it is not difficult to emerge. An anonymous, yet able surgeon whose pupil I was, on and off, at the start of my professional career, pronounced the following judgement:

> "Doctor, when you know your trade and know why you do things one way rather than another, you can go wherever you like."

It is equally true that many Italians have the defect of overrating everything that is produced abroad and of underrating everything produced in Italy, thus confirming the old adage that 'no man is a prophet in his own land'.

Regional anesthesia is a vast, continuously developing science, because it is constantly being enriched both as a result of the discovery of new drugs and as a result of the development of new techniques. In parallel with the technological progress made over the last two decades, there has been a substantial upsurge of literature in specialist and non-specialist journals, monographic studies, and treatises regarding regional anesthesia. The present volume helps the reader to familiarize himself with the current state of the art of the subject. Its aim is to provide both a summary of what one needs to know and an open window on a world no longer destined to be a domain reserved only to a few specialists dedicated to orthopedic anesthesia, but rather the common heritage of many others who use their anesthetic skills for vascular surgery or for reconstructive plastic surgery or surgery of the hand.

Anesthesia of the Upper Limb, first published in Italian on the occasion of the centenary (1911–2011) of the execution of the first two types of percutaneous brachial plexus block (Hirschel's axillary block and Kulenkampff's supraclavicular block), presents itself as a book with an admirable typographical layout, aimed not only at expert anesthetists, but also at postgraduate students lacking specific know-how who have just completed their undergraduate courses and set out on the task of acquiring the basic knowledge indispensable for their specialist training.

A book can express two fundamental, didactic options, one more extensive in scope and with greater in-depth detail, and the other, no less complete, but more agile and essential. The authors of this volume have succeeded in producing a commendable fusion of these two qualities and, while being fully aware that most of what they were saying had already been written, they have often succeeded in dealing with the various topics in a simple, laid-back manner, in such a way as to make for enjoyable reading.

Rome

Prof. Rodolfo Proietti
Director of the Postgraduate School of
Anesthesiology and Resuscitation
Catholic University of the Sacred Heart

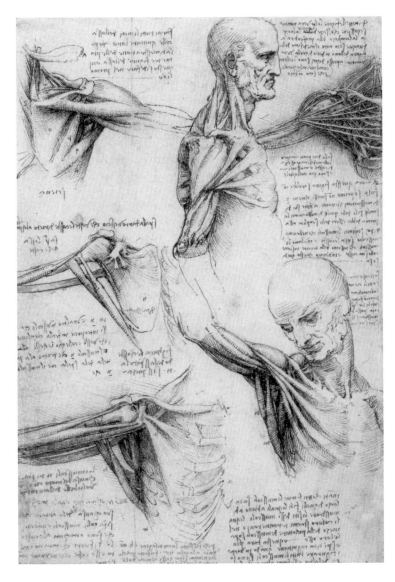

Leonardo Da Vinci "Study of head and shoulder" 1509–1510

Preface

The second decade of the last century was a magical time for regional anesthesia of the upper extremity. It was the period that witnessed the advent of the four most important percutaneous brachial plexus block techniques: Hirschel's axillary technique on July 18 and Kulenkampff's supraclavicular technique on October 7, Kappis posterior approach in 1912 followed by Barny's infraclavicular approach in 1914.

The centenary of these first two percutaneous brachial plexus blocks coincided with the publication in Italian of this monographic study, which, in addition to tracing the evolution of the various block techniques that followed the first two in the course of time, focuses on the more modern methods, particularly with a view to their safety.

The aim of this volume is to present the fruit of a 100 years' experience in the field of the regional anesthesia of the upper limb, it being understood that these 100 years not only represent the historical period dating from the execution of the first two blocks to the present day, but also the sum total of the years of study, application, and experience that each of the three authors has spent in this extraordinary branch of anesthesiology.

Regional anesthesia presents indubitable advantages in almost all branches of surgery, because it combines perfect anesthesia with long-lasting postoperative analgesia and above all, if applied to orthopedic traumatology, it affords the best prophylaxis of reflex sympathetic dystrophy.

Anesthesia of the upper extremity came strongly to the fore with the advent, on the one hand, of hand surgery and, on the other, of arthroscopic and prosthetic surgery of the shoulder.

Particular care has been taken in the chapters on the anatomy and topographic anatomy of the region where the brachial plexus originates and develops, providing an adequate complement of iconographical material, ably assisted in this by Eduard Egarter Vigl, an anatomist of the Munich School, and Head of the Institute of Pathological Anatomy of Bolzano Regional Hospital, famous worldwide for his studies and research regarding the Similaun mummy. We believe, in fact, that a sound knowledge of anatomy is fundamental for the anesthetist who has to penetrate tissues, fascias and muscles, avoiding vessels, meninges and serosas, despite being equipped with two important instruments such as electrical nerve stimulation and ultrasound. The closing decade of the twentieth century witnessed a major revolution in electrostimulation, which definitively supplanted the old method of paresthesias provoked by nerve puncture. Above all, with the paresthesia system it was difficult to establish exactly which nerve was being stimulated, even in a calm, compliant patient. The sensation provoked was generally strong, unpleasant, and approximate.

> "Neurostimulation is a unique instrument because it clearly reveals the direct relationship between anatomy and physiology," said Alain Borgeat, speaking about electrical nerve stimulation as applied to the axillary block: "... neurostimulation is a wonderful teaching tool; within two minutes you can demonstrate the triple innervation of the thumb—abduction, radial nerve, adduction, ulnar nerve, and opposition, median nerve. No resident will ever forget such a picture ..."

In the third millennium the great novelty consists in the use of ultrasound guidance which, with the perfecting of the technology, is increasingly proving to be more precise, particularly as regards its resolution capability. This is a technique capable of visualizing the various nerves, which is unquestionably extremely helpful, without, however, being able to analyze them, and this constitutes one of its limitations. For this reason, the anesthetist is obliged to resort to the simultaneous use of the electrostimulator, also because, in most ultrasound appliances in use in the departments, the visualization is still two-dimensional, which may lead to a substantial parallax error, and the resolution capacity is not always optimal. To conclude, we agree with Admir Hadzic when he says...

> "electrostimulation and ultrasound guidance are complementary, and not two mutually exclusive technologies".

This book is also designed above all for a readership of young colleagues in the hope that it will help them to master the difficult art of regional anesthesia, despite being applied to a limited sector of the human body. In any event, the chapters on conscious sedation, on the use of perineural adjuvants, and on postoperative analgesia in all its forms are also applicable to other sectors of regional anesthesia. We have sought to give this book a fundamentally didactic slant, with the result that certain concepts or procedures may seem boringly repetitive in different chapters, but this is intentional—*repetita iuvant* ('repetition helps'). We have, however, also attempted to adopt a narrative approach in certain chapters so as to render the account simpler, more attractive, and therefore easier to memorize. We hope that, just as we enjoyed ourselves writing this book, so our readers will enjoy reading it.

Fernando Alemanno
Mario Bosco
Aldo Barbati

Acknowledgments

The authors wish to thank:

Professor Carlo D. Franco, Doctors Elfriede Prinnegg, Marta Putzu, James Oscar Quinto and Ann Davies for their critical revision of a number of chapters;

Doctors Philipp Agostini, Guido Botter, Claus Pfundmair, and Ludwig Rogg for their important bibliographical contribution; Ms. Francesca Alemanno, Lara Botticini, Carla Di Bella, Roberta Gnali, Gabriella Marinoni, and Mr. Simone Tomasotti for their invaluable iconographic contribution.

Contents

1. **Anatomy of the Brachial Plexus** 1
   F. Alemanno and E. Egarter Vigl

2. **Topographical Anatomy** 19
   F. Alemanno and E. Egarter Vigl

3. **Anatomy of the Cervical Plexus** 37
   F. Alemanno and E. Egarter Vigl

4. **The Anesthetic Line** 41
   P. Grossi

5. **Electrical Nerve Stimulation and Percutaneous Identification of the Target** 45
   L. Perotti, M. Allegri, A. Matteazzi and P. Grossi

6. **Supraclavicular Brachial Plexus Block Techniques** 55
   F. Alemanno

7. **Ultrasound-Guided Interscalene and Supraclavicular Blocks** 117
   Astrid U. Behr

8. **Complications of Supraclavicular Techniques** 141
   F. Alemanno

9. **Infraclavicular Brachial Plexus Block** 157
   M. Bosco and A. Clemente

10. **Axillary Brachial Plexus Block** 185
    M. Bosco and A. Clemente

11. **Truncular Blocks** 207
    A. Barbati

12. **Intravenous Retrograde Anesthesia** 225
    M. Raffa, M. Greco and A. Barbati

13	**Sedation in Regional Anesthesia**	231
	F. Alemanno and F. Auricchio	

14	**Perineural Adjuvants for Postoperative Analgesia**	253
	F. Alemanno	

15	**Postoperative Analgesia**	261
	F. Coluzzi	

16	**Stellate Ganglion Block**..........................	279
	F. Alemanno and B. Westermann	

Contributors

F. Alemanno Institute of Anesthesiology, Resuscitation and Pain Therapy, University of Verona, Verona, Italy

M. Allegri Anesthesia, Resuscitation and Pain Therapy Service, IRCCS Policlinico San Matteo, Pavia, Italy

F. Auricchio Anesthesia and Resuscitation Service, Bolzano Regional Hospital, Bolzano, Italy

A. Barbati Pain Therapy Service, Padre Pio Hospital, Mondragone, Caserta, Italy

Astrid U. Behr Department of Medicine DiMed, Anaesthesiology and Intensive Care Unit, University of Padua, Padua, Italy

M. Bosco Department of Anesthesiology and Critical Care Medicine, Catholic University of the Sacred Heart, Rome, Italy

A. Clemente Anesthesiology, Intensive Care and Pain Therapy Service, IRCCS-Immacolata Dermopathic Institute (I.D.I.), Rome, Italy

F. Coluzzi Department of Medico-Surgical Sciences and Biotechnologies, Faculty of Pharmacy and Medicine, Sapienza University, Rome, Italy

E. Egarter Vigl Institute of Pathological Anatomy, Bolzano Regional Hospital, Bolzano, Italy

M. Greco Simple Operative Unit, Resuscitation and Intensive Care, P.O. Ariano Irpino, Avellino Local Health Authority, Avellino, Italy

F. Grossi Pain Therapy and Regional Anesthesia Service, IRCCS Policlinico San Donato Milanese, Milan, Italy

A. Matteazzi Pain Therapy and Regional Anesthesia Service, IRCCS Policlinico San Donato Milanese, Milan, Italy

L. Perotti Anesthesia, Resuscitation and Pain Therapy Service, IRCCS Policlinico San Matteo, Pavia, Italy

P. Pippa Department of Anesthesia and Resuscitation, Orthopedic Traumatology Centre, University of Florence, Florence, Italy

A. Polletta San Filippo Neri Hospital, Rome, Italy

M. Raffa Complex Operative Unit, Anesthesia and Resuscitation, P.O. Ariano Irpino, Avellino Local Health Authority, Avellino, Italy

B. Westermann Division of Anesthesiology and Pain Medicine, Jeroen Bosch Ziekenhuis, Hertogenbosch, The Netherlands

Anatomy of the Brachial Plexus

F. Alemanno and E. Egarter Vigl

The brachial plexus is formed by the anterior divisions (ventral rami) of the somatic nerves C5, C6, C7, C8 and T1. It may also receive contributions from C4 which gives a branch to C5 and from T2 which gives a branch to T1. If this contribution is mainly or exclusively from C4, the plexus is defined by Winnie as 'prefixed', whereas when it comes largely or solely from T2, the plexus is defined as 'postfixed'.

Since all supraclavicular blocks are more effective on the cranial metameres of the plexus and may be inefficacious on the caudal ones, the prefixed brachial plexus condition is favourable for the purposes of shoulder surgery. Unfortunately, these configurations are unpredictable.

The brachial plexus is made up of roots, trunks, divisions and cords. When it comes to understanding the anatomy of the brachial plexus, that is, the disposition of its constituent elements, by far the clearest explanation is that provided by Testut, which we cite at some length here below (for the sake of greater clarity, we have taken the liberty of changing a few of the terms used in the old nomenclature, replacing them with terminology in current usage).

'The five anterior rami (anterior divisions of the spinal nerves constituting the roots of the brachial plexus; Editor's note), on emerging from the intervertebral foramina and the intertransverse spaces, behave as follows:

The fifth cervical nerve root, descending steeply laterally and obliquely, merges with the sixth root at an acute angle to form a single trunk, the upper primary trunk, which immediately splits into an upper and lower branch; the result is a capital X on its side (✕).

Likewise, the first thoracic nerve root ascends obliquely and merges with the eighth cervical root, the direction of which is almost horizontal; another trunk, the lower primary trunk, is thus formed which also divides into an upper and lower branch, producing another capital X on its side (✕), lower than the first one.

Between the two horizontal exes (✕) runs the seventh cervical nerve root, horizontally and in isolation, as far as the level of the first rib, where it splits into two branches, forming a sort of capital Y on its side (≺); the upper branch merges with the upper bifurcation of the X above, while the lower branch merges with the lower bifurcation of the X below.

The divisions of the primary trunks unite to form the three cords, namely the lateral, medial and posterior cords, which emit the terminal branches (nerves; Editor's note) of the brachial plexus.

F. Alemanno (✉)
Institute of Anesthesiology, Resuscitation and Pain Therapy, University of Verona, Verona, Italy
e-mail: fernando@alemannobpb.it

E. Egarter Vigl
Institute of Pathological Anatomy, Bolzano Regional Hospital, Bolzano, Italy

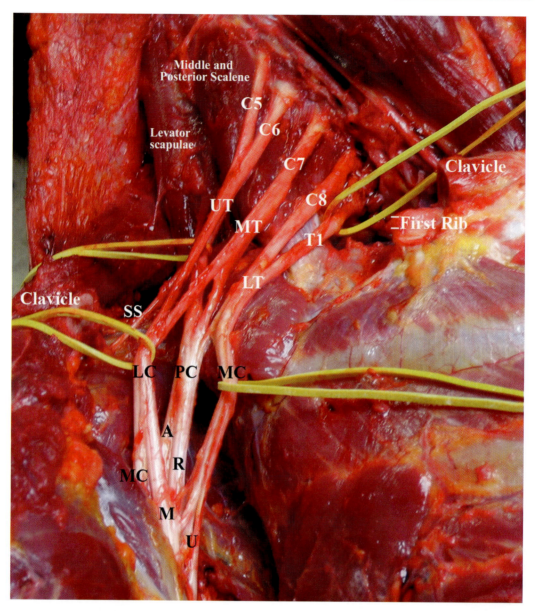

Fig. 1.1 *C5, C6, C7, C8, T1*: Brachial plexus roots; *UT, MT, LT* upper, middle and lower trunks; *SS* suprascapular nerve; *LC, MC, PC* lateral, medial and posterior cords; *A* axillary (or circumflex) nerve; *R* radial nerve; *MC* musculocutaneous nerve; *M* median nerve; *U* ulnar nerve. The clavicle, first rib, anterior scalene and the clavicular head of the sternocleidomastoid muscle have been removed

The above description, which is undoubtedly simple and schematic, is the description to be found in almost all textbooks, but is rarely observed in anatomical preparations, the actual anatomical make-up of the brachial plexus being much more complicated (Fig. 1.1).

1.1 Anatomical Disposition and Relationships

We shall now see where and how these nerves are placed in the cervico-thoracic area.

The cervical roots of the plexus, C5, C6, C7 and C8, pass behind the vertebral artery and after settling into their specific gutter on the respective transverse processes they are directed downwards and laterally towards the first rib, where they unite to form the trunks. The anterior division of the somatic nerve T1 (thoracic root of the lower primary trunk), on the other hand, passes in front of the neck of the first rib and then travels superiorly and laterally to join the root C8 at the level of the shallow groove the plexus itself produces in the first rib.

The trunks of the plexus are situated in the short tract between the inner edge of the anterolateral part of the first rib and the anterior edge of the clavicle. Just after emerging at the level of the anterior edge of the clavicle, the distal divisions of the trunks unite, as mentioned above, to form the three cords of the brachial plexus.

At this point, however, some further clarification is needed: whereas the proximal branches (roots) of the two X's are orientated vertically, the distal branches of the two X's and those of the Y (rami) descend obliquely and pass below the clavicle in the direction of the axilla, turning 90° clockwise on the right and counterclockwise on the left, the upper branches, thus becoming anterior and the lower branches posterior, respectively. In practice, on the way towards the thoraco-coracoid groove, the upper branches of the X's and the Y pass in front of the lower branches, whose position is no longer inferior but becomes posterior.

Therefore, to form the cords, the distal branches of the X's and Y (the rami of the brachial plexus) unite; the anterior divisions (initially superior) of the upper and middle trunks merge to form the lateral cord; the anterior division (initially superior) of the lower trunk forms the medial cord; and the posterior divisions of the three trunks (initially inferior) form the posterior cord (Fig. 1.2).

The lateral and medial cords supply the innervation of the volar (or flexor) side of the upper limb, and the posterior cord innervates the dorsal (or extensor) side.

The cords, once formed, are located, in their course towards the axilla, in the gutter between the coracoid process and the first ribs of the chest wall, covered by the pectoralis minor muscle, where they can be reached by the various infraclavicular block techniques.

The lateral and medial cords give rise to two branches that merge to form the median nerve: the lateral cord branching off to form the musculocutaneous nerve directly and the medial cord branching off to form the ulnar nerve. The posterior cord, after emitting a branch that forms the axillary nerve, terminates by forming the radial nerve (Table 1.1 and Fig. 1.2).

The spatial configuration of the brachial plexus can be compared to that of a right-angled triangle, the height of which corresponds to the line joining the five intervertebral foramina from which its roots emerge, the base of which lies on the plane of the upper surface of the first rib, and the lower apex of which is situated in a position corresponding to the axilla. At the point of transition from the neck to the thoracic region, the brachial plexus crosses the scalene triangle. The latter, formed by the anterior scalene muscle medially and by the middle scalene muscle laterally, has as its base the anterolateral portion of the first rib which is characterized by three more or less accentuated transverse grooves, produced by the subclavian vein (medial in relation to the scalene triangle), more laterally by the subclavian artery, and even more laterally by the brachial plexus (both within the triangle). The vein and artery are separated by Lisfranc's tubercle onto which the anterior scalene muscle inserts. The scalene triangle can be compared to a triangular ladder, the base of which is situated on the anterolateral portion of the first rib and the apex of which abuts upon the sixth cervical vertebra. On the basis of anatomical measurements we have made, the base lies at a distance of about 4.5–6 cm from the cervical spine according to the build of the individual (Fig. 1.3).

At the level of the scalene triangle, the plexus is invested by the middle cervical fascia which also invests the carotid neurovascular bundle

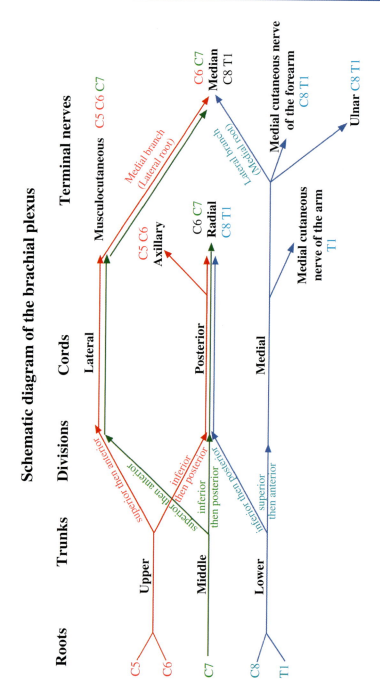

Fig. 1.2 Schematic representation of the brachial plexus and its terminal branches. Unfortunately, the diagram on paper gives only a rather flattened two-dimensional view of the spatial projection of the various elements so we have tried to help out by adding the toponomastics

1 Anatomy of the Brachial Plexus

Table 1.1 Roots and trunks contribute to the formation of the various terminal nerves

Brachial plexus nerves				
Upper primary trunk	C5 C6			
Middle primary trunk	C7			
Lower primary trunk	C8 T1			
Terminal nerves	Trunks:	Upper	Mid	Lower
Axillary nerve (deltoid m.)		C5–6		
Musculocutaneous nerve (biceps m.)		C5–6		
Median nerve (flexor carpi radialis m. and pronator muscles)		C5–6	C7	C8
Radial nerve (triceps m. extensor muscles of the forearm and abductor pollicis m.)		C5–6	C7	C8–T1
Ulnar nerve (flexor carpi ulnaris m. and adductor pollicis m.)				C8–T1
Medial cutaneous nerve of the forearm				C8–T1

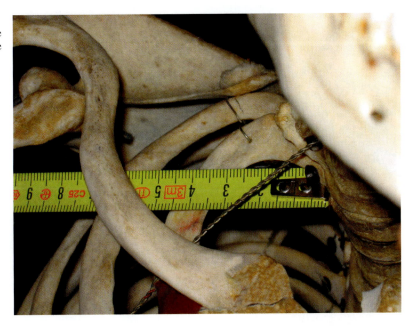

Fig. 1.3 Distance of the base of the scalene triangle (anterolateral portion of the first rib) from the cervical spine. The distance ranges from 4.5 to 6 cm (the height of the skeleton examined was 150 cm)

(Fig. 1.4a). Proceeding laterally, the fascia terminates enveloping the omohyoid muscle. This muscle crosses the area of the scalene triangle with a variable disposition, sometimes being mostly retroclavicular (Fig. 1.4c), sometimes crossing the upper part of the triangle (Fig. 1.4a), and sometimes lying in an intermediate position between the two (Fig. 1.4b). The transverse cervical artery of the scapula and the superficial cervical artery, branches of the subclavian artery, cross the plexus from bottom to top passing thence into the neurovascular bundle.

On emerging from the scalene triangle, the brachial plexus, before penetrating below the clavicle, from which it is separated by the subclavius muscle, passes above the first rib and comes into contact with the superior digitation of the serratus anterior muscle (Fig. 1.5).

Beneath the clavicle, the cords of the brachial plexus, travelling in the direction of the axilla, run in the groove bounded by the coracoid apophysis and by the first thoracic ribs, covered by the pectoral muscles and separated from the shoulder joint by subscapularis muscle tendon,

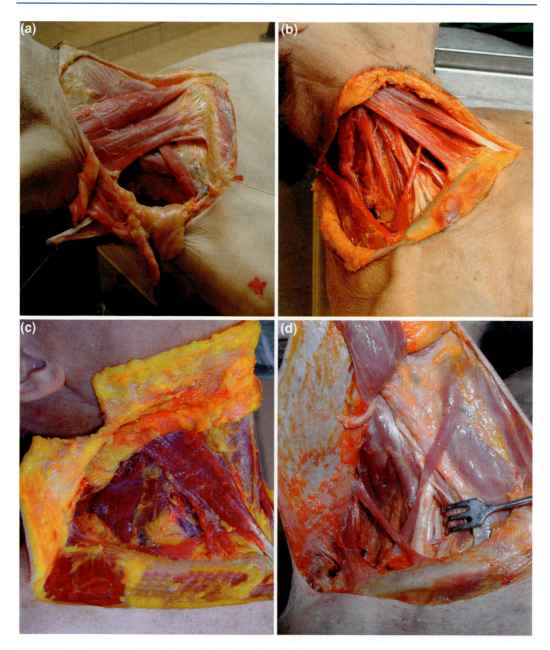

Fig. 1.4 In panels (**a**) and (**b**), the omohyoid muscle presents a regular trend and, as in the treatises on topographical anatomy, it divides the supraclavicular triangle into the two omotrapezius and omoclavicular triangles; in panel (**c**), the lateral belly, in contrast, is almost hidden behind the clavicle. In panel (**d**), the two heads—sternal and clavicular—of the sternocleidomastoid muscle—have been disinserted and the muscle has been raised to reveal the intermediate tendon and the insertion of the medial belly of the omohyoid muscle on the hyoid bone

which, together with the serratus anterior muscle, forms the groove that accommodates the neurovascular bundle of the axilla. Their anatomical disposition in the area between the lower edge of the clavicle and the upper border of the pectoralis minor muscle is the classic

1 Anatomy of the Brachial Plexus

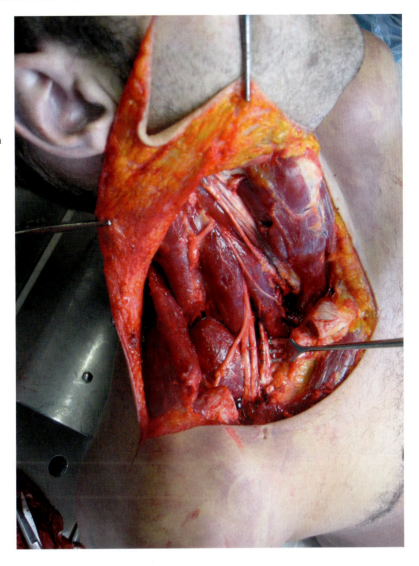

Fig. 1.5 Brachial plexus resting on the superior digitation of the serratus anterior muscle, the supraclavicular nerve that traverses the muscle horizontally, and the phrenic nerve adhering to the anterior scalene muscle, medially to which runs the vagus nerve

nerve–artery–vein disposition, proceeding in a lateromedial direction. The posterior cord is the deepest and most external; this is followed by the lateral cord, the position of which is more superficial and intermediate than that of the other two. Lastly, the medial cord is the closest to the artery, which becomes anterior to it at the point where the entire neurovascular bundle descends below the pectoralis minor muscle.

At the level of the lower border of the pectoralis minor muscle, the three cords give rise to the terminal nerves of the brachial plexus.

As regards the relationships with the artery, the latter is situated medially and slightly anterior to the plexus in the scalene triangle, behind the clavicle and at the infraclavicular level (in the thoraco-coracoid groove), it is again situated anterior to the plexus; in the axilla, it mostly passes between the two branches that converge to form the median nerve and then continues posterior to the nerve.

The anastomosis with the sympathetic system is formed by one or two ramuscules that run from the fifth and sixth cervical nerve roots to the middle cervical ganglion and by another four ramuscules that run from C6, C7, C8 and T1 to the vertebral nerve which is an efferent branch of the stellate ganglion. This anastomosis explains the Bernard-Horner syndrome, one of the most characteristic and most frequent side effects of supraclavicular blocks.

We shall now divide the nerves arising from the brachial plexus into two groups—collateral and terminal.

1.2 Collateral Nerves of the Brachial Plexus

An initial, gross topographical classification distinguishes between the collateral branches of the brachial plexus according to whether they originate above, at or below the level of the clavicle.

In view, however, of the variable lengths of the roots, the trunks themselves and the distal division branches (anterior and posterior) and the variability of the position of the clavicle itself in relation to the first rib, depending on the constitutional shape and size of the thorax (which vary according to the various types of individual, ranging from Stiller's asthenic habitus type to the weight-lifter type), we believe it is easier to distinguish between the collateral nerves of the brachial plexus according to whether they arise from the roots, the trunks or the cords.

Among those generally defined, on the basis of the initial classification, as supraclavicular, we therefore distinguish between those that arise from the roots (nine in number) and those arising from the trunks (only two). Of the latter two nerves, only the suprascapular nerve—the most distal—carries sensory fibres, which innervate the shoulder.

The supraclavicular nerves are therefore practically all motor nerves and would not appear to play any role in sensory anesthesia, save for the fact that it is precisely the motor nerves that are stimulated electrically and thus lead us to understand, as a function of the twitch evoked, what the position of the needle tip is and what nerve it corresponds to. Moreover, in certain surgical procedures, as in the case of shoulder surgery, blockade of the motor nerve with consequent muscle relaxation is particularly useful.

We shall now see, proceeding in a distal direction, where the various nerves arise and in which spinal metameres they originate.

1.2.1 Nerves Arising from the Roots

The first nerves arising from the roots of the brachial plexus are all motor nerves. These are: The collateral nerves for the longus colli muscle, the paravertebral muscle, also innervated by the roots of the cervical plexus (thus by C2–C6) and the scalene muscles: anterior (C4–C6), middle (C3–C8) and posterior (C6–C8).

These are immediately followed by the long thoracic nerve (C5–C6–C7) that innervates the serratus anterior muscle and is situated posterior to the plexus, skirting the posterior scalene muscle, and then proceeds laterally, supplying a twig to each digitation of the serratus anterior muscle.

The dorsal scapular nerve arising from C4 or C5 and innervating the levator muscle of the scapula (also called the angular muscle of the scapula) and sometimes also the rhomboid muscle; it also follows the posterior scalene muscle in its course. When this nerve is stimulated, it causes the raising of the shoulder, which may also be erroneously interpreted as a contraction of the deltoid muscle. It may be stimulated directly if the needle tip is in a fairly posterior position to the plexus, or via the root C5 in the paravertebral techniques.

The nerve of the rhomboid muscle arising from C4 or C5.

The phrenic nerve root arising from C5 (the phrenic nerve is formed by three roots, C3, C4 and, of course, C5).

1.2.2 Nerves Arising from the Trunks

- The nerve to the subclavius muscle (C5–C6), which arises from the upper trunk in an anterior direction abutting upon the anterior scalene

muscle, runs parallel to the phrenic nerve, which it supplies with an anastomotic branch.
- The suprascapular nerve. This nerve also arises from the upper trunk in a posterior direction, which, however, immediately becomes parallel to the plexus but on a more superficial plane and then dorsally passes below the omohyoid and trapezius muscles, and finally inserts into the coracoid notch, enclosed superiorly by the transverse ligament. It innervates the supraspinatus and infraspinatus muscles. It is the only nerve originating above the clavicle endowed with sensory fibres arising from the shoulder joint. In the supraclavicular brachial plexus block techniques, stimulation of the suprascapular nerve should not be regarded as valid because after a few millimetres from its origin it abandons the neurovascular bundle and travels for a distance of a few centimetres parallel to the plexus with the result that one is much more likely to stimulate it outside rather than inside the bundle.

1.2.3 Nerves Arising from the Cords

From the lateral cord:
1. nerve of the pectoralis major muscle, arising from C5, C6, C7, C8, T1, is anastomosed to the pectoralis minor nerve that departs from the medial cord. Its direction is anterior.
   From the medial cord:
1. pectoralis minor nerve, arising from C6, C7, C8, T1, is anastomosed to the pectoralis major nerve;
2. medial cutaneous nerve of the arm (exclusively sensory), arising from C8 to T1.
   From the posterior cord:
1. upper subscapular nerve, arising from C5, C6 (innervates the subscapular muscle);
2. lower subscapular nerve, arising from C8 to T1 (innervates the subscapular muscle);
3. nerve of the dorsalis major muscle, arising from C7, C8;
4. nerve of the teres major muscle, arising from C7, C8.

From the topographical point of view, the collateral nerves arising from the brachial plexus, according to the direction they take after their origin, can be subdivided into three groups: anterior, posterior and inferior (or descending).

The nerves belonging to the anterior group are three in number:
1. nerve to the subclavius muscle (arising from the upper trunk);
2. nerve of the pectoralis major muscle (arising from the lateral cord);
3. nerve of the pectoralis minor muscle (arising from the medial cord).

There are seven nerves, all motor nerves, in the posterior group:
1. suprascapular nerve (the only one endowed with sensory fibres), arising from the upper trunk;
2. the dorsal scapular nerve or nerve of the levator (or angular) muscle of the scapula, arising from the roots C4 and C5;
3. nerve of the rhomboid muscle, arising from the roots C4 and C5;
4. upper subscapular nerve, arising from the posterior cord (C5–C6);
5. lower subscapular nerve, arising from the posterior cord (C8–T1);
6. nerve of the dorsalis major muscle, arising from the posterior cord (C7–C8);
7. nerve of the teres major muscle, arising from the posterior cord (C7, C8).

There are only two nerves belonging to the inferior or descending group:
1. nerve of the serratus anterior muscle or long thoracic muscle, arising from the roots C5, C6, C7;
2. medial cutaneous nerve of the arm, exclusively sensory, arising from the medial cord (C8–T1).

1.3 Terminal Nerves of the Brachial Plexus

The six terminal nerves of the brachial plexus all arise in the axillary cavity.

1.3.1 The Axillary or Circumflex Nerve (C5–C6)

This nerve is so named because it envelops the posterolateral part of the neck of the humerus describing a curve with anterosuperior concavity. It splits off from the posterior cord at the point where the posterior cord ends giving way to the radial nerve. Some authors, perhaps rightly, consider it to be a posteriorly directed collateral branch of the posterior cord. It accompanies the posterior circumflex artery (branch of the axillary artery), entering a quadrangular space bounded by the humerus laterally, by the long head of the triceps brachii muscle medially, by the teres minor muscle superiorly and by the teres major muscle in its lower part; it then insinuates itself between the humerus and the deltoid muscle.

At the level of the quadrangular space described here above, it emits two collateral branches, namely the nerve of the teres minor muscle (motor) and the lateral cutaneous nerve of the arm (sensory), the latter descending alongside the posterior border of the deltoid muscle and going on to supply fibres to the skin of the shoulder and the lateral surface of the arm. The multiple terminal branches basically provide motor fibres for the deltoid muscle, but also sensory fibres for the shoulder joint.

1.3.2 The Radial Nerve (C6–C7–C8–T1)

The radial nerve originates as the continuation or terminal branch of the posterior cord from the point of origin of the axillary nerve. It innervates the triceps brachii muscle and the extensor muscles of the forearm. The sensory component consists in sensory fibres that supply the dorsal and radial part of the hand, the posterior surface of the forearm and the proximal posterolateral part of the arm.

In the axilla, it is situated posteriorly to the axillary artery and anteriorly to the subscapularis muscle and to the aponeurosis of the latissimus dorsi and teres major muscles. It descends posteriorly between the triceps vastus lateralis and vastus medialis muscles, passing behind and around the humerus in the musculospiral groove, accompanied by the deep humeral artery and vein, and covered by the long head of the triceps muscle. It then comes to rest on the anterolateral surface of the humerus, inserting between the anterior brachialis muscle (which remains medial) and the supinator longus muscle (which remains lateral), again accompanied by the humeral vessels.

Collateral Branches of the Radial Nerve
The radial nerve emits eight collateral branches:
1. The medial cutaneous branch (sensory). This branch is the first to depart from the nerve and innervates the skin of the posterior region of the arm as far as the olecranon process;
2. superior and inferior branches supplying the long head of the triceps brachii muscle, from the upper portion of the latter to the tendon that inserts on the olecranon;
3. the vastus medialis muscle nerve, supplying the muscle of the same name;
4. The vastus lateralis muscle nerve and the nerve of the anconeus muscle innervating the respective muscles. This is a fairly long nerve that departs from the radial nerve at the level of the spiral groove of the humerus. It innervates the triceps vastus lateralis muscle with its collateral branches and the anconeus muscle with its terminal branch;
5. The dorsal and lateral cutaneous branch of the forearm. This originates in the lower part of the spiral groove of the humerus and supplies the skin of the dorsal region of the forearm as far as the carpus;
6. a thin branch supplying the anterior brachial muscle. It is present in 75 % of cases;
7. The supinator longus muscle nerve. It originates below the previous nerve and innervates the muscle of the same name;
8. the extensor carpi radialis longus nerve, innervating the muscle of the same name.

Terminal Branches of the Radial Nerve

Above the fold of the elbow, the radial nerve emits two terminal branches one anterior and cutaneous, and the other posterior (profound muscular branch).

Anterior or Cutaneous Branch

This is the thinner of the two. Basically, it receives fibres from C6, but also from C5 to C7. It innervates the dorsal skin of the hand and the first three fingers as far as the first interphalangeal joint.

Proceeding towards the periphery, it can be seen medial to the supinator longus muscle and lateral to the radial artery. After descending beyond two-thirds of the forearm, it receives an anastomotic branch from the musculocutaneous nerve, travels laterally and dorsally and then moves closer to the surface, perforating the antebrachial aponeurosis (brachioradialis fascia) at the level of the posterior border of the supinator longus muscle, ultimately trifurcating into a lateral branch, a middle branch and a medial branch.

The lateral branch prolongs the direction of the nerve from which it originates along the radial margin of the hand, constituting the radial dorsal digital nerve of the thumb; it emits a ramus innervating the skin of the thenar eminence and the abductor pollicis brevis muscle (also innervated by a twig from the median nerve).

The middle branch at the level of the first interosseous interdigital space divides to form a lateral ramus that constitutes the dorsoulnar digital nerve of the thumb and a medial ramus supplying the skin of the dorsal part of the first phalanx of the index finger.

The medial branch receives anastomotic fibres from the ulnar nerve and then goes on to innervate the skin of the dorsal surface of the hand and the first phalanx of the index and middle finger.

Posterior or Muscular or Profound Branch

This branch receives fibres from C6, C7 and sometimes also from C8. It immediately emits the nerve of the extensor carpi radialis brevi muscle and then proceeds laterally and dorsally, emitting the supinator brevis nerve that perforates the muscle of the same name and innervates it. It reaches the dorsal surface of the forearm, describing a half spiral around the neck of the radius and then inserts between the muscles of the superficial layer and those of the deep layer, innervating them with many branches. In this way, the extensor digitorum muscle, the extensor digiti minimi muscle and the anterior cubital muscle are innervated by the dorsal branches. The anterior branches, by contrast, proceed to the muscles of the deep layer and, particularly, to the abductor pollicis longus muscle, to the extensor pollicis brevis muscle and to the extensor indicis muscle. The posterior branch terminates finally with the interosseous dorsal nerve of the forearm, which is adjacent to the interosseous membrane and is a satellite nerve of the dorsal interosseous artery. On reaching the radiocarpal zone, it passes beneath the dorsal ligament of the carpus together with the tendons of extensor digitorum muscle. Lastly, it redistributes on the back of the hand to the radiocarpal, carpal and carpo-metacarpal articulations and, even more distally, to the metacarpal interosseous spaces and phalangeal articulations.

1.3.3 The Musculocutaneous Nerve (C5–C6–C7)

The lateral cord of the brachial plexus divides and gives rise to the musculocutaneous nerve and to a more medial branch that continues as the lateral root of the median nerve.

The musculocutaneous nerve (both motor and sensory) innervates the biceps, coracobrachialis and brachialis muscles; it then extends down into the forearm with only the sensory fibres that constitute the lateral cutaneous nerve of the forearm. In the axilla, it descends obliquely and laterally, perforates the coracobrachialis muscle, placing itself first between the biceps and the anterior brachial muscle and then between the biceps and the brachioradialis muscle. On reaching the fold of the elbow, it becomes more superficial, perforating the superficial aponeurosis, where, as the lateral antebrachial cutaneous nerve of the forearm, it supplies the lateral surface of the forearm.

Its collateral branches emitted before perforating the superficial aponeurosis are the coracobrachialis nerve, the biceps nerve and the anterior brachial nerve, innervating the respective muscles.

The only terminal branch is the lateral cutaneous nerve of the forearm which divides into a dorsal and a volar branch; the terminal filaments of the dorsal branch extend as far as the first metacarpus and the first interosseous space. The volar branch, on the other hand, after emitting an anastomotic branch to the radial nerve at the wrist, terminates, accompanying the radial artery, at the radiocarpal articulation.

1.3.4 The Median Nerve (C6–C7–C8–T1)

The median nerve originates from the lateral and medial cord. These two roots straddle the axillary artery and merge on its ventral surface. The nerve then closely follows the course of the artery when it becomes the brachial artery and provides motor branches to the flexor and pronator muscles of the forearm. It provides the sensory innervation of the volar side of the hand as far as the lateral sagittal half of the 4th finger, the ulnar nerve being responsible for the medial half of the 4th finger and the sensory innervation of the whole of the little finger.

Thus, the lateral cord of the brachial plexus divides and gives rise, as we have seen, to the musculocutaneous nerve and to a more medial branch that becomes the lateral root of the median nerve.

The medial cord of the brachial plexus divides and gives rise medially (as we shall see) to the ulnar nerve and to the medial cutaneous nerve of the forearm, and laterally to the medial root of the median nerve.

The two roots of the median nerve, the lateral one from the lateral cord and the medial one from the medial cord, merge in a **V** shape to form the nerve that, once formed, transforms the **V** into a **Y**. The axillary artery lies on the bisector of the **V** and posterior to it.

The position of the nerve in the arm is somewhat medial to the biceps; it runs along the border of the latter, accompanied by the brachial artery.

At the elbow, the nerve is located medially to the brachial artery. In the forearm, immediately after the bifurcation of the brachial artery into the radial and ulnar arteries, the nerve crosses ulnar artery anteriorly, placing itself in the middle of the volar surface of the forearm between the flexor digitorum profundus and flexor digitorum superficialis muscles, thus acquiring the name of median nerve as a result of its position.

At the level of the carpus, the median nerve is located lateral to the flexor digitorum muscle tendon; it then passes through the carpal tunnel, on exiting from which it emits its terminal branches.

Collateral Branches of the Median Nerve
Whereas, at the level of the arm, the median nerve does not emit any collateral branches with the exception of an anastomotic branch that connects it to the musculocutaneous nerve, after the elbow, it emits several collateral branches. These are as follows:
1. the small articular branches destined to innervate the volar surface of the elbow;
2. the nerve of the pronator teres muscle;
3. anterior muscular branches also to the pronator teres muscle, to the palmaris longus and brevis muscles and to the flexor digitorum superficialis muscle;
4. posterior muscular branches that travel to the flexor pollicis longus muscle and to the two radial bundles of the flexor digitorum profundus muscle;
5. the volar interosseous nerve of the forearm destined to innervate the flexor pollicis longus muscle, the flexor digitorum profundus muscle and the pronator quadratus muscle;
6. the palmar cutaneous nerve which departs from the median nerve just above the carpus, insinuates itself between the palmaris longus and brevis muscles and then divides into two

cutaneous branches, one lateral to innervate the thenar eminence and the other palmar to innervate the middle palmar region.

Terminal Branches of the Median Nerve

The median nerve emits its terminal branches posteriorly to the volar annular ligament of the carpus.

These branches are six in number and, proceeding from the radius to the ulna, are designated by progressive Roman numerals, as people used to do in the first half of the last century with the offspring of large families:

1. The first branch is the shortest and travels laterally, forming a concave curve superiorly. At the level of the thenar eminence, it trifurcates into a branch to the abductor pollicis brevis muscle, a branch to the flexor pollicis brevis muscle and a branch to the opponens pollicis muscle.
2. The second branch follows the course of the flexor pollicis longus tendon, becoming the radial digital nerve of the thumb.
3. The third branch, with a course similar to the first, becomes the ulnar digital nerve of the thumb.
4. The fourth branch, after emitting a twig for the first lumbrical muscle, divides and forms the volar digital nerve and the dorsal digital nerve of the index finger.
5. The fifth branch, with a course corresponding to the second interosseous space, after emitting a twig for the second lumbrical muscle, divides and forms the volar ulnar digital nerve of the index finger and the volar radial digital nerve of the middle finger.
6. The sixth branch, with a course corresponding to the third interosseous space, after receiving an anastomotic twig from the ulnar nerve, divides and forms the volar ulnar digital nerve of the middle finger and the volar radial digital nerve of the ring finger.

In conclusion, the median nerve is a mixed motor and sensory nerve. Its motor branches innervate the muscles of the volar region of the forearm except for the anterior cubital muscle and the ulnar head of the flexor digitorum profundus muscle innervated by the ulnar nerve. At the palmar level, they innervate the first two lumbrical muscles and the muscles of the thenar eminence, except for the adductor pollicis muscle and the medial fasciculus of the flexor pollicis brevis muscle, innervated by the ulnar nerve.

The sensory fibres innervate the volar surface of the thenar eminence, the volar surface of the index finger and the radial half of the ring finger and the respective dorsal parts of the third and second phalanges.

1.3.5 The Ulnar Nerve (C8–T1)

The ulnar nerve is the major terminal continuation of the medial cord, which ends immediately after making its contribution to the median nerve. The ulnar nerve originates from the medial cord just below the lower border of the pectoralis minor muscle. It innervates the ulnar flexor muscle of the carpus, the ulnar head of the flexor digitorum profundus muscle, and the lumbrical muscles with the exception of the first two. It supplies sensory fibres to the skin of the little finger and to the medial part of the fourth finger.

The medial cord of the brachial plexus, as we have seen, divides and gives rise laterally to the medial root of the median nerve, and medially to the ulnar nerve and the medial cutaneous nerve of the forearm.

Comparative anatomy teaches us that, in felines and ruminants, that is, animals that notoriously do not habitually swing to and fro on lianas, the ulnar and median nerve are fused, whereas, in monkeys, the ulnar nerve is more developed than the median nerve and serves a larger area, there being a prevalence of gripping (a function proper to the 4th and 5th fingers), due to these animals' climbing habit, over prehensility (a function proper to the first, second and third fingers).

In its descent from the axilla, the ulnar nerve follows a course parallel, but posterior to the median nerve. At the elbow, it passes into the olecranon fossa covered by the ligament of the same name. The result is that the nerve enters a kind of osteofibrous tunnel. At this level, the nerve is easily detectable both by palpation and by eliciting with slightly more pressure the characteristic paraesthesia with which everyone is familiar. Only a few milliliters of anesthetic suffice to block it, making sure, however, that the needle bevel remains outside the tunnel, and otherwise, there is a risk of ischaemizing the nerve.

In the forearm, the nerve passes between the flexor digitorum profundus muscle and the pronator quadratus muscle, which remain posterior, and is covered anteriorly first by the anterior cubital muscle and then by the antebrachial aponeurosis. At a distance of approximately ten centimetres from the elbow, the ulnar nerve meets the ulnar artery which then accompanies it as far as the wrist, remaining lateral to it throughout.

At the wrist, on the contrary, the ulnar nerve remains anterior to the annular ligament of the carpus, inserting itself between the pisiform and hamate bones, again accompanied laterally by the ulnar artery.

1.3.6 Collateral Branches of the Ulnar Nerve

- articular branches originating at the level of the olecranon fossa and going on to innervate the elbow joint;
- muscular branches innervating the anterior cubital muscle and the flexor digitorum profundus muscle;
- an anastomotic branch to the medial cutaneous nerve of the forearm.

The dorsal cutaneous nerve of the hand, which originates at a distance of approximately 5 cm from the wrist, runs posterior to the ulna, inserting itself between the latter and the tendon of the flexor carpi ulnaris muscle. It then trifurcates into the dorsal ulnar digitorum nerve of the little finger, the dorsal radial digitorum nerve of the same finger and a twig to the dorsal skin of the first phalanx of the ring finger.

Terminal Branches of the Ulnar Nerve

At the level of the wrist, the ulnar nerve emits its two terminal branches: the superficial branch and the deep branch.

Superficial Branch (Mixed)

In its course, this branch innervates the skin of the hypothenar eminence, the palmar cutaneous muscle and the flexor brevis muscle of the little finger. It then divides into a medial branch, which becomes the medial volar digital nerve of the little finger, and a lateral branch that passes via the fourth interosseous space, ultimately dividing into the radial volar digital nerve of the little finger and the ulnar volar digital nerve of the ring finger.

Deep Branch (Motor)

This branch originates laterally to the piriform bone and after passing medially around the hamate bone travels towards the radius, remaining deep in the volar region, thus forming a large loop, from the distally disposed convex part of which emerge the branches innervating the hypothenar eminence (in particular, the adductor brevis muscle, and the flexor and opponens muscles of the little finger) as well as twigs innervating the third and fourth lumbrical muscles and all the interosseous muscles. The terminal portion of the deep branch innervates the adductor pollicis muscle and the medial bundle of the flexor pollicis brevis muscle (as we have already seen, the lateral bundle is innervated by the median nerve).

1.3.7 The Medial Cutaneous Nerve of the Forearm (C8–T1)

The medial cutaneous nerve of the forearm and the medial cutaneous nerve of the arm, often a collateral branch of the former, originate from the medial cord, the former as a terminal nerve and the latter as a collateral branch. These are sensory nerves whose course runs parallel and posterior to the ulnar nerve. The medial cutaneous nerve of the forearm innervates the medial part of the forearm as far as the wrist. The medial cutaneous nerve of the arm innervates the medial part of the arm and is the most caudal nerve of the brachial plexus, running and resting upon the surface of the first fasciculus of the serratus anterior muscle.

The medial cutaneous nerve of the forearm originates from the medial root of the median nerve and therefore from the medial cord of the brachial plexus. It immediately assumes a posterolateral position in relation to the axillary artery. It arises from the superficial fascia of the arm at the point where the basilic vein perforates the fascia to become the axillary vein, that is, approximately between the lower two-thirds and the upper third of the arm.

At the same level, the medial cutaneous nerve of the arm arises, innervating the skin of the medial surface of the arm as far as the elbow.

Just before the epitrochlea, the medial cutaneous nerve of the forearm divides into a posterior and an anterior branch. The posterior branch innervates the dorsal skin of the ulnar region as far as the wrist. The anterior branch divides into several branches that enter into contiguous relationships with the basilic vein and then distributes progressively distally to the skin of the anteromedial region of the forearm as far as the wrist.

The medial cutaneous nerve of the arm often originates independently of the two confluent branches departing from C8 to T1 and then anastomoses with the intercostobrachial nerve from T2.

1.4 Contribution of the Intercostal Nerves to the Brachial Plexus

Generally speaking, a thoracic spinal nerve, once formed, divides at its origin into a posterior division, which serves the dorsal muscles, and an anterior division that forms the actual intercostal nerve. The latter, among the various collateral branches, emits lateral cutaneous branches and anterior cutaneous branches, both of which have a sensory function. The lateral cutaneous branches of the first and second intercostal nerves contribute sensory fibres to the brachial plexus.

The first intercostal nerve is relatively thin in that it mostly contributes to forming the lower primary trunk of the brachial plexus. It is apparently devoid of the lateral cutaneous branch because its sensory fibres have been redirected to forming, in succession, the lower primary trunk, the medial cord of the plexus and the medial root of the median nerve, from which the medial cutaneous nerve of the forearm originates.

The lateral cutaneous branch of the second intercostal nerve, instead of innervating the thoracic skin, enters the axilla where it is called the intercostobrachial nerve, also forming an anastomosis with the medial cutaneous nerve of the arm; sometimes another anastomotic branch connects it to the caudal root of the lower primary trunk formed by the first thoracic nerve. Lastly, with its terminal twigs, it supplies the skin of the medial region of the arm.

The third intercostal nerve, with its lateral cutaneous branch, may also make an anastomotic contribution to the intercostobrachial nerve. For the above reasons, the second and third intercostal nerves have been, respectively, named the first and second intercostobrachial nerves.

1.5 Connections with the Sympathetic System

The brachial plexus is connected to the cervical sympathetic chain via two grey rami communicantes, which run from C5 and C6 to the middle cervical ganglion and via another four rami, which run from C6, C7 and C8 and from the white ramus communicans of T1 to the stellate ganglion. All these are therefore afferent branches (to the ganglion). The efferent branches from the middle cervical ganglion are the thyroid branches that form the thyroid plexus around the inferior thyroid artery, the cardiac branches that form the middle cardiac nerve (cardioaccelerator) and the anastomotic branch to the inferior laryngeal nerve (recurrent nerve).

A first group of efferent nerves from the stellate ganglion follows the vessels and supplies the upper limb.

A second efferent group forms the so-called vertebral nerve or, better, vertebral plexus, following the artery of the same name and insinuating itself with its branches in the foramina of the transverse processes of the cervical vertebrae.

A third group, with an inferomedial course, forms the inferior cardiac nerve (cardioaccelerator) after connecting via an anastomosis to the middle cardiac nerve.

This should come as no surprise because in the embryo, the heart is originally located in the cervical region and only later migrates into the thorax followed by its own innervation.

This anatomical disposition may contribute to the onset of Bezold-Jarisch syndrome in the eventuality of involvement of the cardiac nerves in brachial plexus block.

The white ramus communicans that runs from T1 to the stellate ganglion also carries the motor fibres that innervate the ciliary muscle of the iris, and the thin muscular fibres of Tenon's capsule and the tarsus palpebrae. These fibres originate from the lateral column of the spinal cord, enter the first thoracic nerve and then, via the white ramus communicans, reach the stellate ganglion and go on, via the intermediate sympathetic longitudinal cord, to reach the eyeball. This explains the onset of Claude Bernard-Horner syndrome in cases of blockade of the sympathetic component. In this syndrome, palpebral ptosis is due to plegia of the tenuous smooth muscle fibres of the tarsus palpebrae, which leads to a reduction in the palpebral rim; miosis is due to plegia of the ciliary muscle, and enophthalmos is due to plegia of the tenuous smooth muscle fibres of Tenon's capsule which, inserting on the circumference of the eyeball and wrapping themselves around it, no longer maintain ocular tension.

On the contrary, in case of hyperthyroidism, sympathetic hypertone gives rise to an increase in the tension of Tenon's capsule and the tarsal fibres with consequent exophthalmos.

Peripheral neurosurgical procedures have demonstrated that the second and third thoracic ganglions contribute to the sympathetic innervation of the upper limb. In fact, when these ganglions are removed thoracoscopically, stable results may be achieved in the treatment for various ischaemic diseases of the upper limb or in the case of axillary and/or palmar hyperhydrosis.

Also of interest are the anatomical relationships of the paravertebral sympathetic chain. The latter lies on the deep (or paravertebral) cervical fascia in a medial position in relation to the anterior tubercles of the transverse processes. Actually, it is the paravertebral fascia itself which splits and endows the sympathetic chain with a tenuous investing layer; at the cervical level, it is covered by the carotid artery, the internal jugular vein and the vagus nerve which constitute the neurovascular bundle of the neck and lastly by a muscular plane consisting basically in the sternocleidomastoid muscle. The posterior border of this muscle affords the most direct access route to the sympathetic chain, although the simplest access technique is Moore's two-finger technique, applied at the level of the anterior border of the muscle.

Bibliography

Alemanno F, Capozzoli G, Egarter-Vigl E, Gottin L, Bartoloni A (2006) The middle interscalene block: cadaver study and clinical assessment. Reg Anesth Pain Med 31:563–568

Alemanno F, Egarter Vigl E (2010) Lesioni nervose. In Pippa P, Busoni P (eds) Anestesia Locoregionale, Verduci Editore, p 44

Bairati A (1974) Anatomia umana: sistema nervoso periferico, organi di senso, sistema tegumentario, vol III. Minerva Medica, Torino

Chiarugi G, Bucciante L (1972) Istituzioni di anatomia dell'uomo. Vallardi Editore, Milano

Herbert L (2000) Lehrbuch Anatomie. Urban and Fischer, Auflage-München-Jena

Moore DC (1969) Anestesia regionale. Piccin Editore, Padova

Netter FH (1983) Atlante di anatomia fisiopatologia e clinica, Sistema Nervoso, vol 7, Ciba-Geigy Edizioni

Schiebler TH, Schmidt W (1999) Anatomie: Zitologie, Histologie, Entwicklungsgeschichte, makroskopische und mikroskopische Anatomie des Menchen. Springer, New York

Sieglbauer F (1935) Lehrbuch der normalen Anatomie des Menschen: Urban & Schwarzenberg; Berlin, Wien, Auflage 3

Sobotta J, Becher H (1974) Atlante di anatomia dell'uomo, USES—Edizioni Scientifiche, Firenze

Testut L (1942) Anatomia umana, Miologia, libro terzo. UTET, Torino

Testut L (1943) Anatomia umana, Sistema nervoso periferico, libro sesto. UTET, Torino

Von Lanz T, Wachssmuth W (1973) Anatomia pratica: Arto superiore Vol. I, Parte III. Piccin Editore, Padova

Waldeyer A, Mayet A (1976) Anatomie des Menschen. Walter de Gruyter Verlag, Berlin-New York

Winnie AP (1984) Tecniche perivascolari di blocco del plesso brachiale. Verduci Editore, Roma

Topographical Anatomy

2

F. Alemanno and E. Egarter Vigl

2.1 The Supraclavicular Region

The supraclavicular region has a triangular shape, and for this reason, it is also called the supraclavicular triangle, bounded by the sternocleidomastoid muscle, the trapezius muscle and anteriorly by the clavicle. The latter is a long, relatively flattened bone, that connects the scapula via the acromial process to the manubrium sterni. It presents a double curvature, one curve medial and anteriorly convex, and the other lateral and posteriorly convex which gives it the appearance of a capital S on its side, or a kind of 'chicane', whose point of transition from one curve to the other corresponds approximately to its midpoint. The upper surface, which is fairly flat laterally, becomes more rounded in the medial portion; it is covered by skin, by the platysma muscle and by the supraclavicular nerves, which are sensory branches of the cervical plexus.

The clavicle is fairly smooth in its middle part and presents rough areas at the ends for the insertion of the deltoid and trapezius muscles laterally and the clavicular head of the sternocleidomastoid muscle medially. The underside presents a rough surface for the insertion, proceeding mediolaterally, of the costoclavicular ligament, the subclavius muscle and the two coracoclavicular ligaments (conoid and trapezoid). In the middle part of the lower surface, there is a foramen for the nutrient artery of the bone. The anterior edge is the insertion site for the pectoralis major muscle medially and the deltoid muscle laterally. As stated above, the posterior edge and the upper surface of the bone are the insertion sites for the clavicular head of the sternocleidomastoid muscle medially and the trapezius and deltoid muscles laterally. The middle portion of the posterior edge is connected anatomically with the lateral belly of the omohyoid muscle, with the scalene muscles and with the subclavian artery and vein.

The posterior convexity of the lateral portion of the clavicle is modelled by the combined linear forces produced by the trapezius and deltoid muscles. The anterior convexity of the medial portion, on the other hand, is modelled by the linear force of the pectoralis major muscle, poorly contrasted by the linear force of the clavicular head of the sternocleidomastoid muscle.

Like all the long bones of the body, the clavicle presents two apophyses and a diaphysis. Of these, only the diaphysis is part of the supraclavicular region.

The supraclavicular region may take on the appearance of a groove lying right behind the clavicle, and for this reason, it is called the supraclavicular groove or fossa. Its size is inversely proportional to the subject's muscular development. It is fairly deep in thin people, but

---

F. Alemanno (✉)
Institute of Anesthesiology Resuscitation and Pain Therapy, University of Verona, Verona, Italy
e-mail: fernando@alemannobpb.it

E. Egarter Vigl
Institute of Pathological Anatomy, Bolzano Regional Hospital, Bolzano, Italy

may be very small if the musculature is well developed, to the point, in fact, of becoming almost virtual if hypertrophic trapezius and sternocleidomastoid muscles come into contact with one another.

If the subject turns his head towards the opposite side examined and his arm is pulled downwards, the lateral apophysis of the clavicle rotates slightly downwards, the fossa becomes shallower, and the organs it contains become more superficial. On the other hand, when the head is bent downwards and turned slightly towards the side being examined, the muscles relax and it proves easier to palpate the region, thus detecting the pulse of the subclavian artery and sometimes, medially to the latter, also the Lisfranc's tubercle, at the point of insertion of the anterior scalene muscle.

2.1.1 Superficial Planes of the Supraclavicular Region

The superficial planes of the supraclavicular region are constituted by the skin and, only in its anterior inferomedial part, by the platysma, whose tenuous bundles, contained in a splitting of the superficial cervical fascia, insert in the

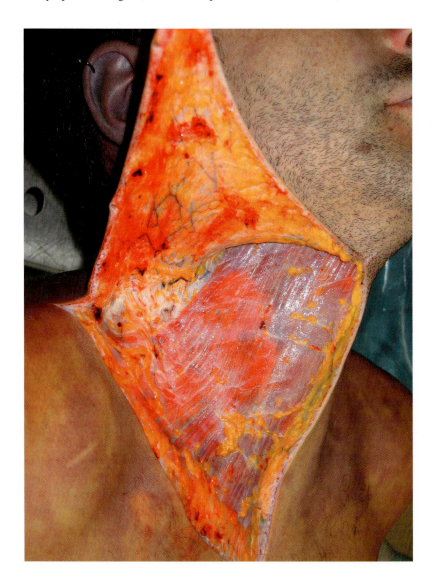

Fig. 2.1 Superficial planes of the supraclavicular region

dermis. The subcutaneous connective tissue may be abundant or scarce (Fig. 2.1).

At a deeper level, the superficial cervical fascia, after splitting to enclose the sternocleidomastoid muscle and the thin fibres of the platysma, reunites to invest the posterior portion of the supraclavicular fossa and then splits again, on coming into contact posteriorly with the anterior border of the trapezius muscle. Superficial nerves and vessels are also present. The nerves are almost exclusively sensory; only the platysma is served by motor muscles. The small-calibre arteries are branches of the superficial cervical artery or the suprascapular artery. The small-calibre veins, which are extremely variable, converge on the external jugular vein. A thin layer of areolar adipose tissue separates the middle cervical fascia from the superficial cervical fascia; this layer accommodates the path of the external jugular vein. This vein, almost always visible at first sight or when palpating the subclavian artery (Fig. 2.2), is characterized by considerable variability.

The *external jugular vein* is formed by the confluence of the superficial temporal vein and the internal maxillary vein; it descends approximately along the line that runs from the angle of the mandible to the midpoint of the clavicle; it crosses the sternocleidomastoid muscle obliquely and then perforates the middle cervical fascia at the level of the medial angle of the supraclavicular triangle (formed by the anterior border of the trapezius muscle, by the posterior border of the sternocleidomastoid muscle and bounded in its lower part by the posterior edge of the clavicle) (Fig. 2.4); it then passes anteriorly to the anterior scalene muscle and finally merges into the subclavian vein laterally to the confluence of the latter with the internal jugular vein. The middle cervical fascia at this point may appear to be reinforced by Dittel's falciform fold; this closely resembles the same anatomical disposition that exists at the point where the saphenous vein joins the femoral vein.

During its course, the external jugular vein receives numerous tributaries, the most important of which—because they are to be found in the context of the omoclavicular triangle (Fig. 2.4)—are the transverse scapular vein and

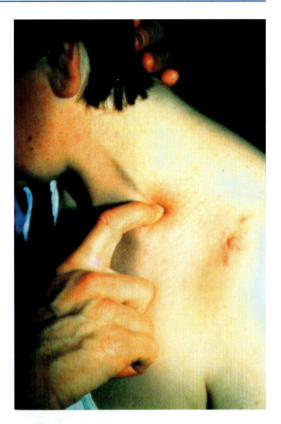

Fig. 2.2 External jugular vein is evident, compressed by the anesthetist's index finger in the act of detecting the pulse of the subclavian artery

the transverse cervical vein, corresponding to the respective arteries of the same name.

The external jugular vein has been proposed by Rucci as an alternative landmark if the pulse of the subclavian artery is not detectable. Sometimes, it may be absent or double, in which case the indication may be misleading, in that the anesthetist does not know which of the two it refers to.

2.1.2 The Sternocleidomastoid Muscle

The sternocleidomastoid muscle (SCM) is the most evident muscle in the neck region. Its shape is roughly rectangular, and in actual fact, the muscle consists of two overlapping muscular branches or heads, the sternal and the clavicular head (Fig. 2.3).

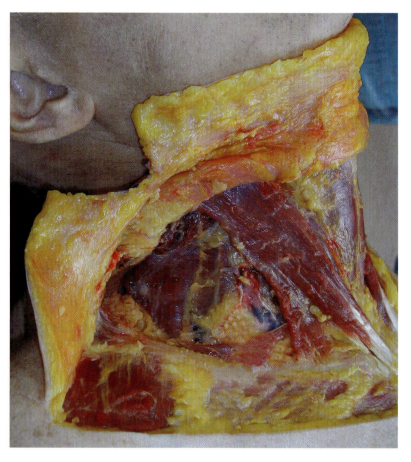

Fig. 2.3 On removing the platysma, the anatomical pathologist exposes the sternal and clavicular insertion of the sternocleidomastoid muscle. Note that the omohyoid muscle is partly hidden behind the clavicle

Proceeding upwards, the sternal head becomes broader and at the same time thinner and then inserts on the lateral surface of the mastoid process and on the lateral margin of the upper nuchal line. Contraction of the muscle causes the subject's head to rotate towards the opposite side. The clavicular muscular head, which is deeper, inserts on the medial fourth of the clavicle and mainly runs below the sternal head, mostly attaching itself to the apex and anterior margin of the mastoid process; less often, following the muscle bundles of the sternal head, it inserts, like the latter, on the lateral margin of the upper nuchal line. Contraction of this muscle causes the ipsilateral flexion of the head of the body.

In the classic rheumatic torticollis syndrome, it is mostly only the superficial sternal muscular bundle that is involved, that is, the one that inserts on the manubrium sterni.

The sternocleidomastoid muscle is situated below the platysma which, however, does not cover the more distal part of the sternal head or the upper third of the muscle. Immediately below the platysma, the superficial cervical fascia, on reaching the level of the sternocleidomastoid muscle, splits in order to envelop it. The sternocleidomastoid muscle therefore presents an external surface, mostly covered by the platysma or by the skin, and an internal surface that is in relation to the intermediate portion of the omohyoid muscle, with the middle cervical fascia, with the common carotid artery, with the internal jugular vein, with the vagus nerve and, deeper down, with the cervical sympathetic chain. It presents an anterior and a posterior border. The latter is an important landmark for the anesthetist because behind it lies the branches of the superficial cervical plexus.

The superficial cervical fascia, which adheres reasonably well to the muscle in the paramastoid region, adheres less effectively to the rest of the muscle on proceeding distally, mainly taking on the function, above the omohyoid muscle, of investing the neurovascular bundle of the neck (carotid artery, internal jugular vein and vagus nerve).

On the posterior plane of the sternocleidomastoid muscle and the superficial cervical fascia, proceeding from the omohyoid muscles on both sides, and anterior and inferior to the latter, a musculo-aponeurotic plane can be seen, formed by the two omohyoid muscles and the middle cervical fascia. This structure, with its trapezoidal appearance, has the hyoid bone as its upper base, the clavicles and the sternum as its lower base, and the two omohyoid muscles as its sides. The middle cervical fascia, after enveloping the posterior margin of the two muscles, terminates at this point.

The innervation of the sternocleidomastoid muscle is supplied by the accessory nerve and the third cervical somatic nerve.

Below the superficial planes described, we find two very important anatomical elements, namely the omohyoid muscle and the middle cervical fascia; on removing, the latter the neurovascular bundle of the neck is revealed (carotid artery, internal jugular vein, vagus nerve).

2.1.3 The Omohyoid Muscle

The omohyoid muscle (or scapular hyoid muscle) is a muscle composed of two muscle bellies, one superior (or anterior) and the other inferior (or posterior or lateral), separated by an intermediate tendon, which create an anteromedially convex arch. The middle cervical fascia extends between the omohyoid muscles on either side and is delimited by them.

The upper belly inserts on the lateral portion of the hyoid bone and on its greater horn. The lower belly inserts on the upper edge of the scapula close to the coracoid notch; it traverses the lower part of the supraclavicular triangle (formed by the posterior border of the sternocleidomastoid muscle, by the anterior border of the trapezius muscle and by the posterior edge of the clavicle), dividing the supraclavicular triangle—in a highly variable manner positionally—into two other triangles, one larger, posterior triangle also known as the omotrapezoid triangle (of little importance for our purposes), and a smaller anteromedial triangle, also known as the omoclavicular triangle (Fig. 2.4). The latter is bounded by the lower border of the omohyoid muscle, by the posterior border of the sternocleidomastoid muscle and by the posterior edge of the clavicle. This second triangle is much more important because it corresponds to the neurovascular bundle of the supraclavicular fossa (brachial plexus, subclavian artery).

Occasionally, the omoclavicular triangle proves to be virtual, as the omohyoid muscle is partly hidden behind the clavicle (Fig. 2.3). In this case, the muscle needs to be removed if the anatomical pathologist wishes to expose the neurovascular bundle or displaced by the surgeon attempting to reach the subclavian artery.

In the supraclavicular region, the omohyoid muscle is normally to be found below the platysma and in turn covers the scalene triangle.

Both the muscle bellies are innervated by the descending branch of the hypoglossal nerve which, after anastomosis to the descending branches of C1, C2 and C3 to form the hypoglossal nerve loop, thus supplies them with innervation from the anterior divisions of the first three cervical nerves.

The function of the omohyoid muscle is unclear, as is the significance of the intermediate tendon. A hypothesis has been advanced, not shared by all, that contraction of this muscle may increase the radius of curvature of its arch, thus subjecting the middle cervical fascia to tension and keeping the large veins of the neck open and so favouring blood leakage during inspiration. As far as the intermediate tendon is

Fig. 2.4 Supraclavicular triangle is divided by the omohyoid muscle into the respective omotrapezoid and omoclavicular triangles, the latter being particularly interesting anesthesiologically. Posterior to the omohyoid muscle, in the omotrapezoid triangle, we note the *upper* digitation of the serratus anterior muscle, the middle scalene muscle, and the levator scapulae muscle

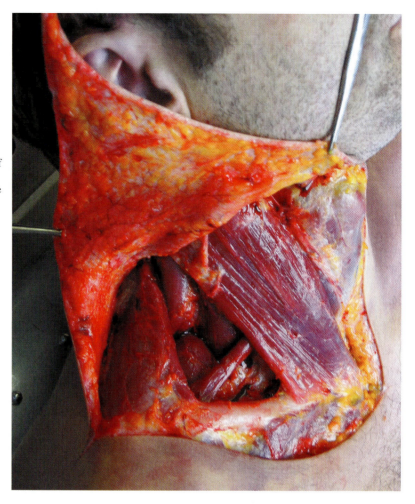

concerned, its significance may have to do with some ancestral aponeurotic reinforcement at the intersection of the first cervical rib.

2.1.4 The Scalene Triangle and Surrounding Area

When the omohyoid muscle and the middle cervical fascia are removed, the supraclavicular fossa is visible with its irregular and poorly defined walls, revealing the true characteristic of this anatomical entity, namely that of actually being a transition zone between the chest, neck and upper limb, via which transit vessels running from the chest to the neck and upper limb, and others that run from the neck and upper limb to the chest, and nerves travelling from the neck to the upper limb and chest, all of which endowed with lymph nodes, loose cellular tissue and adipose tissue.

The supraclavicular fossa is triangular and pyramidal in shape; its base coincides with the superior aperture of the thorax and the plane of the upper surface of the first rib. From its posteromedial border, and above it, the series of transverse processes of the cervical vertebrae constitutes the medial dihedral angle of the pyramid. It is from this angle that the two walls—medial and posterior—of the pyramid depart, formed, respectively, by the anterior scalene muscle and the middle scalene muscle. The lateral wall is formed by the skin, subcutaneous areolar tissue, platysma, superficial cervical fascia, omohyoid muscle and middle cervical fascia.

The base of this pyramid, as we have said, consists in the transverse plane corresponding to the upper surface of the first rib and the first thoracic vertebra. At its lateral apex, the base dwindles, without any very precise outline, and merges into the apex of the armpit. Nor could this be otherwise, in view of the fact that the lateral apical zone constitutes an area of transition for all the neurovascular elements of the upper limb.

The *first rib* bounds the superior aperture of the thorax, occupied by the apex of the lung and by the pleural dome with its suspensory system (Zuckerkandl's membrane) consisting of tenuous fibromuscular bundles.

On upper surface of the first rib two gutters and a shallow track can be noted. Of the two gutters, the posterior one has been excavated by the subclavian artery, and the shallower, anterior one by the subclavian vein. They converge in the vicinity of the lateral edge of the rib, while, in the vicinity of the medial edge, they are separated by the Lisfranc's tubercle which constitutes the caudal osseous insertion of the anterior scalene muscle. The track, which is shallower than the two gutters and positioned posterior to them, is produced by the brachial plexus.

The point where the trapezius, levator scapulae and sternocleidomastoid muscles unite is the apex of the pyramid described above. At this same point, the superficial cervical fascia fuses with the deep cervical fascia.

The contents of the supraclavicular fossa consist of vessels, lymphatic vessels and connective tissue.

The *subclavian artery* is the most representative vessel. On the right side of the body, it originates from the brachiocephalic trunk or innominate artery, corresponding on the surface of the body to the sternoclavicular joint; on the left side of the body, it arises directly from the aorta, corresponding on the skin to the upper surface of the clavicle, at a distance of three centimetres lateral to the sternoclavicular joint.

The subclavian artery presents a prescalene portion (situated medial to the scalene muscles) which travels upwards from its origin anteriorly and laterally and surrounds the pleural dome before crossing the first rib; at this point, its imprint is immediately visible lateral to the Lisfranc's tubercle (interscalene portion); it then passes below the clavicle (clavicular portion) where it changes its name, becoming the axillary artery. Seven collateral arteries arise from the subclavian artery:

- the vertebral artery and the inferior thyroid artery with an ascending course;
- the internal mammary artery and the supreme intercostal artery with a descending course;
- the deep cervical artery with a posterior course towards the nape of the neck;
- the suprascapular artery and the transverse artery of the neck, which are of specific interest to us, present a lateral course crossing the supraclavicular fossa and then travelling towards the scapula. The suprascapular artery passes close to the posterior margin of the clavicle at a distance of about half a centimetre from it; the transverse artery of the neck, of fairly large calibre, crosses in front of the brachial plexus and often in front of or between its cords. It is the transverse cervical artery, in addition to the subclavian artery from which it originates, that may be exposed to puncture and the source of haematoma formation in supraclavicular brachial plexus block techniques.

As regards the relationships of the subclavian artery at the interscalene level, it occupies the medial angle of the scalene triangle (Fig. 2.5), separated medially from the subclavian vein by the interposition of the anterior scalene muscle. It is in relation to the phrenic nerve which runs adhering to the surface of this muscle before penetrating into the thorax. Posterolaterally, it is in relation to the brachial plexus. It is also in relation to the external jugular vein which, before blending into the subclavian vein, passing in front of or laterally to the anterior scalene muscle, crosses the artery perpendicularly. It is also in relation to the structures that invest the supraclavicular fossa, with the middle cervical fascia, with the omohyoid muscle, with the superficial cervical fascia, with the platysma, with the subcutaneous areolar tissue and with the skin.

2.1.5 The Scalene Muscles

Despite the name, these muscles have nothing to do with a ladder (Italian 'scala'), since the name derives etymologically from the Greek 'σκαληνός' which means unequal. There are three scalene muscles—anterior, middle and posterior—which connect the first two ribs to the cervical vertebrae.

The Anterior Scalene Muscle

This muscle inserts cranially on the anterior tubercles of the transverse processes of the sixth, fifth, fourth and third cervical vertebrae. These four heads unite to form the actual muscle body that inserts on the Lisfranc's tubercle at the level of the upper surface of the first rib. The anterior scalene muscle is in relation medially to the subclavian vein which is separated from the subclavian artery precisely by the insertion of the muscle. The subclavian artery is situated laterally to the muscle and separates it from the brachial plexus despite the close contiguity of the two (Fig. 2.5).

The phrenic nerve, adhering in its upper part to the lateral surface of the muscle, then to its anterior surface and lastly to its medial border, before penetrating into the thorax, traverses it obliquely in a lateromedial downward direction. The anterior scalene muscle, moreover, is also in relation to the lateral belly of the omohyoid muscle which traverses it at various levels—the position of the muscle being extremely variable—before disappearing with its intermediate tendon beneath the sternocleidomastoid muscle.

The Middle Scalene Muscle

This muscle inserts on the posterior tubercles of the transverse processes of the last six cervical vertebrae and on the posterior borders of their respective grooves (from which the somatic nerve emerges). Its insertion on the first rib is not as characteristic as that of the anterior scalene muscle, but consists in a rough area located

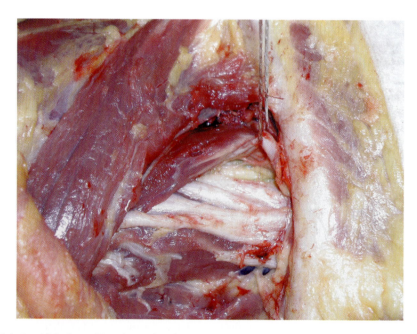

Fig. 2.5 Right brachial plexus. To enhance its visualization, the subclavian artery has been suspended by a thread. To be noted medial to it is the anterior scalene muscle and laterally the lower trunk of the brachial plexus. On the border between the anterior scalene and the sternocleidomastoid muscle, we see the phrenic nerve adhering to the anterior surface of the anterior scalene muscle. At the level of the middle scalene muscle, the suprascapular nerve is visible, severed during the dissection

on the upper surface of the rib, posteriorly to the shallow track produced by the brachial plexus and to the gutter produced by the subclavian artery. As a variant, it may also insert on the second rib.

The middle scalene muscle is fundamentally in relation to the anterior scalene muscle, together with which it bounds the scalene triangle, formed by the two scalenes, which splay out lower down at an acute angle, with the first rib as the base. The brachial plexus, which crosses the triangle in the direction of the axilla, is separated from the anterior scalene muscle by the interposition of the subclavian artery and as a result is closer to the middle scalene muscle (Fig. 2.5).

The Posterior Scalene Muscle

Situated posterolaterally in relation to the middle scalene muscle, the posterior scalene muscle inserts cranially on the posterior tubercles of the transverse processes of the fourth, fifth and sixth cervical vertebrae, and sometimes from the fifth to the seventh. It then travels downwards, laterally and posteriorly to the middle scalene muscle, passing above the first rib and going on to insert in a rough portion of the edge of the second rib (Fig. 2.6).

It may often be fused with the middle scalene muscle, with which it appears to form a single body, despite dividing caudally into two bundles that insert, the anterior one on the first rib, and the posterior one on the second rib.

The posterior scalene muscle enters into a relationship dorsally with the levator scapulae muscle, while its costal insertion is covered by the first two digitations of the serratus anterior muscle.

Innervation

The anterior and middle scalene muscles are innervated by thin nerve branches stemming from the anterior divisions of the third, fourth, fifth and sixth cervical nerves. The posterior scalene muscle is innervated by thin nerve filaments stemming, instead from the posterior divisions of the third, fourth, fifth, sixth and seventh cervical nerves.

2.1.6 The Shoulder Muscles

The muscular apparatus of the shoulder girdle is notoriously composite and complex; numerous muscles contribute to its stability and its functions. These muscles, in the eventuality of arthroscopic surgery under regional anesthesia, are not always adequately relaxed when they are not voluntarily activated by the patient, possibly in an attempt to change what may be an uncomfortable position. This may create difficulties for the surgeon. Moreover, a number of these muscles, if stimulated outside the neurovascular bundle, move the shoulder, simulating contraction of the deltoid muscle and creating the illusion of stimulating the brachial plexus.

But let us proceed in an orderly fashion, describing here below the most important muscles and their innervation.

The Deltoid Muscle

The deltoid muscle, triangular in shape, envelops the shoulder joint externally, inserting, from front to back, on the lateral third of the clavicle, on the acromion and on the scapular spine. These distinct bundles, converging laterally and inferiorly, insert on the deltoid tuberosity of the humerus.

It is innervated by one of the terminal branches of the brachial plexus, the axillary or circumflex nerve (C5–C6). The function of the deltoid muscle is to raise the upper limb and abduct it. With its action alone, however, the arm would never be raised above the horizontal plane. The raising of the upper limb is due to the scapula and to its muscles, which, with a rotatory movement, anteriorize the inferior angle and raise the lateral angle, that is, the glenoid cavity. The twitch of the deltoid muscle, in addition to that of the biceps and triceps muscles, is optimal for brachial plexus blocks performed for shoulder surgery.

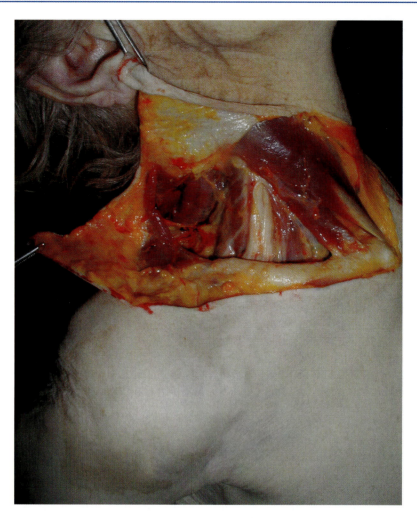

Fig. 2.6 Enigma as to whether the posterior scalene muscle exists as an entity in itself or whether it is fused with middle scalene muscle, in which case the term 'posterior scalene muscle' is used to refer to the two fused muscles as a single muscle, can be clarified with the wisdom of Solomon by saying that the two muscles are mainly fused in their cranial part but separated in their caudal part, so that each reaches its own point of insertion, that is, the first rib in the case of the middle scalene muscle, and the second rib in the case of the posterior scalene muscle. Nevertheless, there are many cases in which they remain separated throughout their entire course from the insertion on the transverse processes as far as their respective costal insertions. The two muscles, though adhering to one another, are separated by their respective perimysial sheaths. Moreover, the innervation itself separates them, the middle scalene muscle, like the anterior scalene muscle, being innervated by the anterior branches of the cervical nerves, whereas the posterior scalene muscle is innervated by the posterior branches of the same nerves

The Rotator Cuff

There are four muscles that form the rotator cuff: the supraspinatus, infraspinatus, subscapularis and teres minor muscles. They constitute the 'roof' of the glenohumeral joint.

The Supraspinatus Muscle

It extends from the supraspinatus fossa of the scapula to the head of the humerus. It inserts medially on the periosteum of the fossa of the same name and then passes beneath the acromioclavicular joint to insert finally on the greater tuberosity of the humerus (trochite). In its proximal part, it is covered by the trapezius muscle. It is innervated by the suprascapular nerve. Its arm-raising action is similar to that of the deltoid muscle. Moreover, it draws the head of the humerus towards the glenoid cavity of the scapula, at the same time slightly rotating the arm externally.

The Infraspinatus Muscle

Situated on the posterior surface of the scapula, this muscle presents a greater consistency and power than the previous one. It inserts on the medial part of the infraspinatus fossa and extends towards the glenohumeral joint, the muscle dividing into three bundles, the upper, middle and lower bundles, which converge on the joint itself. Here, it inserts on the greater tuberosity of the humerus (trochite). It is innervated by the suprascapular nerve. This muscle, too, draws the head of the humerus towards the glenoid cavity and imparts a slight external rotation movement to the arm.

N.B. If the suprascapular nerve is stimulated electrically, with consequent contraction of the supraspinatus and infraspinatus muscles, this sets the shoulder in motion by simulating contraction of the deltoid muscle. Now the suprascapular nerve, which is also part of the brachial plexus, abandons the neurovascular bundle very proximally, running for almost its entire extent outside the latter (Fig. 2.5), and therefore, when the suprascapular nerve is stimulated, there is a very strong likelihood that this will take place outside the bundle, giving rise to twitches which are unreliable for the purposes of anesthesia. However, the operator only needs to rest the hand not accompanying the needle on the skin of the shoulder, previously thoroughly disinfected, in order to perceive or not the twitches of the deltoid muscle, even when delivering a low current intensity with the electrical nerve stimulator (0.3 mA).

The Subscapularis Muscle

Situated on the anterior surface of the scapula, this muscle occupies the entire subscapular fossa and inserts medially on the medial border of the latter. From here, its bundles are directed obliquely upwards until they reach the lesser tuberosity of the humerus on which they insert. A number of bundles also insert on the crest of the trochine. Innervation of the muscle stems from two roots of the brachial plexus (C5 and C6) from which derive the superior subscapular nerve for the upper muscular bundles and the inferior subscapular nerve (C5-C7) for the lower bundles.

Its action is threefold:
1. It adducts the humerus.
2. It draws the head of the humerus towards the glenoid cavity.
3. It rotates the humerus internally with an antagonist action to that of the supraspinatus and infraspinatus muscles. In practice, it adducts and internally rotates the arm.

The Teres Minor Muscle

The constitutionally rather frail teres minor muscle inserts on the axillary edge of the scapula and then travels towards the lower part of the greater tuberosity of the humerus (trochite). It is innervated by a branch of the axillary or circumflex nerve (C5–C6), which innervates the deltoid muscle. Its action is similar to that of the infraspinatus muscle: It draws the head of the humerus towards the glenoid cavity, at the same time rotating the arm externally.

The Teres Major Muscle

The teres major muscle is tougher than the teres minor. It inserts medially on the inferior angle of the scapula, and after passing in front of the neck of the humerus, it reaches the posterior border of the biceps groove in which it inserts. It is innervated by the teres major nerve, a branch of the lower subscapular nerve (C5–C7). Its action moves the arm posteriorly and medially; in practice, it adducts and internally rotates the arm. It exerts a synergistic action with the latissimus dorsi muscle. It is activated in the retroversion of the arm.

The Trapezius Muscle

Despite the name, however you look at it, partially or as a whole, its shape is triangular. It inserts on the middle third of the superior nuchal line, on the external occipital protuberance, on the spinal processes of C6 and C7, and of the first ten thoracic vertebrae, and on the respective supraspinous ligaments. From these medial insertions, the upper bundles insert laterally on the lateral third of the posterior edge of the clavicle, the middle bundles on the medial edge of the acromion and on the posterior edge of the scapular spine and the lower bundles on the medial part of the scapular spine. The superoanterior border of the muscle, together with the sternocleidomastoid muscle and the clavicle, bounds the region known as the supraclavicular region. Like the sternocleidomastoid muscle, the trapezius muscle is innervated by the spinal accessory nerve and by a number of branches of the cervical plexus (C2–C4). Contraction of the muscle causes lifting of the shoulder.

The Levator Scapulae Muscle

The levator scapulae muscle inserts on the transverse processes of the first two cervical vertebrae, on the posterior tubercles of the transverse processes of the third and fourth cervical vertebrae and distally on the superior angle and medial edge of the scapula. It is in relation to the sternocleidomastoid muscle, the trapezius muscle, by which it is covered, and with the skin of the upper portion where it is not covered by the trapezius muscle. In turn, it covers the splenius muscle. It is in relation anteriorly to the posterior scalene muscle (Fig. 2.7).

The levator scapulae muscle belongs to the same muscle group as the upper portion of the serratus anterior muscle, with which it is sometimes united. It is innervated by the levator scapulae nerve (C4–C5). Its action consists in raising the medial angle of the scapula, thus bringing about the lowering of the shoulder. Contracting bilaterally, it extends the neck, and contracting unilaterally, it bends the neck on the same side. It also intervenes in forced inspiration.

The Splenius Muscle

The splenius muscle is located below the sternocleidomastoid and trapezius muscles. Chiarugi describes this muscle as two distinct muscles: the splenius capitis and splenius cervicis muscles.

The Splenius Capitis Muscle

From the mastoid process and the lateral half of the superior (or highest) nuchal line, the splenius capitis muscle travels downwards, inwards and posteriorly and inserts on the spinous processes of the seventh cervical vertebra and the first two thoracic vertebrae.

The Splenius Cervicis Muscle

This muscle originates on the posterior part of the transverse process of the atlas and the epistropheus and sometimes of the third cervical vertebra, then travels obliquely downwards medially and posteriorly and inserts on the spinous processes of the third, fourth and fifth thoracic vertebrae. The splenius cervicis muscle is innervated by the dorsal branches of the cervical nerves and particularly by the dorsal branch of the second cervical nerve, the greater occipital nerve, or Arnold's nerve. Its action serves to extend, tilt, and laterally rotate the head.

The Rhomboid Muscle

Its name is due to its rhomboid or lozenge-like shape. It inserts proximally on the supraspinous ligament between the sixth and seventh cervical vertebrae and on the spinous processes of the seventh cervical and first four thoracic vertebrae. Distally, it inserts on the medial edge of the scapula.

2 Topographical Anatomy

Fig. 2.7 From *right* to *left*, we note the anterior scalene muscle, the brachial plexus, the two scalene muscles (middle and posterior, fused cranially), the omohyoid muscle (transfixed by the first needle), the levator scapulae muscle, the splenius cervicis muscle (transfixed by the second needle), and the splenius capitis muscle

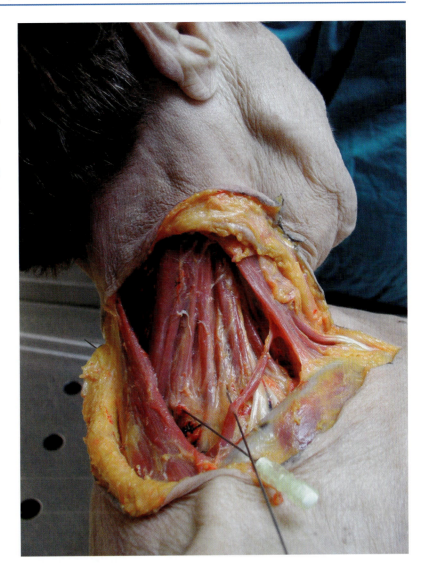

It is innervated by the rhomboid nerve, a collateral branch of the brachial plexus (C4–C5). Contraction of this muscle gives rise to a rotatory movement of the scapula to such an extent that the inferior angle of the latter is adducted and the lateral angle lowered, and with it the entire shoulder.

The Serratus Anterior Muscle

The serratus anterior muscle inserts on the medial edge of the scapula and, adhering tightly to the ribs from the first to the tenth, performs its function of keeping the scapula pressed against the rib cage. In cases of hypotrophy, it favours the so-called winged scapula phenomenon. It is normally divided into three portions:

- The upper portion which is directed slightly obliquely, downwards and forwards and which inserts with two digitations on the first and second ribs.
- The middle portion which inserts along the entire anterior length of the medial edge of the scapula and on the second, third and fourth ribs with a slightly oblique direction upwards and forwards.
- The lower portion which, from the inferior angle of the scapula, inserts on the fifth to the

tenth ribs with an oblique direction downwards and from back to front.

We will deal here only with the first portion which is topographically related to the brachial plexus.

As the first two digitations adhere tightly to the first two ribs, they present a convex upper surface and a concave lower surface. They are in relationships to the subscapularis, supraspinatus, infraspinatus, rhomboid, levator scapulae and the middle and posterior scalene muscles; with the brachial plexus which, on exiting from the scalene triangle, comes to rest on them; and with the suprascapular nerve, which, on abandoning the neurovascular bundle, crosses the muscle and proceeds towards the scapula (see Fig. 1.5 Anatomy).

It may fuse abnormally with the levator scapulae muscle whose muscular group it is part of. It is innervated by the long thoracic nerve (C5–C6). It has two functions:
1. It keeps the scapula pressed against the thorax and rotates it upwards, thus raising the shoulder.
2. It functions as an accessory respiratory muscle.

2.1.7 The Cervical Fasciae

European treatises normally describe three cervical fasciae: the superficial fascia, the middle fascia, and the deep fascia. In English-language texts, the three fasciae are simply lumped together as the deep (or prevertebral) cervical fascia. This constitutes a source of considerable confusion. For our part, we will refer to the classic description furnished by Testut, whose textbooks have served for the training of several generations of European anatomists.

The Superficial Cervical Fascia

The superficial cervical fascia, situated more or less at subcutaneous level, completely encircles and envelops the neck like a thin orthopaedic collar. On the median anterior raphe, it presents the cervical linea alba. From there, passing laterally, it encounters the sternocleidomastoid muscle (SCM); it splits to enclose the SCM and then recomposes itself at the level of the posterior border. It then invests the supraclavicular triangle (constituted by the anterior border of the trapezius muscle, by the posterior border of the sternocleidomastoid muscle and by the clavicle), where, on encountering the anterior border of the trapezius muscle, it splits to envelop the muscle and attach itself finally to the spinous processes of the cervical vertebrae and the first dorsal vertebrae. Between the superficial cervical fascia and the skin are inserted the platysma and the external jugular vein, which is situated beneath the platysma. In actual fact, both the external jugular vein and the platysma itself are enveloped by a splitting of the fascia.

From the internal surface of the superficial cervical fascia, at the level of the anterior border of the trapezius muscle, departs an interesting septum called the vertebral extension (or vertebral septum or cervical extension) which runs in an anteromedial direction towards the scalene muscles and in turn splits into a posterior lamina, which, after enveloping the middle and posterior scalene muscles, attaches itself to the posterior tubercles of the transverse processes, and an anterior lamina which, enveloping the anterior scalene muscle, attaches itself to the anterior tubercles of the transverse processes, fusing with the deep cervical fascia on the anterior surface of the muscle (Fig. 2.8).

"Between these two laminae there is an important space, the intermediate space of the scalene muscles, where the subclavian artery and the nerve trunks giving rise to the brachial plexus are to be found" (Testut).

The two vertebral extensions, right and left, of the superficial cervical fascia divide the cross section of the neck into two distinct regions: one anterior, the neck region, and the other posterior, the nuchal region.

The Middle Cervical Fascia

The middle cervical fascia, which is trapezoidal in shape, lies between the upper border of the omohyoid muscle on one side and that on the

2 Topographical Anatomy

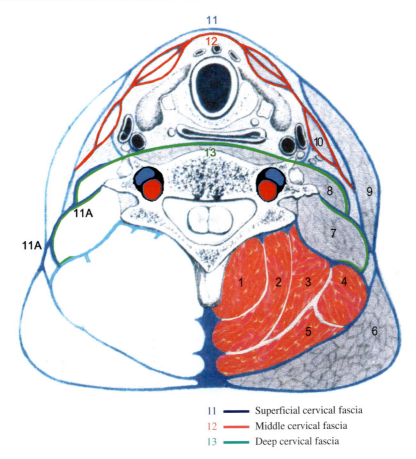

11	▬▬▬	Superficial cervical fascia
12	▬▬▬	Middle cervical fascia
13	▬▬▬	Deep cervical fascia

Fig. 2.8 Cross section of the neck at the sixth cervical vertebra level. *Pink* muscles from *left* to *right*: *1* muscles of the paravertebral groove; *2* semispinal muscle of the head (or musculus complexus major); *3* longissimus muscle of the head (or musculus complexus minor); *4* levator scapulae muscle; *5* splenius muscle; *6* trapezius muscle (*grey*); *7* middle and posterior scalene muscles; *8* anterior scalene muscle; *9* sternocleidomastoid muscle; *10* omohyoid muscle; *11* superficial cervical fascia (*sky blue*) enveloping the sternocleidomastoid muscle; *11A* vertical extension of the superficial cervical fascia; *12* middle cervical fascia (*red*) which envelops and departs from the omohyoid muscles, from which it attaches laterally to the superficial cervical fascia at the level of the medial surface of the SCM muscle and medially to the deep cervical fascia; *13* deep cervical fascia (*green*)

opposite side (Fig. 2.9). It invests the omoclavicular triangle and then goes on to insert on the posterior edge of the clavicle where it fuses with the fascia of the subclavius muscle.

The upper base constituted by the hyoid bone is fairly short; the lower base, on the other hand, is very long, extending across from one coracoid notch to the other; in resting conditions, the two sides, constituted by the left and right omohyoid muscles, present an arch-like appearance, tending to become more rectilinear in the presence of contraction of the two muscles.

The middle cervical fascia is covered by the superficial cervical fascia from which it is separated by a thin layer of loose cellular connective tissue; in turn, with its internal surface, it invests the larynx, the body of the thyroid gland, the trachea, the pharynx, the oesophagus and the neurovascular bundle of the neck (formed by the common carotid artery, by the internal jugular vein and by the vagus nerve). The paravertebral sympathetic chain is located posteriorly and in a more medial position, in contact with the deep (or prevertebral) cervical fascia.

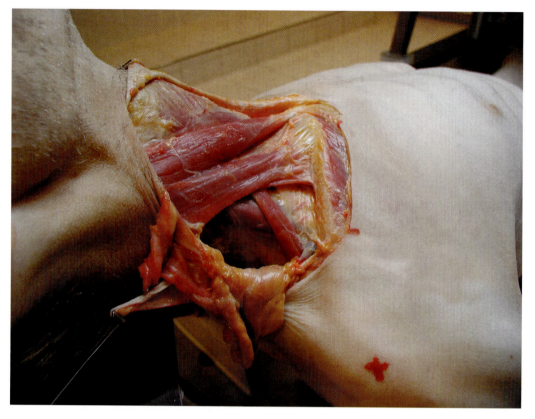

Fig. 2.9 Part of the middle cervical fascia which departs from the anterior border of the omohyoid muscle. It disappears under the SCM, going over to the contralateral omohyoid muscle and superiorly to the hyoid bone

The middle cervical fascia, on reaching the level of the subhyoid muscles medially, splits and envelops them, and then recomposes itself and encounters its contralateral equivalent on the midline.

The Deep (or Prevertebral) Cervical Fascia

The deep cervical fascia is attached, proceeding from top to bottom, to the occipital bone and to the transverse processes of the cervical vertebrae; here, it is juxtaposed to the anterior surface of the anterior scalene muscle where it fuses with the superficial cervical fascia, whose anterior vertebral extension lamina envelops the muscle; it is also attached to the costal processes of the first thoracic vertebrae where it dwindles and disperses in the loose cellular tissue of the posterior mediastinum. With its posterior surface, it is also in relation to the prevertebral muscles: the longus colli and the major and minor anterior rectus muscles; more anteriorly, it is in relation to the pharynx, oesophagus, the neurovascular bundle of the neck (invested by the middle cervical fascia) and the paravertebral sympathetic chain which it envelops by splitting. Only the superior cervical ganglion is not contained in the splitting, thus proving less adherent to the fascia.

For anesthesiological purposes, it is important to note:
- that the fasciae of the scalene muscles are formed by the splitting of the vertebral extension of the superficial cervical fascia which at this level fuses and continues with the deep cervical fascia;
- that the latter, after fusing at this level with the superficial cervical fascia—driven in the embryogenetic phase of development by the nerve rudiments which on progressing toward the periphery then go on to form the brachial

plexus—constitutes an authentic sheath around the plexus that extends, encircling and accompanying the various elements—roots, trunks, and cords. This sheath is fairly thick proximally at the level of the deep cervical fascia. Compartments are thus formed, by and large one for each nerve trunk, but not always communicating with one another, which may limit the spread of the anesthetic;

- that the paravertebral sympathetic chain is situated close to the deep cervical fascia or prevertebral aponeurosis; this may constitute a cleavage plane that communicates with the thoracic cavity (see the section on Bezold-Jarisch syndrome in Chap. 8).

2.1.8 Gale E. Thompson and Duane H. Rorie

Quite apart from all the treatises of anatomy, more or less exhaustive in their descriptions, the study by Thompson and Rorie entitled 'Functional anatomy of the brachial plexus sheaths', published in *Anesthesiology* in 1983, remains a classic for anesthesiological purposes. The article clearly outlines the structure and conformation of the neurovascular bundle.

The authors adopt a study method combining the use of anatomical dissection, histological preparations and X-rays obtained using contrast media. The radiological study was conducted on ten volunteers and the anatomical study on three cadavers. The histological preparations stained with haematoxylin and eosin showed that the connective tissue forming the fibrous fringes presents a denser consistency proximally at its origin, on abandoning the deep cervical fascia, and progressively becomes more loosely organized distally. At each level, the authors noted that the connective tissue that makes up the sheath of the neurovascular bundle extends inwards, forming septa between the various components of the plexus: The consistency of these septa is entirely similar in terms of thickness and density to the sheath enveloping the bundle. Thus, the neurovascular bundle appears as a multicompartmental structure. The various compartments would appear to be well defined at the axillary level and to present greater communication at the proximal level.

These interfascial septa, on the one hand, limit the transverse spread of anesthetic from one compartment to another and, on the other hand, explain why the anesthetic solution spreads easily in a longitudinal direction up and down the nerve. This would account for the fact that sometimes the anesthesia may be well induced on one nerve (generally, one which, when stimulated, presents twitches or paraesthesia; editor's note), but insufficient or even totally absent on another.

Four years later, B. L. Partridge et al., in a study conducted on eighteen cadavers and published in *Anesthesiology* in 1987, demonstrated that, also at the axillary level, there is communication between the various compartments and therefore that there is no need for multiple injections.

Bibliography

Brizzi F, Casini M, Castorina S, Franzi AT, Levi AC, Lucherini A, Maritozzi G, Miani A, Pacini P, Renda T, Ruggeri A, Santoro A, Soscia A (1998) Anatomia topografica – Testa-collo. Edi-Ermes, Milano

Chiarugi G, Bucciante L (1972) Istituzioni di anatomia dell'uomo. Vallardi Editore, Milano

Dalens B (1995) Anestesia loco-regionale dalla nascita all'età adulta. Fogliazza Editore, Milano

Hafferl AW (1989) Lehrbuch der topographischen Anatomie. Thiel von Springer Gmbh

Netter FH (1985) Atlante di anatomia fisiopatologia e clinica. Edizioni CIBA-GEIGY, Varese

Partridge BL, Katz J, Benirschke K (1987) Functional anatomy of the brachial plexus sheaths: implications for anesthesia. Anesthesiology 66:743–747

Pernkopf E (1960) Topographische Anatomie des Menschen. Urban & Schwarzenberg, Wien

Rucci FS et al (1992) Il decorso della vena giugulare esterna quale punto di repere di superficie nel blocco perivascolari succlavio. Minerva Anestesiol 58:397–401

Sobotta J, Becher H (1974) Atlante di anatomia dell'uomo. USES – Edizioni Scientifiche, Firenze

Testut L, Jacob O (1977) Trattato di anatomia topografica. UTET, Torino

Testut L (1943) Anatomia umana. UTET, Torino

Thompson GE, Rorie DK (1983) Functional anatomy of the brachial plexus sheaths. Anesthesiology 59:117–122

Anatomy of the Cervical Plexus

F. Alemanno and E. Egarter Vigl

In our anatomical description of the innervation of the supraclavicular region, we cannot neglect to make some mention, however brief, of the cervical plexus. The superior cervical somatic nerves, in fact, in addition to numbering among the terminal nerves as important a nerve as the phrenic nerve, have numerous anastomoses and imbrications sharing territorial competence with the brachial plexus.

The cervical plexus, on the one hand, sends anastomotic contributions to the brachial plexus and, on the other hand, exerts an action complementary to the latter in the sensory innervation of the shoulder and clavicle.

It is formed by the anterior divisions of the first four cervical nerves.

The anterior division of the first cervical nerve emerges at a point above the atlas and below the occipital bone and runs alongside the vertebral artery in the groove produced by the latter in the posterior arch of the atlas; on reaching the point where the vertebral artery exits from the transverse foramen coming to rest on its own dedicated track, it crosses the artery from below, travelling forwards and caudad, and forms an anastomotic loop with an ascending branch of the second cervical nerve.

The anterior divisions of the second, third and fourth cervical nerves, on emerging from their respective intervertebral foramina, proceed along the dedicated tracks of their transverse apophyses, passing behind the vertebral artery. At the lateral ends of the transverse apophyses, they anastomose to one another in the following manner:

- The anterior division of the second nerve pair, at the lateral end of the transverse apophysis of the epistropheus, divides into two branches. One branch, travelling upwards, forms the anastomotic arch with the first nerve, while the other descends forming the second anastomotic arch with the third pair.
- The anterior division of the third nerve pair, at the end of the transverse apophysis of the third vertebra, divides into three branches, the uppermost of which anastomoses with the descending branch of the second nerve, while the lowest anastomoses with the ascending branch of the fourth pair. The middle branch constitutes the cutaneous transverse nerve of the neck.
- The anterior division of the fourth cervical nerve, at the end of the transverse apophysis of the fourth vertebra, gives rise to three main branches: An upper branch that anastomoses with the descending ramus of the third nerve, a lower branch that constitutes the anastomotic contribution to the brachial plexus and

F. Alemanno (✉)
Institute of Anesthesiology Resuscitation and Pain Therapy, University of Verona, Verona, Italy
e-mail: fernando@alemannobpb.it

E. Egarter Vigl
Institute of Pathological Anatomy, Bolzano Regional Hospital, Bolzano, Italy

lastly a branch that constitutes the main root of the phrenic nerve.

Thus, the three anastomotic arches that unite the first, second, third and fourth anterior divisions of the first four spinal nerves constitute the cervical plexus. The five superficial or cutaneous branches and the ten deep or muscular branches originate from the five anterior divisions, before emitting the anastomoses, and from the anastomotic arches.

In order not to get involved in a long and rather pedantic description of the fifteen nerve branches of the cervical plexus, we will deal here only with the five superficial or cutaneous branches, these being relevant to the subject we are addressing, leaving the description of the other nine (except for the phrenic nerve) to the treatises of anatomy.

3.1 Superficial or Cutaneous Branches

All the superficial branches, to become such, present a monotonic behaviour: They run caudad and laterally, reaching the posterior border of the sternocleidomastoid muscle. On reaching the latter, they then travel cephalad, horizontally, or obliquely caudad to reach their respective areas of competence.

3.1.1 Cutaneous or Transverse Nerve of the Neck

This nerve often originates at the point where the two anastomotic branches—superior and inferior—of the anterior division of the third nerve separate, so much so that at times it seems as if the nerve trifurcates *ad modum tridentis* (like a trident). It emerges behind the posterior border of the sternocleidomastoid muscle and, after passing beneath the external jugular vein, travels on the lateral surface of the muscle, in a medial direction, innervating the suprahyoid, infrahyoid and carotid regions with two terminal branches; it gives off an anastomosis with a cervical twig of the facial nerve. Its cranial branch (resting upon and parallel to the auricular nerve) reaches the edge of the mandible, its imbrications overlapping the territory of competence of the mandibular branch of the trigeminal nerve. It innervates the skin caudad as far as the jugular region.

3.1.2 Auricular Nerve

The auricular nerve, which is of no interest for our purposes, but which we describe for the sake of completeness, originates from the anastomosis of the second and third nerve pairs. It emerges from the posterior border of the sternocleidomastoid muscle, a few centimetres above the cutaneous nerve of the neck. It adheres to the lateral surface of the muscle, proceeds cephalad and innervates the outer ear.

3.1.3 Lesser Occipital Nerve

The lesser occipital nerve, also called the mastoid branch, arises from the second and third cervical nerves. It emerges from the posterior border of the sternocleidomastoid muscle slightly above the auricular branch, ascends along the posterior border of the muscle and distributes to the mastoid and occipital regions and to the posterior part of the temporal region.

This, then, is the lesser occipital nerve, but what about the greater occipital nerve? This is the question that comes to the mind of the reader whose memories of anatomy have begun to fade. The greater occipital nerve or Arnold's nerve is not part of the cervical plexus because it is formed by the posterior branch of the second cervical nerve. It emerges beneath the posterior arch of the atlas, surrounds the lower border of the inferior oblique muscle of the head and then travels cephalad crossing the trapezius muscle and becoming subcutaneous in the occipital region, medially to the lesser occipital nerve, where its terminal branches innervate all the skin of this region.

3 Anatomy of the Cervical Plexus

3.1.4 Supraclavicular Branches

These branches, which are variable in number, arise from the third loop of the cervical plexus and from the anterior division of the fourth pair. United initially in a single trunk—the supraclavicular ramus as it is more properly called—from which the supra-acromial nerve also originates the supraclavicular rami branch out while still beneath the sternocleidomastoid muscle, but emerge, closely grouped together, from its posterior border, just behind the external jugular vein. They divide into an anterior group that straddles the vein, proceeding caudad and forwards, following the two heads of the muscle, and another group with a distinctly lower course towards the middle third of the clavicle. They pass beneath the platysma and after perforating it become more superficial, innervating the skin of the supra- and infraclavicular region at the level of the middle and medial third of the clavicle as far as the lateral border of the pectoralis major muscle (Fig. 3.1).

3.1.5 The Supra-Acromial Branch

This branch, which is important for the purposes of complete anesthesia of the shoulder, originates from the fourth cervical nerve sharing a

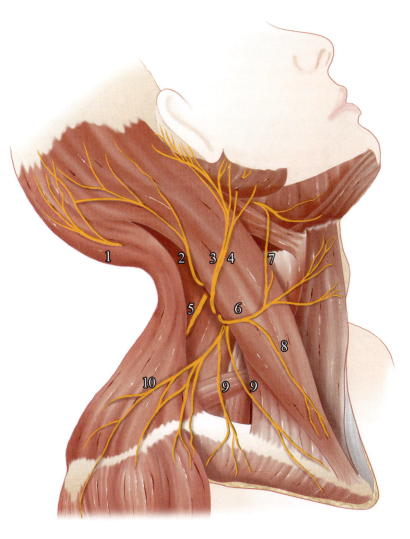

Fig. 3.1 Anatomical illustration of the distribution of the superficial cervical plexus. *1* Greater occipital nerve, which is not part of the brachial plexus; *2* lesser occipital nerve; *3* great auricular nerve; *4* cranial branch of the cutaneous nerve of the neck (parallel to the great auricular nerve); *5* accessory nerve, *6* cutaneous or transverse nerve of the neck; *7* its anastomotic loop with a cervical twig of the facial nerve; *8* caudal branches of the cutaneous or transverse nerve of the neck; *9* supraclavicular nerves innervating the skin of the middle and medial third of the clavicle; *10* supra-acromial branch

common trunk with the supraclavicular nerve that originates from the same cervical nerve, so much so that Bairati describes it as the lateral branch of the supraclavicular nerve.

This branch, too, emerges from beneath the posterior border of the sternocleidomastoid muscle, after which it runs laterally and caudad, passing in front of the external surface of the trapezius muscle. It then proceeds in the subcutaneous tissue, branching out at the level of the lateral third of the clavicle, to the entire shoulder.

3.2 The Phrenic Nerve

We have said that the deep cervical branches are of little interest anesthesiologically, but we cannot refrain from describing the phrenic nerve, which is involved in a substantial percentage of cases in which supraclavicular brachial plexus block techniques are performed, sometimes constituting a major complication.

The largest and most exhaustive monographic study in this connection is the one published by Luschka in the second half of the nineteenth century, which is still valid today (human anatomy does not change in the course of time).

The main root of the phrenic nerve is constituted by the anterior division of the fourth cervical nerve pair with a contribution from the branches of the anterior division of the third and fifth cervical pairs.

The phrenic nerve, emerging from the apex of the scalene triangle, adheres to and runs obliquely across the anterior surface of the anterior scalene muscle (Fig. 1.5). After travelling over the surface of the muscle in an inferomedial direction, it reaches the medial angle formed by the anterior scalene muscle and the first rib where it enters the thorax.

We will limit ourselves to describing the relationships, which the phrenic nerve has in the neck region, because it is in this region that the proximal brachial plexus block techniques are applied.

The phrenic nerve proceeds transversely for a short distance in a medial and oblique caudal direction through the space containing the neurovascular bundle of the brachial plexus, emerging from it at the level of the upper angle of the scalene triangle. It appears, adhering to the anterior surface of the anterior scalene muscle, covered by the splitting of the middle cervical fascia that envelops the omohyoid muscle. It is in the segment that crosses the upper part of the space described by Winnie that the phrenic nerve is involved in the block, all the more so, the more the needle tip lies in a paracervical position. Descending, it reaches the medial border of the anterior scalene muscle, and approaching the subclavian artery, it crosses the superficial cervical artery and the transverse cervical artery posteriorly; it then inserts itself between the subclavian artery, located deeper down, and the subclavian vein (located more superficially); proceeding then in an oblique, posterior direction, it reaches the anteromedial portion of the pleural dome, gaining access to the thoracic cavity.

The phrenic nerve, on a more superficial plane, is first crossed by the omohyoid muscle and then invested by the middle cervical fascia; finally, it is covered by the sternocleidomastoid muscle. Its entry point into the thorax corresponds to the interstice between the two heads of the sternocleidomastoid muscle.

Bibliography

Bairati A (1974) Anatomia umana, vol 3. Sistema nervoso periferico, organi di senso, sistema tegumentario. Minerva Medica, Torino

Chiarugi G, Bucciante L (1972) Istituzioni di anatomia dell'uomo. Vallardi Editore, Milano

Lippert H (2000) Lehrbuch Anatomie. Urban & Fischer, München-Jena

Schiebler TH, Schmidt W (1999) Anatomie: Zitologie, Histologie, Entwicklungsgeschichte, makroskopische und mikroskopische Anatomie des Menchen. Springer, Berlin, New York

Sieglbauer F (1935) Lehrbuch der normalen Anatomie des Menschen. vol 3. Auflage Urban & Schwarzenberg; Berlin

Sobotta J, Becher H (1974)Atlante di anatomia dell'uomo. USES—Edizioni Scientifiche, Firenze

Testut L (1943) Anatomia umana. UTET, Torino

Von Luschka H (1853) Der Nervus Phrenicus des Menschen, Tübingen

The Anesthetic Line

P. Grossi

The evolution of regional anesthesia techniques over the years has witnessed the alternation of a whole series of extremely heterogeneous approaches to the nerve structures. The aim of these procedures was to reconstruct, by means of cutaneous landmarks, the course of the underlying nerves which were then located with various systems, ranging from the eliciting of paresthesias to the more recent electrical nerve stimulation and ultrasound methods, so as to be able to perform the anesthetic block with a needle located close to the target.

In clinical practice, it is important to reduce to a minimum the attempts to locate the nerve by means of the needle, also in view of the discomfort that this kind of exploration causes the patient.

The reduction in the time taken to find the nerve and the attempts at exploration are closely related to the recognition of fixed anatomical landmarks common to all patients, analysis of which makes it possible to identify a point on the skin at which the needle needs to be inserted in order to reach the target nerve situated in depth.

Grossi, in 2003, for the purposes of making anesthetic block techniques safer, more accurate and more reproducible, developed the concept of the "anesthetic line", an important aid in the search for the best means of locating the nerve structures targeted in the block.

This is achieved by identifying cutaneous anatomical landmarks which may be some distance from the area of the block and not directly involved in it, but which lie over the course of the targeted nerve structures and represent an alignment with the latter in what is a theoretical "anesthetic line", that highlights, at the cutaneous level and on the frontal plane, the course of the underlying nerve structures in depth.

It thus proves possible to obtain an anatomical guide for the introduction of the needle.

Similar reasoning prompted Bazy (1914) in the early years of the twentieth century to propose tracing a line from Chassaignac's tubercle to the apex of the coracoid process of the scapula.

The concept of an anesthetic line merely reflects an anatomical virtual observation or visualization of the cranio-caudal longitudinal course of the nerve structure which, when the patient assumes given positions aimed at highlighting the anatomical landmarks, makes it possible to represent the nerve structure in a rectilinear manner and therefore in a configuration more easily accessible from the outside with a needle.

In the specific case of upper limb blocks, when the patient is positioned with the head turned towards the opposite side to the block and with the arm slightly abducted, it clearly emerges that the various anatomical landmarks enable the plexus to be visualized as a rectilinear structure (Fig. 4.1).

P. Grossi (✉)
Pain Therapy and Regional Anesthesia Service,
IRCCS, Policlinico San Donato Milanese, San
Donato Milanese, MI, Italy
e-mail: pagrossi@fastwebnet.it

4.1 The Anesthetic Line for the Upper Limb

The anesthetic line is obtained by placing the patient in the supine position with the head turned towards the side opposite to the side to be blocked and with the upper limb abducted 45° to the trunk.

We thus have a common starting position for all blocks of the upper limb, allowing good visualization of the following landmarks (Fig. 4.1):

- the apex of the scalene triangle, Chassaignac's tubercle;
- the midpoint of the clavicle;
- the deltopectoral groove, highlighting the coracoid process and the profile of the rib cage;
- the pulse of the axillary artery at the armpit;
- possibly, the medial epicondyle of the elbow, if the block is performed at the midhumeral level.

In this situation, we may note that the various cutaneous landmarks follow a linear route that departs from the apex of the scalene triangle and proceeds as far as the point where the axillary artery pulse is palpated at the armpit. This line can be extended as far as the medial epicondyle of the elbow in the case of blocks performed at the midhumeral level.

This expedient, which enables the anesthetist to "visualize" a three-dimensional structure such as the brachial plexus in terms of a two-dimensional frontal view, that is to say a line on the skin, allows both complete appreciation of the course of the underlying nerve structure and the choice of a variety of different approaches,

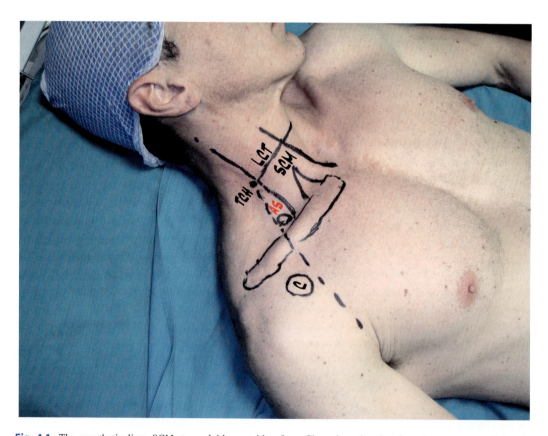

Fig. 4.1 The anesthetic line: *SCM* sternocleidomastoid muscle; *AS* subclavian artery pulse; *TCH* Chassaignac's tubercle; *C* coracoid apophysis; *LCT* transverse cricoid line. The anesthetic line is the *dashed line* that departs from Chassaignac's tubercle and passes tangential to the subclavian artery pulse; it passes over the midpoint of the clavicle and then proceeds tangentially also to the coracoid apophysis, finally reaching the axillary fold

which will vary according to the different inclinations and directions of the needle when performing the block.

One advantage of the anesthetic line consists in the possibility of selecting the dermatomes and blockable areas, performing an injection in a cranial or caudal direction.

4.1.1 The Anesthetic Line and Interscalene Approach

After the classic positioning of the patient, the anesthetic line is traced on the skin connecting the various landmarks.

The base of the needle is placed at the level of the midpoint of the clavicle, and the tip is directed craniad parallel to the course of the anesthetic line. In this way, the tip of the needle should lie at the level of the groove formed by the scalene triangle, approximately 2 cm below the classic entry point of the Winnie's technique.

After puncturing the skin, the progression of the needle in this direction enables it to reach the nerve bundle containing the brachial plexus in a targeted manner.

The concurrent use of electrical nerve stimulation permits the correct placement of the needle in the vicinity of the nerve bundles of the plexus. At a depth of approximately 1–2 cm, it will be possible to evoke the twitch of the deltoid muscle usually regarded as satisfactory for locating the brachial plexus.

The volume of anesthetic necessary for the block is 30–40 ml.

With this approach, the vascular structures are further away from the needle tip and a pleural puncture is a very rare occurrence.

Potential effects on the phrenic nerve, however, are present, as in other types of interscalene approach with variable clinical manifestations in all cases.

One hypothetical complication that may occur if the needle progresses too deeply is the accidental injection of local anesthetic into the epidural space. This type of complication, however, is not typical of this approach but has been reported as a result of interscalene blocks performed with the classic technique.

4.1.2 The anesthetic Line and Infraclavicular Approach

The infraclavicular approach with the aid of the anesthetic line is based on a modified version of the Raj's technique.

The approach to the brachial plexus by the infraclavicular route is characterized by the introduction of the stimulating needle (at least 10 cm long) at a point lying at a distance of approximately 3 cm from the midpoint of the clavicle (at the level of the coracoid process) on a line traced as an extension of the posterior border of the sternocleidomastoid muscle, which crosses the clavicle at the midpoint and extends as far as the armpit at the point where the pulse of the axillary artery is detectable. Ideally, this line represents, on the skin, the course of the deep underlying brachial plexus.

The anesthetic line is traced with the patient in the basic supine position.

The patient is then positioned with the upper arm abducted 45°.

After accurately locating the coracoid process and the deltopectoral groove, the anesthetist proceeds, after inducing a local anesthetic skin wheal, to introduce the needle, which, for the technique involving a single administration, is performed in a vertical direction perpendicular to the course of the anesthetic line. At a depth of 4–8 cm, depending upon the patient's constitution, it will be possible to locate the plexus by evoking the typical peripheral twitches which may include the contraction of the biceps muscle due to stimulation of the musculocutaneous nerve which is still a part of this area.

The total volume of anesthetic necessary for the block is 30–40 ml.

Two possible complications are associated with this approach, namely the risk of pleural or arterial puncture. On the basis of the data reported in the literature, however, the incidence of these complications would not appear to be very significant.

Bibliography

Bazy L (1917) Chapter. In: Pauchet V, Sourdat P, Laboure J (eds) L'Anesthésie Regionale. G. Doine et Cic, Paris, pp 222–225

Grossi P (2003) The anesthetic line: a guide for new approaches to block the brachial plexus. Reg Anaesth Pain Med 7(2):56–60

Raj PP, Montgomery SJ, Nettels D et al (1973) Infraclavicular brachial plexus block. A new approach. Anesth Analg 52:897–904

Winnie AP (1979) Factors influencing the distribution of local anesthetics in the brachial plexus sheath. Anesth Analg 58:225

Electrical Nerve Stimulation and Percutaneous Identification of the Target

L. Perotti, M. Allegri, A. Matteazzi and P. Grossi

5.1 Introduction

The execution of a peripheral block requires a procedure that permits accurate identification of the nerve structures. The identification of a nerve or a nerve plexus for the purposes of performing a regional anesthetic block is done by means of invasive or non-invasive techniques using needles or other specific instruments.

These procedures entail the use of a needle which, via direct mechanical stimulation or via the impulses generated and conducted by an electrical nerve stimulator, make it possible to locate the target nerve structure by evoking paraesthesias and/or motor responses.

With the appropriate technique, the evoked responses attest to the correct positioning of the needle tip in relation to the target of the block.

When an electrical stimulation is applied, a weak direct current is supplied to the tip of the needle by means of a current generator called nerve stimulator, which delivers square wave current. This current gives rise to a depolarization of the nerve fibres close to the point from which the current wave is administered (in this specific case, the needle tip).

Electrical nerve stimulation (ENS) works on the basis of the principle according to which it is possible to apply, in a targeted manner and in the immediate vicinity of the nerve structure, a series of electrical stimuli which, by stimulating the motor fibres, cause the contraction of the muscles innervated by these fibres.

In other words, if an electrical impulse passes through the needle used for the block and if the needle is close to the motor fibres of the nerve, a depolarization is produced capable of causing a motor contraction (called twitch) in the muscular district innervated by the nerve stimulated; this contraction enables the anesthetist to identify exactly which nerve fibres are involved.

The correct execution of regional anesthesia with ENS requires compliance with a set of rules which are summarized in the 10 commandments listed below.

L. Perotti
Anesthesia, Resuscitation and Pain Therapy Service,
IRCCS Foundation, Policlinico San Donato Milanese, San Donato Milanese (MI), Italy

M. Allegri (✉)
Anesthesia, Resuscitation and Pain Therapy Service,
IRCCS Policlinico San Matteo, Pavia, Pavia, Italy
e-mail: massimo.allegri@unipv.it

A. Matteazzi
Pain Therapy and Regional Therapy Service,
IRCCS, Policlinico San Donato Milanese, San Donato Milanese (MI), Italy

P. Grossi
Pain Therapy and Regional Anesthesia Service,
IRCCS, Policlinico San Donato Milanese, San Donato Milanese (MI), Italy

5.2 Ten Commandments for the Use of ENS

1. A thorough knowledge of (1) anatomy, (2) the course, relations and cutaneous ramifications of the nerve structures and (3) the dermatomere and myomere subdivisions.
2. Choose the approach to the nerve structures carefully in relation to the anatomical area of interest and the type of surgery to be performed.
3. Position the neutral electrode at a distance of at least 20 cm from the stimulating needle.
4. Avoid positioning the indifferent electrode on the course of the nerve to be blocked.
5. Use low-intensity current when eliciting the twitches so as to guarantee patient comfort.
6. Use the minimum stimulus intensity necessary to obtain the strongest twitch (0.5 mA). This rule enables one to reach the correct distance between the needle and the nerve.
7. Always seek the "best twitch" before proceeding to inject the local anesthetic; that is to say the twitch corresponding to the sensory area wherein the surgery will be performed.
8. In case of multiple blocks, first locate the nerve or part of the brachial plexus most involved in the surgical site (e.g. for surgery of the foot, first perform the sciatic nerve block followed by the femoral nerve block; invert these procedures for knee surgery).
9. After the first injection of local anesthetic, complete the block by searching for the accessory nerve branches, avoiding introducing the needle into the anesthetized area.
10. Always perform the Raj test.

5.2.1 The Raj Test

Once the nerve root has been located, 2 ml of anesthetic solution is injected, while maintaining the electrical stimulation unaltered.

The following situations may arise:
(a) the peripheral twitches are interrupted: *correct location*;
(b) the peripheral twitches persist: *needle positioned in the pre-fascial area*. In the event of pre-fascial injection, the needle must be withdrawn and repositioned in search of the best twitch;
(c) the peripheral twitches persist and the patient experiences intense paraesthesia along the nerve: *perineural injection*. In the event of perineural injection, the procedure must be suspended immediately and the needle repositioned;
(d) the peripheral twitches persist and the patient complains of intense pain and immediate anesthesia of the nerve trunk involved: *intraneural injection*. In the event of intraneural injection, the procedure must be definitively suspended.

5.3 Electrical Nerve Stimulation

In excitable cells, the electrical stimulation induced by the electrical nerve stimulator is capable of depolarizing the cell membrane.

The action potential is generated on condition that the stimulating current reaches a certain threshold intensity (I) for a certain amount of time (t) and that the intensity is reached rapidly.

A particular intensity–duration curve, and therefore, a particular "rheobase" and "chronaxie" characterize the various types of excitable cells.

The characteristic intensity–duration curve is very steep for stimuli of brief duration. In other words, both stimuli which are very intense but have a duration below a certain value (temporal threshold, chronaxie) and stimuli which have a very long duration, but an intensity lower than the rheobase, do not excite the cell.

The decisive factors in nerve stimulation are as follows:

5.3.1 Rheobase

The term "rheobase" refers to the minimum direct current intensity, applied for an indefinite period of time, capable of producing an action potential:

$$\delta(t) \to \omega$$

5.3.2 Chronaxie

"Chronaxie" refers to the minimum amount of time needed to produce an impulse with a current intensity double that of the rheobase. This parameter provides a measure of the excitability of the fibre.

5.4 Variability of Nerve Fibre Responses

The nerve fibres, that supply the musculoskeletal innervation and those that conduct sensitivity and nociception, considerably differ in terms of size, conduction velocity, refractory period and myelination.

Since the excitation threshold is lower in large-calibre myelin fibres, we have a situation whereby, on increasing the stimulus intensity, the nerve fibres are activated in the following order:

$$A\alpha, A\beta, C, A\delta \text{ and } C$$

A suitably modulated electrical stimulation is therefore capable of evoking a painless motor response without stimulating the $A\delta$ and C-fibres.

It is equally important to stress that local anesthetics block the conduction of the non-myelinated nerve fibres (C-fibres) first and then that of myelinated fibres of larger calibre.

It is therefore possible to perform selective blocks of mixed nerves in conditions of substantial safety with only minimal patient discomfort.

5.4.1 Characteristics of the Electrical Stimulus

The electrical stimulus is characterized by the following:

- waveform;
- duration;
- frequency;
- intensity.

Currently, most authors agree that direct current impulses with a square waveform, generated by constant current stimulators, are optimal.

The stimulus duration is measured in milliseconds (ms), the frequency in Hertz (Hz) and the intensity in milliamperes (mA). Some electrical nerve stimulators of the latest generation measure the charge delivered rather than the current intensity; in this case, the measurement unit is the nC (nanocoulomb) which represents the product of the current intensity and the duration of the stimulus.

The ideal duration of the stimulus, bearing in mind the intensity–duration curve of the normal muscle, is 0.3 ms which corresponds to the rheobase value; the most commonly used stimulation frequency is 2 Hz. The ideal stimulus intensity, with a duration of 0.3 ms, is 1–1.5 mA for the approach phase to the nerve, with a gradual reduction to 0.5–0.4 mA in the nerve location phase (see ten commandments).

5.5 Electrical Nerve Stimulators

The latest generation of electrical nerve stimulators have continuous control of the current setting and the current actually delivered to the nerve; they are also equipped with automatic compensation circuits for any variations in electrical resistance.

The parameters influencing the electrical stimulation activity are as follows:

5.5.1 Rheobase

As described above, the term rheobase corresponds to the minimum direct current intensity capable of exciting the cell if applied for an indefinitely long period:

$$\delta(t) \to \omega$$

5.5.2 Frequency

This value can be reduced to as little as 1 Hz for nerves of larger calibre or for blocks performed on fractured limbs, or increased to 3–4 Hz for nerve endings that are particularly thin and difficult to locate.

5.5.3 Stimulus Intensity

If the product of current intensity and the stimulus duration is used, the recommended values are 300–600 nC for the exploratory phase and 150 nC for the location phase.

5.5.4 Coulomb's Law and Ohm's Law

On the basis of Coulomb's law and Ohm's law, the current intensity that flows in a medium (intensity at the distance r from the electrical source) is inversely proportional to the square of the distance from the source and directly proportional to the constant depending on medium and the intensity of the source. Intensity, in turn, is directly proportional to voltage and inversely proportional to resistance.

The resistance can also be defined by a formula in which it is directly proportional to the specific resistance and length of the conductor and inversely proportional to the cross section of the conductor.

Thus, the estimate of the electrical charge that effectively reaches the nerve is influenced by numerous variables, in that it is conditioned by the substantial variability of the human body and by the different tissue resistances that the needle encounters during its progression.

Schematically, the stimulation can be represented as a closed electrical circuit formed by the human body, the exploratory needle (positive pole) and the neutral electrode placed on the skin (negative pole). In clinical practice, one variable always encountered consists in the distance between the stimulating needle and the cutaneous electrode, which cannot be determined exactly in advance.

5.5.5 Cutaneous Variability

The cutaneous variability is influenced by the different composition of the tissue layers the needle passes through, the distance and the reciprocal position of the electrodes.

5.5.6 Electrode-to-Needle Distance

According to a number of authors, the optimal positioning of the cutaneous electrode should be not less than 15–20 cm from the needle entry point, in a position opposite the course of the nerve. In this way, almost all the current delivered will invest the nerve and will be rapidly discharged onto the neutral electrode, reducing to a minimum the dispersion towards the rest of the body and making it possible to reduce the current intensity necessary to locate the nerve structure.

5.5.7 Hypothetical Complications of Electrical Nerve Stimulation

The harmful effects of ENS may be the following:
1. electrochemical effects;
2. Joule effects related to heat production;
3. traumatic injuries.

Current studies, however, appear to confirm the efficacy and safety of the procedure. The use of insulated needles and adequate stimulation parameters renders the Joule effect practically negligible, and the risk of electrical nerve injury practically nil.

What remains, as in the techniques involving paraesthesia, are possible direct traumatic injuries to the nerve. Such events, however, are limited thanks to the electrical stimulation which affords better perception of the approach of the needle to the target nerve.

5.6 Other Methods for Performing Peripheral Nerve Blocks

5.6.1 Percutaneous Electrical Nerve Stimulation

The traditional methods for performing peripheral nerve blocks are based on the identification of anatomical landmarks. These landmarks constitute an approximate starting point for invasive exploration with the needle.

The aim of the needle exploration may be anatomical (e.g. palpation of the axillary artery or ultrasound imaging) or functional (sensory response to mechanical stimulation, e.g., paraesthesia or motor response to the electrical stimulation of the nerve).

Recent studies have addressed the development of a procedure that permits ENS via the percutaneous route.

Unlike the ultrasound method based on the visualization of the target structures, percutaneous electrical stimulation uses as its functional endpoint the motor or sensory response to electrical stimulation of the underlying nerve. Percutaneous electrical stimulation is used to determine the exact point of insertion of the needle at the cutaneous level so as to reduce the invasive search for the nerve through exploration in depth.

Ganta et al. have studied the use of an electrocardiographic electrode for performing an interscalene block. The electrode, coupled to the electrical nerve stimulator, was positioned on the skin to locate the optimal access point.

Urmey proposes the use of a percutaneous exploratory electrode capable of facilitating the identification of the interscalene groove in patients with difficult anatomy.

The use of percutaneous stimulation to elicit a sensory response (paraesthesia) in case of electrical stimulation of a purely sensory nerve (lateral femoral cutaneous nerve) has been reported by Shannon et al.

Urmey and Grossi have recently described a technique called Percutaneous Electrode Guidance (PEG). PEG uses percutaneous electrical stimulation for the non-invasive pre-location of the target nerve or nerve plexus. Unlike the percutaneous techniques described above, PEG employs a special transcutaneous electrode equipped with a fine metal tip (less than 1 mm). The electrode is designed to furrow the skin and subcutaneous tissues in the direction of the nerve, so as to reduce the electrical tissue resistance as well as the distance from the target nerves. The electrode is electrically shielded and sterile.

This technique has recently been perfected and simplified, though conserving the original concept. The tip of the stimulating needle is used both as a cutaneous electrode and as an invasive electrode. The needle tip is enclosed in a rounded, non-conductive, sterile plastic shell that transforms the needle tip itself into a smooth cutaneous electrode. Once located the exact cutaneous entry point, the needle can then pierce the shell to perforate the skin and reach the target nerve.

5.6.2 Scientific Basis as a Guide to Percutaneous Electrical Nerve Stimulation

The ability to stimulate a peripheral nerve or nerve plexus electrically is as follows:
1. directly proportional to the electrical current intensity (I), that is to say the amperage applied to the stimulating electrode or to the needle;
2. proportional to the duration of the impulse of the square wave current generated by the electrical nerve stimulator;
3. inversely proportional to the electrode-to-nerve distance;
4. inversely proportional to the electrical impedance of the tissue interposed between the electrode and the target nerves.

5.6.3 Current Flow (Amperage)

The use of high amperages for stimulating peripheral nerves (2–5 mA) makes it possible to elicit a motor response at a greater distance from the nerve. In view of the fact that the electrode progressively approaches the nerve, the motor response to the electrical stimulation can be achieved by progressively reducing the amperage.

A motor response to stimulation with currents below 0.5 mA and conventional impulse durations of 0.1–0.2 ms indicates that the needle tip is very close to the nerve structure. The relationship between current flow (I), voltage (V) and tissue resistance (R) is governed by Eq. 5.1.

$$I = V/R \qquad (5.1)$$

Starting the search for the nerve structure at a high amperage, whether with a percutaneous or invasive approach maximizes the sensitivity (ability to elicit a motor response).

This principle is normally used for monitoring the neuromuscular junction during general anesthesia, delivering very high currents ($\sim$50 mA) via cutaneous electrodes; for this application, the specificity of the technique is obviously of minor importance.

For peripheral nerve blocks, on the other hand, currents of 2–5 mA increase the sensitivity but the maximum specificity is achieved at very low current values (<0.5 mA).

5.6.4 Duration of the Electrical Impulse

What is meant by the duration of the electrical impulse is the duration, expressed in milliseconds, of the square wave of the periodic impulse delivered by the electrostimulator for the purposes of stimulating the nerve or nerve plexus.

On increasing the duration of the electrical impulse, the total flow of electrons, calculated as the area under the curve, also increases. Increasing the duration of the electrical impulse also increases the nerve stimulation capacity in a manner directly proportional to the increase in impulse duration itself (maintaining the other variables unchanged).

Similarly, the current flow (amperage), at high impulse durations (0.3–1.0 ms), corresponds to a greater sensitivity of the technique for the initial pre-location of the nerve with the percutaneous or invasive approach. Conversely, a lower impulse duration (e.g. 0.1 ms) minimizes the specificity of the technique as regards the final invasive location of the nerve or nerve plexus.

5.6.5 Electrode-to-Nerve Distance

The distance (in the formula here below, the length L) between the electrode (needle tip) and the target nerve is one of the main factors capable of influencing the possibility of obtaining a motor response to the electrical stimulation at a precise electrical current and impulse duration. This relation is governed by Eq. 5.2.

$$R = pL/A \qquad (5.2)$$

where R is the electrical resistance, p is the tissue resistivity, L is the electrode-to-nerve distance and A is the conduction area.

Thus, on the basis of the two equations, it emerges that a greater current flow is needed to stimulate a nerve at a certain distance. The inverse proportion of this property is exploited when a stimulating needle is used to perform a nerve block.

Since the motor response diminishes on increasing the distance between the electrode (needle tip) and the nerve structure, obtaining a motor response at very low amperages and impulse durations indicates that the needle tip is very close to the target nerve.

By the same token, it may be noted that a higher current is required for a smaller conductive area.

Therefore, stimulation with a small electrode (needle tip) increases the specificity and indicates proximity to the nerve.

Therefore, for the purposes of percutaneous stimulation, which occurs at a greater distance compared to the classic invasive techniques, a greater electrical current and/or impulse duration is required. For locating a nerve or nerve plexus percutaneously at a relatively low amperage (2–5 mA), it is useful to reduce the electrode-to-nerve distance by compressing the skin layers and subcutaneous tissues towards the target nerve and to employ a needle tip electrode in order to maximize the specificity.

5.6.6 Electrical Impedance of the Tissue

The last variable that influences the ability to elicit a motor response to electrical stimulation of the nerve is the electrical impedance of skin and the underlying tissues. In general, higher the water:lipid ratio of the tissue, lower will be its electrical impedance. The skin is characterized by very high electrical impedance. Performing a skin incision serves to reduce the electrical impedance, or, expressed conversely, to increase the conductivity of the tissues, facilitating the elicitation of a motor response at a given amperage and impulse duration.

5.6.7 Frequency of the Electrical Impulse

The frequency (f) of the square wave electrical impulse generated by the electrical nerve stimulator is usually set at 1 or 2 Hz.

Increasing the frequency to 2 Hz may facilitate a more rapid and constant feedback, albeit at the expense of slightly greater patient discomfort. Any further increase in the stimulation frequency makes the procedure even more uncomfortable. The frequencies that induce tetanus (usually set at 50 or 100 Hz on the stimulators currently available on the market) are very painful and therefore should not be used for locating the nerve targets.

5.6.8 Principles of Percutaneous Electrode Guidance

Percutaneous electrode guidance (PEG) enables the anesthetist to optimize the above-mentioned variables in such a way as to perform percutaneous stimulation and therefore pre-location of the nerve target at relatively low amperages (<5 mA). The use of a smooth-tip electrode makes it possible to indent the skin without causing the patient too much discomfort. Indenting the skin reduces to a minimum the distance between the exploratory electrode and the nerve, reducing the electrical impedance by compressing the underlying tissues, thus increasing the electrical conductivity.

Contrary to the traditional method, where a brief impulse duration is preferable for the precise location of the nerve structures by means of the needle tip, cutaneous stimulation with PEG presents the advantage of employing longer impulse durations (0.2–1.0 ms). Longer impulse durations enable motor responses to be elicited at lower amperages. Furrowing the skin (in some cases several centimetres are required) brings the cutaneous electrode close to the nerve or nerve plexus. Since most of the location process is done by the probe, which indents the skin towards the nerve structure, the needle tip usually works in very close proximity to it.

5.6.9 Early Clinical Experience with the PEG Technique

Urmey and Grossi have reported the first clinical cases of peripheral blocks or plexus blocks performed using the PEG technique. These authors used a cylindrical cutaneous electrode with a conductive metal tip measuring 1 mm in diameter. After positioning the probe and furrowing the skin above the target nerve, specific motor responses were sought. At the point of the maximum motor response with the minimum amperage of the cutaneous probe (2 Hz, 0.2 ms), the electrical nerve stimulator was switched off and a stimulating needle (B. Braun, Melsungen, Germany) was introduced through the probe and directed towards the nerve. This procedure was used initially on 7 patients. Since the nerves were pre-located with a cutaneous electrode, the needle was introduced in all cases with an initial amperage of 0.5 mA (normally acceptable as an endpoint). Only in one case was it necessary to increase the needle amperage up to more than 0.5 mA. The target nerves were easily found within a few seconds of starting the cutaneous exploration with the surface electrode.

The minimal percutaneous stimulation current expressed in mA is directly related to the measured depth of the needle (beyond the tip of the probe). The maximum depth to which the needle was inserted in these patients was 2 cm. In this way, the technique is more useful for superficial nerve or plexus blocks, including brachial plexus blocks, midhumeral blocks, wrist blocks, femoral nerve blocks, popliteal blocks and posterior tibial nerve blocks.

A further breakthrough in ENS has been made by the studies of Urmey and Grossi on the combined and sequential use of stimulation waves. In fact, by generating a sequence of stimulations, it proves possible to modulate the approach of the needle to the target nerve. This procedure is called sequential electrical nerve stimulation (SENS). It uses a sequence of stimuli of varying duration including not only careful stimulation at 0.1 ms but also stimulations of longer duration (0.1, 0.3 and 1.0 ms generated with a frequency of 3 Hz). At greater distances, only impulses of long duration will bring contraction of the muscles, while impulses of 0–1 ms duration will induce a motor response only when the needle is close to the nerve. The result is that only the presence of all the stimuli in succession will indicate that the needle is in the immediate vicinity of the target nerve structure.

This system is currently under study, but would appear to be an additional aid for the accurate location of the nerve structures with the maximum safety and efficacy; it affords reliable visual feedback regarding the position of the needle and reduces the need to vary the settings of the electrical nerve stimulator during the nerve location phase.

5.6.10 Ultrasound-Guided Regional Anesthesia

With the aid of ultrasound techniques, it proves possible to visualize not only the correct positioning of the needle close to the target nerve, but also the spread and distribution of the local anesthetic around the nerve, thus reducing the drug dose necessary for performing the nerve block.

Whenever a perineural catheter is positioned, one should assess whether the catheter is placed correctly in relation to, and in the vicinity of, the nerve to be blocked.

Lastly, it is possible to avoid the most common complications, including the intravascular administration of anesthetic, epidural or subarachnoid puncture, haematoma formation as a result of accidental vascular puncture and nerve injury.

Ultrasound guidance is useful for facilitating the execution of peripheral and central blocks and affords direct visualization of the target point, the adjacent structures and the spread of local anesthetic.

The advantages also include a reduction in the complication rate and the rapid onset of the block. In addition, the use of ultrasound may make it possible to modify and adapt pre-existing techniques on the basis of the direct anatomical evidence.

Although regional anesthesia has become increasingly safe over the years, we are witnessing a growing number of reports regarding the complications of regional techniques (haematoma, neuropathic pain, puncture of the dura mater, etc.). In recent years, many authors have suggested that the use of ultrasound may permit better location of the peripheral nerves, by improving the technique and its application and reducing side effects.

5.6.11 Execution Technique

To achieve appropriate image resolution for the execution of a nerve block, it is necessary to use high-impedance ultrasound probes.

Most nerve blocks require frequencies ranging from 10 to 14 MHz. Broadband transducers with a 5–12 MHz or 8–14 MHz band afford excellent resolution of the superficial structures in the higher frequency range and good penetration depth at lower frequencies. Linear probes are known to be more efficacious as a means of representing peripheral nerve anatomy. Modern ultrasound software, moreover, enables the technical limitations of the procedure to be overcome with the aid of computerized processing capable of enhancing the quality of the images obtained.

The connective tissue within the nerve fibres reflects the ultrasounds in an anisotropic manner: the angle and intensity of the reflection depend on the angle at which the ultrasound beam meets the longitudinal axis of the nerve. Consequently, linear transducers with a parallel emission band are more advantageous than those with divergent sound waves.

Recent studies have demonstrated the advantages afforded by the use of ultrasonography in regional anesthesia as compared to conventional techniques based on the use of electrical nerve stimulators and loss of resistance.

The positioning of the needle can be done without evidence of muscle contraction provoked by the electrical nerve stimulator, which is a distinct advantage for patients with limb problems (fractures) that limit their range of movement and for amputees. In addition, the ability to visualize accessory nerve branches not otherwise capable of being located with the classic techniques guarantees the possibility of optimal anesthetic planning with the possible use of tourniquets.

An advantage is also obtained as compared with the classic technique in patients with anatomical variants, in obese patients and in those with a long history of diabetes or peripheral neuropathy.

The use of ultrasound in nerve blocks was described for the first time by La Grange et al. in 1978 where ultrasound was used for supraclavicular brachial plexus blocks.

Clearly, an optimal distribution of local anesthetic around the nerve is indispensable for the success of the procedure. With the ultrasound-guided approach, the distribution of the anesthetic solution around the nerve can be observed. Ultrasound guidance also provides information about the anatomical relationships between the nerve structures themselves and the surrounding vascular structures, thus reducing the possibility that some of the most feared complications may occur, namely intraneural and intravascular injection.

In addition, we should consider that the amount of drug used can be reduced as a result of the direct visualization of its distribution, which is a particularly important factor in the case of multiple blocks.

Another advantage reported in the literature is the possibility of repeating the block if this should prove necessary.

Ultrasound guidance has furnished appreciable advantages in the execution of nerve blocks of both the upper and lower limbs. For example, in the case of supraclavicular brachial plexus blocks, a reduced risk of pneumothorax and a more rapid execution of the block have been reported. In the case of the use of US guidance for the execution of anesthetic blocks of the lower limb, easier identification of the sciatic and popliteal nerves has been reported.

Ultrasonography, thanks to the possibility of visualizing the patient's anatomy, makes regional anesthesia techniques safer in the case of patients presenting anatomical variants or alterations in the area involved in the execution of the block and permits the direct visualization of the devices used in regional anesthesia, such as needles or perineural catheters, thus optimizing their use and making it safer.

Bibliography

ENS and PEG

Douglas Ford J, Pither C, Raj Prithvi P (1984) Comparison of insulated versus uninsulated needles for locating peripheral nerves with a peripheral nerve stimulator. Anesth Analg 63:925–928

Duprè LJ (1992) Neurostimolateur en anesthésie Locorégionale. Cahiers d'Anesthésiologie 40(7):503–510

Ganta R, Cajee R, Henthorn R (1993) Use of transcutaneous nerve stimulation to assist interscalene block. Anesth Analg 76:914–915

Pither C, Raj PP, Douglas JF (1985) The use of peripheral nerve stimulators for regional anesthesia. A review of experimental characteristics, technique and clinical applications. Reg Anesth 10:49–58

Shannon J, Lang S, Yip R (1995) Lateral femoral nerve block revisited: a nerve stimulator technique. Reg Anesth 20:100–104

Smith BE (1990) The role of electrical nerve stimulation in regional anesthesia. Anesth Crit Care 1:234–238

Urmey W, Grossi P (2003) Percutaneous electrode guidance (PEG) and subcutaneous stimulating electrode guidance (SSEG): modifications of the original technique. Reg Anesth Pain Med 28:253–255

Urmey W, Grossi P (2002) Percutaneous electrode guidance (PEG): a noninvasive technique for prelocation of peripheral nerves to facilitate nerve block. Reg Anesth Pain Med 27:261–267

Urmey W (2010) Electrical stimulation and ultrasound in regional anesthesia. Eur J Pain Supplement 4(4):319–322

Urmey W (1996) Upper extremity blocks. In: Brown D (ed) Regional anesthesia and analgesia. WB Saunders, Philadelphia, pp 254–278

Ultrasound-guided regional anesthesia

Aromaa U, Lahdensuu M, Cozanitis DA (1997) Severe complications associated with epidural and spinal anaesthesias in Finland 1987–1993. A study based on patient insurance claims. Acta Anaesthesiol Scand 41(4):445–452

De Tommaso O, Caporuscio A, Tagariello V (2002) Neurological complications following central neuraxial blocks: are there predictive factors? Eur J Anaesthesiol 19(10):705–716

Denny NM, Harrop-Griths W (2005) Location, location, location! Ultrasound imaging in regional anaesthesia. BMJ, pp 94: editorial I

Grau T, Leipold RW, Horter J, Conradi R, Martin EO, Motsch J (2001) Paramedian access to the epidural space: the optimum window for ultrasound imaging. J Clin Anesth 13:213–217

Gray AT, Schafhalter-Zoppoth I (2003) Ultrasound guidance for ulnar nerve block in the forearm. Reg Anesth Pain Med 28(4):335–339

Greher M, Kirchmair L, Enna B et al (2004) Ultrasound-guided lumbar facet nerve block: accuracy of a new technique confirmed by computed tomography. Anesthesiology 101(5):1195–1200

Greher M, Scharbert G, Kamolz LP et al (2004) Ultrasound-guided lumbar facet nerve block. Anesthesiology 100:1242–1248

Horlocker TT (2000) Complications of spinal and epidural anesthesia. Anesthesiol Clin North America 18(2):461–485

Kirchmair L, Entner T, Kapral S, Mitterschiffthaler G (2002) Ultrasound guidance for the psoas compartment block: an imaging study. Anesth Analg 94:706–710

La Grange P, Foster PA, Pretorius LK (1978) Application of the Doppler ultrasound blood flow detector in supraclavicular brachial plexus block. Br J Anaesth 50:965–967

Marhofer P, Greher M, Kapral S (2005) Ultrasound guidance in regional anesthesia. Br J Anaesth 94:7–17

Minville V, Zetlaoui PJ, Fessenmeyer C, Benhamou D (2004) Ultrasound guidance for difficult lateral popliteal catheter insertion in a patient with peripheral vascular disease. Reg Anesth Pain Med 29(4):368–370

Moen V, Dahlgren N, Irestedt L (2004) Severe neurological complications after central neuraxial blockades in Sweden 1990–1999. Anesthesiology 101(4):950–959

Peterson MK, Millar FA, Sheppard DG (2002) Ultrasound-guided nerve blocks. Br J Anaesth 88(5):621–624

Puolakka R, Haasio J, Pitkanen MT et al (2000) Technical aspects and postoperative sequelae of spinal and epidural anesthesia: a prospective study of 3,230 orthopedic patients. Reg Anesth Pain Med 25(5):488–497

Sandhu NS, Capan LM (2002) Ultrasound-guided infraclavicular brachial plexus block. Br J Anaesth 89:254–259

Schafhalter-Zoppoth I, Gray AT (2004) Ultrasound-guided nerve block in the presence of a superficial ulnar artery. Reg Anesth Pain Med 29(3):297–301

Schafhalter-Zoppoth I, McCulloch CE, Gray AT (2004) Ultrasound visibility of needles used for regional nerve block: an in vitro study. Regional Anesth Pain Med 29(5):480–488

Sinha A, Chan VWS (2004) Ultrasound imaging for popliteal sciatic nerve block. Reg Anesth Pain Med 29(2):130–134

Spence BC, Sites BD, Beach ML (2005) Ultrasound-guided musculocutaneous nerve block: a description of a novel technique. Reg Anesth Pain Med 30(2):198–201

Supraclavicular Brachial Plexus Block Techniques

F. Alemanno

> *If there are many ways of performing the same operation, that means than none of them is really just what the doctor ordered.*
>
> Livio Zava, General Surgeon, Treviso, 1967.

6.1 A Little Bit of History

What we mean by the term "supraclavicular techniques" is those techniques whose entry point is located above the clavicle, be it in the immediate vicinity of the latter (these are mainly perivascular techniques such as the Kulenkampff technique) or closer to the vertebral column (such as Kappis posterior approach or Winnie's interscalene technique).

The supraclavicular brachial plexus block techniques are the most complete form of regional anesthesia of the upper limb, their efficacy extending from the shoulder to the hand.

It is no accident that historically, of the first three brachial plexus blocks, two were performed at a level above the clavicle, namely the Kulenkampff technique (1911) and Kappis posterior approach (1912), the exception being Hirschel's axillary approach (1911).

1911 was an exceptional year for regional anesthesia of the upper limb; it was the year that witnessed the advent of the two most important percutaneous brachial plexus block techniques, that is to say Hirschel's percutaneous axillary block and, a few months later, Kulenkampff's supraclavicular block.

Since 1911, that is, when Dietrich Kulenkampff, a physician working at the Royal Hospital in Zwickau, Germany, described his technique, *Die Anästhesierung des Plexus brachialis* (Anesthesia of the brachial plexus) destined to remain a basic reference work for several generations of anesthetists, many other methods have been proposed, with variable popularity ratings and often short-lived in their diffusion and application.

Kulenkampff conceived and developed a technique, which the First World War promoted in the field. Despite the risk of pneumothorax, it long remained the most commonly performed technique, albeit with a number of variants, up until 1970, when Winnie introduced his interscalene block technique. Kappis technique did not enjoy the same measure of success, because it was too painful for the patient, and presented the additional risk of subarachnoid injection or injection into the vertebral artery. Also Santoni's similar technique, which appeared 4 years later, failed to solve the problems, possibly multiplying them fivefold by inserting the needle at five different points. It was thanks to the work of Pasquale Pippa that this approach was subsequently revised and re-proposed according to modern concepts and methods.

However, in the half century following the advent of the Kulenkampff technique, the risk of pneumothorax prompted many anesthetists to favour Hirschel's axillary block, which was undoubtedly safer, even if more limited as regards the extent of the territory to be anesthetized.

F. Alemanno (✉)
Institute of Anesthesiology, Resuscitation and Pain Therapy, University of Verona, Verona, Italy
e-mail: fernando@alemannobpb.it

Winnie's interscalene technique, when it was first introduced in 1970, found favour with many anesthetists because it solved the problem of what was the most feared complication, namely pneumothorax. His great merit was that he emphasized and publicized the concept of the anatomical space constituted by the neurovascular bundle. The technique presents the risk of subarachnoid injection or injection into the vertebral artery. Accidental puncture of the vertebral artery, particularly in young subjects, can cause spasm of the vessel with aspiration of a small amount of blood. With the injection of the anesthetic, however, the spasm is resolved and there is a risk of producing local anesthesia of the brain via the basilar artery, which is the clinical equivalent of an intravenous injection of thiopentone, with, in addition, the risk of convulsions.

Brown's plumb-bob method appeared on the scene in 1993. This is an attractive technique and is apparently easy to perform; it presents a potential risk of pneumothorax with an incidence, as reported by the author, ranging from 0.5 to 5 % (in expert hands, the incidence is at the low end of the range). Another possible complication is block of the phrenic nerve.

Alemanno's technique came in the wake of personal experience of two cases of pneumothorax (both in the space of a week) in the 'seventies, and an injection of 2 ml of mepivacaine into the vertebral artery in the 'eighties.

The idea is to cannulate the neurovascular bundle with the needle directed roughly from the midpoint of the clavicle towards C7, thus taking a horizontal or slightly rising path.

For this reason, the risk of pneumothorax is obviated, as is that of accidental subarachnoid injection or injection into the vertebral artery on account of the safe distance between the entry point and the vertebral column.

Kulenkampff, Kappis, Winnie, Brown, etc… but what about before? It all began in the early 1880s with the use of cocaine as a surface anesthetic by the Viennese ophthalmologist Karl Köller at a suggestion of Sigmund Freud, and with his collaboration.

The anesthetic was applied by instillation onto the conjunctiva for the performance of minor surgery. The communication regarding this use of cocaine as an anesthetic was made at the Heidelberg Congress of Ophthalmology on 15 September 1884; this was followed by a practical demonstration *in corpore viri* (what we would nowadays simply call a workshop) instilling 20 % cocaine onto the conjunctiva of a volunteer.

Dr. Noyes, an American, on returning to New York after the congress published a report on the matter in *The Medical Record* in October 1884. The news spread rapidly and this was followed by extensive use of the procedure which gave rise to a substantial consumption of cocaine, with a consequent rise in price from 2.5 to 6.5 dollars per gram. The drug had previously been used, from the pharmaceutical point of view, only in what was called *Vin Mariani (*Mariani's coca wine) for helping alcoholics to kick their drinking habit. Alcohol addicts were happy to abandon alcohol and rapidly replace it with the new beverage!

In November 1885, William Stewart Halsted, a surgeon working at the Roosevelt Hospital in New York performed the first nerve block of the cutaneous branch of the ulnar nerve under direct vision on his assistant, John Hall, who volunteered to undergo the procedure. Various other anesthetic block techniques (under direct vision) were performed on various nerves; in addition to the ulnar nerve, other nerve structures were targeted including the pudendal nerve, the posterior tibial nerve and the brachial plexus via the supraclavicular route; in the latter case, 0.5 % cocaine was injected directly into the plexus. The incision used in order to reach the plexus was made along the line running from the midpoint of the posterior border of the sternocleidomastoid muscle to the midpoint of the clavicle after infiltrating it with 0.1 % cocaine using a syringe with a long, thin needle. In practice, this was actually a minor surgical operation so as to be able to administer regional anesthesia for the purposes then of performing further surgery.

Since the supraclavicular brachial plexus block techniques are very numerous (numbering more than 20), we will confine our attention to describing those which in our opinion have been characterized by a greater measure of notoriety and/or success.

6.2 Kulenkampff

> Those who see things grow from the very beginning will see them in the most perfect way.
>
> Aristotle

Georg Hirschel in 1911 had just described his percutaneous axillary block when, a few months later, Dietrich Kulenkampff published his percutaneous supraclavicular block technique.

Just as Horace Wells had experimented on himself the anesthetic action of nitrous oxide to relieve the pain of a dental extraction, so Kulenkampff experimented on himself the technique that he then went on to describe and publish, by self-injecting 5 ml of procaine in order to unequivocally understand its effects. After obtaining what was obviously only a partial anesthesia with 5 ml, he then went on to use the technique in clinical practice in his patients, injecting 10 ml initially and 20 ml a few years later, in order to achieve a more complete block of the brachial plexus.

6.2.1 Patient Position

Seated with the head slightly turned to the opposite side (Fig. 6.1).

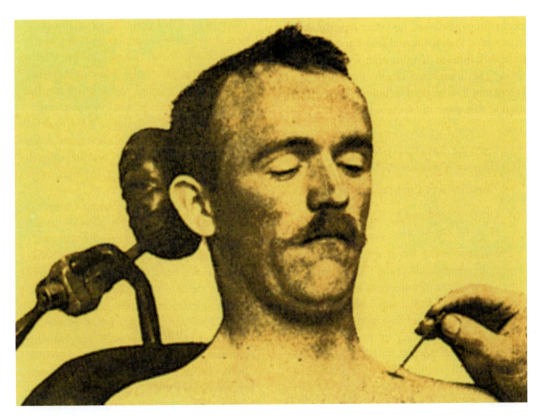

Fig. 6.1 This historic photo clearly shows that, owing to the direction of the needle, the possibility of causing a pneumothorax is very real (by courtesy of Winnie A.P.: *Tecniche Perivascolari di Blocco del Plesso Brachiale*, Verducci Editore, Roma 1984)

6.2.2 Landmarks

1. The pulse of the subclavian artery.
2. The midpoint of the clavicle.

6.2.3 Technique

The puncture is performed laterally to the pulse of the subclavian artery and posteriorly to the midpoint of the clavicle, where the two directions, lateral and posterior, intersect. A thin 4 cm needle is directed caudad posteriorly and medially in relation to the spinous process of T2.

After eliciting the paraesthesia, 20 ml of 2 % procaine is injected. If no paraesthesia is elicited and the needle reaches the first rib, it must be withdrawn and reintroduced more medially, closer to the subclavian artery until paraesthesia is elicited. The anesthetic should not be injected before eliciting well-defined paraesthesia.

But above and beyond any more or less successful explanation, no better description can be provided than the actual first-hand account of the author himself. To this end, we include here below the translation from the German of Kulenkampff's original article along with the original title page in German (Fig. 6.2).

From the Royal Hospital of Zwickau
Director: Professor H. Braun

Anesthesia of the brachial plexus

Dr. D. Kulenkampff
Hospital physician

The recent presentation by Dr, Hirschel regarding anesthesia of the brachial plexus by means of the percutaneous injection of a solution of novocaine-suprarenin prompts me to report here and now on the research I have been undertaking in the same direction. Hirschel has attempted to block the plexus by depositing a bolus of anesthetic at the axillary level. Much more suitable and important for reaching the plexus with a needle without having to fear side effects and complications, however, is the point where the plexus emerges, laterally to the subclavian artery, from the interscalene space and comes to rest on the first rib. Percutaneous anesthesia of nerve trunks is feasible as a rule only if the position of the nerve is defined by bony landmarks capable of serving as a guide to the needle. The sketch reported shows the position of the brachial plexus in relation to the subclavian artery, the clavicle and the first rib, corresponding approximately to the midpoint of the clavicle. At this point, even in obese subjects, the nerve trunks are directed towards the arm, just beneath the skin, and in very closely packed bundles. As the position of the needle is delimited medially by the subclavian artery which can be easily palpated in all individuals, anteriorly by the clavicle and inferiorly by the first rib, the nerves can be reached easily and safely, avoiding the subclavian artery. Moreover, at this point the needle is positioned in the loose connective tissue of the interscalene fossa, where the anesthetic solution spreads easily. We can therefore expect good efficacy as a result of the injection of small amounts of anesthetic.

The injection technique, the course of the procedure and the observations made in experimentation with brachial plexus anesthesia on myself and in surgery on patients are as follows:

First of all, the subclavian artery is localized with the patient possibly in the seated position. This artery is easily detected by means of light palpation. With the patient's head slightly tilted, in many patients the artery is visible, as, moreover, is the interscalene fossa. Almost invariably, this will be the point where an extension of the course of the external jugular vein intersects the clavicle. Immediately lateral to this landmark and abutting upon the upper edge of the clavicle a skin wheal is produced to mark the needle insertion point. A thin needle about 4 cm in length is inserted deep. It is not

Zentralblatt für Chirurgie

herausgegeben von

K. GARRÈ,   **G. PERTHES,**   **E. RICHTER,**
in Bonn,   in Tübingen,   in Breslau.

38. Jahrgang.

VERLAG von JOHANN AMBROSIUS BARTH in LEIPZIG.

Nr. 40.   Sonnabend, den 7. Oktober   1911.

Inhalt.

D. Kulenkampff, Die Anästhesierung des Plexus brachialis. (Originalmitteilung).
1) Versammlung des nordischen chirurgischen Vereins in Stockholm. — 2) Krause u. Garrè, Therapie innerer Krankheiten. — 3) Aievoll, Chirurgische Diagnostik. — 4) Roussy u. Ameuille, 5) Wrede, 6) Gussio, 7) Bernhardt, 8) Green, 9) Tuffier, Zur Geschwulstlehre.
10) Capelle, Knochenbildung in Laparotomienarben. — 11) Jolly, Fettbauch. — 12) Bernheim, Organoskopie. — 13) De Paoli, Kräftigung der Widerstandsfähigkeit des Bauchfells. — 14) Wolff, 15) Sissojeff, 16) Lewit, 17) Berčels, 18) Philip, 19) Fabricius, 20) Carcaterra, 21) Stanton, Zur Appendicitisfrage. — 22) Frattin, 23) Venturi, 24) Lewit, 25) Reich, 26) Cohn, Herniologisches. — 27) Bagger-Jörgensen, 28) Bircher, 29) Fischer, 30) Zweig, 31) Kretschmer, 32) Marcinkowski, 33) Gross, 34) Mayo, Zur Chirurgie des Magens und Duodenum. — 35) Calderara, Gastroenterostomie. — 36) Razzaboni, Enteropexie. — 37) Walzberg, Zur Kasuistik der Erkrankung des Nahrungskanals. — 38) Jakob, Appendikostomie. — 39) Casabona, 40) Boeckel, 41) Ladd, Ileus. — 42) Rochard, Lymphadenome des Darmes. — 43) Waldenström, 44) Lubelsky, Dickdarmkrebs. — 45) Konjetzny, Hirschsprung'sche Krankheit. — 46) Ciechomski, Melanosarkom des Mastdarms. — 47) Krynski, Mesenteriitis fibrosa. — 48) Lindström, 49) Johannsen, Zur Milzchirurgie. — 50) Radziewski, Pankreaschirurgie.

Aus dem Königlichen Krankenstift zu Zwickau.
Direktor: Prof. Dr. H. Braun.

Die Anästhesierung des Plexus brachialis.

Von

Dr. D. Kulenkampff,
Anstaltsarzt.

Hirschel's[1] kürzliche Mitteilung über die Anästhesierung des Plexus brachialis durch perkutane Injektion von Novokain-Suprareninlösung veranlaßt mich, über meine eigenen, in gleicher Richtung angestellten Versuche schon jetzt zu berichten. Hirschel hat den Plexus unter Zuhilfenahme von Stauung in der Achselhöhle zu unterbrechen gesucht. Weit geeigneter zum Treffen mit einer Hohlnadel, ohne daß man Nebenverletzungen zu befürchten braucht, ist aber die Stelle, wo der Plexus nach außen von der Arteria subclavia aus der Scalenuslücke heraustritt und der ersten Rippe aufliegt. Denn die perkutane Anästhesierung von Nervenstämmen ist in typischer Weise in der Regel nur dann sicher ausführbar, wenn die Lage des Nerven durch Knochenpunkte fixiert ist, welche der Hohlnadel als Führung dienen können. Aus umstehender Skizze ergibt sich die Lage des Plexus brachialis zur Subclavia, zum Schlüsselbein und zur ersten Rippe. Sie entspricht ungefähr der Mitte der Clavicula. Hier ziehen auch bei fetten Menschen verhältnismäßig dicht unter der Haut und eng aneinander gelagert die Nerven-

[1] Münchener med. Wochenschrift 1911. Nr. 29.

Fig. 6.2 Original title page of the *Zentralblatt für Chirurgie* Nr. 40, 7 October 1911, with the original article by Kulenkampff on the first page (by courtesy of Gualtiero Bellucci: *Storia della Anestesiologia*. Piccin Editore, Padova 1982)

necessary to press the needle in as far as the first rib. The latter simply represents the lowest point that can be reached. On the other hand, however, it is imperative that the needle should encounter one of the nerves of the arm. Only then will the needle tip lie at the right depth. On touching the nerve trunks, paresthesias and motor reactions are radiated, but no pain is experienced, as I myself was able to confirm. If the direction of the needle is correct, paresthesias will be manifested when the needle has pierced the skin and the superficial and deep fasciae. On no account should one inject the anesthetic before paresthesias have radiated to the arm. The anesthetic solution immediately deprives the nerve trunks of all sensitivity making any proper orientation impossible. A number of instances of anesthesia setting in late and with only a partial effect have taught us that one must above all avoid pressing the needle too low. Complete success depends exclusively on the injection technique, as we have been able to observe in cases in which the procedure was applied twice.

At this point, the first rib, which is particularly wide and flat, runs cephalad and in an almost perfect antero-posterior direction. The needle therefore needs to be inserted in a slightly medial and posterior caudal direction, more or less as if one were aiming to run up against the second or third thoracic spinous process. The plexus is thus reached at a depth of approximately 3 cm. The first rib lies at a slightly lower level. If one runs up against the first rib without touching the plexus, the needle will certainly have been directed too laterally for fear of damaging the subclavian artery. The needle thus needs to be directed more medially until the paresthesia occurs. In adults, we inject 10 cc. of a 2 % solution of novocaine-suprarenin with the usual low suprarenin content of the Novocaine-Suprarenin A tablets manufactured by the Höchster Farbwerke company. Five cc. are sufficient in children. With a 1 % solution we achieved complete anesthesia in one case and a total failure in another. If the anesthesia is retarded in certain nerve areas, the effect can be speeded up by means of light massaging at the injection site.

Paralysis generally sets in immediately after completing the injection and always progresses in the same manner. Initially, the patient perceives a strong heat sensation throughout the arm and in the space of only a few minutes the area of the nerve stimulated with the needle becomes completely numb. Almost simultaneously, the cutaneous area innervated by the musculocutaneous nerve in the ulnar and posterior part of the forearm is anesthetized. The whole of the arm becomes heavy and rapidly loses strength, and the flexion movements of the arm become ataxic. In our cases, anesthesia was established after 15–30 min in the entire arm, with the exception of a triangular area over the deltoid muscle. A strong paresis of all the arm muscles and part of the musculature of the shoulder was observed. In the experiment on myself, I was no longer able to open a door. In some patients the fingers, but also the entire arm, were completely paralyzed. The lateral wall of the armpit was almost always completely insensitive. The small area served by the intercostobrachial nerve and the medial wall of the armpit were anesthetized only in a few rare cases. Furthermore, as in the Heidenhain experiment, the entire arm was hyperemic. The anesthesia generally lasted an hour and a half, and as much as 2–3 h in some cases. Pain at the level of the skin wound generally started to manifest itself only half an hour after the return of sensitivity in the other skin areas. The injection site itself created no problems. I know from my personal experience and from the patients I have questioned in this connection, that the only pain, which cannot really be regarded as such, is that due to the initial skin wheal.

We experimented with the procedure in 25 cases. In 23 patients a hemostatic tourniquet was applied in a proximal position and created not the slightest problem. In one case, about an hour after the start of the surgery, we had to remove the tourniquet because the patient complained of pain due to pressure. In two cases, it didn't need to be used, the anesthesia in any event being complete. In three cases we were able to perform a disarticulation at the level of the elbow in the total absence of pain.

It was possible to detect the nerve trunks and transect them as usual without any kind of painful reaction. We reduced a supracondylar fracture of the humerus almost painlessly in a boy, even though the injection was not perfectly successful owing to the use of a defective syringe. After as little as 10 min the elbow movements that caused the boy a great deal of acute pain no longer produced a reaction, and X-rays were easily obtained. The other cases consisted in phlegmons of tendon sheaths, hand and forearm wounds, and one case of a dislocated fracture of the radius, in which the friction between the two fracture stumps was completely painless.

In three cases we had to administer three cc. of ether, in two of them because we failed to wait long enough and once in the above-mentioned third case in which we removed the hemostatic tourniquet. This was a case of mycosis of the flexor tendon sheath, in which the skin suture was no longer completely painless. The most reliable indicator that anesthesia has been achieved, in addition to the surgery itself, is the patient's ability to support the hemostatic tourniquet. The fact that, in some cases, the hemostatic tourniquet did not cause pain, despite not all the skin areas being anesthetized corresponds to Bier's observation regarding intravenous anesthesia. Bier noted that, in the context of direct anesthesia, the large nerves were insensitive before total insensitivity set in in the areas of indirect anesthesia. Sensitivity tests do not yield reliable results, particularly in our patient population. Moreover, at the level of the upper part of the arm, the area of influence of the cervical nerves (nerves of the superficial cervical plexus, Editor's note), which, however, can be easily anesthetized in case of need by means of subcutaneous injection of anesthetic, varies very considerably. Sometimes the evaluation is made more difficult by the occurrence of hypoanesthesia in some cutaneous areas, which, in any event, is amply sufficient for the surgery. We observed this in some cases in which the puncture and cutting were perceived as a slight burning sensation. The same findings were also reported by Läwen.

The results of our study are therefore as follows: in 15 cases we achieved total anesthesia and sometimes also paralysis of the whole of the arm. In 5 cases there was hypoanesthesia in some cutaneous areas, but sufficient for the surgery, and anesthesia of the remaining operating field. In 5 other cases some cutaneous areas were not anesthetized. The first of these cases refers to the self-experimentation in which I injected myself with only 5 cc., which is insufficient in an adult. In the second case we made an attempt with a 1 % solution. The other three cases referred to the first experiments of other authors and attempts to achieve the best direction of the needle. This also explains the 4 cases in which it proved necessary to inject an additional 10 cc. to obtain complete anesthesia.

Summarizing our experience, then, we can say that if a thin needle is inserted in the manner described here above and a radiating paresthesia is obtained, the

> injection of 10 cc. of a 2 % solution induces safe anesthesia in the whole of the arm. In the proximal third of the arm the spread of the anesthetic varies according to the extent of the supraclavicular nerves and the influence (generally limited) of the intercostobrachial nerve. In case of need, both of these can be easily excluded with a subcutaneous ring injection of the whole arm. Once anesthesia has been obtained, in all cases we apply a hemostatic tourniquet, which, if placed in the vicinity of the area anesthetized, creates no problems. To speed up the onset of anesthesia, in the last two patients, I used the same amount of a 3 % solution. In these two cases it was possible to apply the hemostatic tourniquet after 7 and 8 min, respectively.
>
> I therefore believe that anesthesia of the brachial plexus according to the technique outlined here above represents a typical method which is safe and easy to perform even after only a few attempts. I would say that the experimentation on myself provides sound evidence of this. The anesthesia is useful in all forms of upper limb surgery as far up as the shoulder. I have not yet had the opportunity to experiment with the procedure in cases of dislocation of the shoulder. For operations on the arm general anesthesia has become almost entirely, and venous anesthesia entirely superfluous.

It is curious that every author who has described this technique has done so, making changes to some part or parts of it, either in the form of modifications made by Kulenkampff himself in his subsequent publications or by endowing the description with minor additional expedients, each on the basis of his own point of view and experience. This, of course, has happened for other techniques such as, for instance, the Mulley technique, which, as we shall see, was modified by Hilarowicz.

6.3 Labat Technique (1922)

In the first edition of his book entitled *Regional Anesthesia,* published by Saunders and Co. in 1922, Labat described his brachial plexus block technique.

6.3.1 Patient Position

The position is supine with the arm extended down alongside the body and with the shoulder lowered in order to rotate the clavicle caudad and thus bring the brachial plexus closer to the surface.

6.3.2 Landmarks

1. The pulse of the subclavian artery.
2. The midpoint of the clavicle.

6.3.3 Technique

A skin wheal is induced lateral to the pulse of the subclavian artery, 1 cm above the midpoint of the clavicle. If the subclavian artery pulse cannot be palpated, the skin wheal is simply induced 1 cm above the midpoint of the clavicle.

The patient is instructed to report the paraesthesia when it occurs.

A 5 cm needle is inserted via the skin wheal and is directed caudad and slightly medially towards the first rib. If no paraesthesia occurs, after 3 cm, the needle will come into contact with the first rib; in that case, it must be withdrawn and reinserted in a slightly different direction until paraesthesia occurs; when the latter occurs, 10 ml of anesthetic solution are injected. If no paraesthesia is elicited, it is better not to insist and to deposit the first 10 ml bolus at the level of the first rib.

This first injection, in some ways similar to the Kulenkampff technique, was followed by a second injection, this time orientating the needle towards Chassaignac's tubercle, on reaching which 5 ml of anesthetic is injected.

Lastly, a third injection is performed, reintroducing the needle towards the lateral edge of the first rib where another 5 ml of anesthetic is injected.

To obtain a complete block of the shoulder, Labat, in addition, advised performing a subcutaneous infiltration of the clavicular border and the acromion and a fan-wise infiltration of the thoracic wall of the axilla in order also to anesthetize the intercostobrachial nerve.

6.4 Bonica and Moore Technique (1949)

This is a variant of the Kulenkampff technique, with the addition of two supplementary needle insertions: one in a slightly anterior direction in relation to the first, and the other in a slightly posterior direction.

6.4.1 Bonica's Description

6.4.2 Patient Position

Supine with a small, firm roll between the shoulder blades so as to hyperextend the head.

The head is turned to the opposite side, and slight caudal traction is applied to the limb to be anesthetized.

6.4.3 Landmarks

1. The pulse of the subclavian artery.
2. The midpoint of the clavicle.

6.4.4 Technique

After inducing a skin wheal posterolateral to the pulse of the subclavian artery, a 5 cm 22-G needle is introduced and directed caudad, dorsally and medially towards the spinous process of T3. The needle is advanced slowly until paraesthesia is elicited, and in any case should not be advanced more than 3 cm. At this depth, the needle tip should come into contact with the first rib. At this point, if no paraesthesia has been elicited, the needle must be withdrawn as far as the subcutaneous tissue and reinserted until paraesthesia is registered. When this happens, taking great care to ensure that there is no further shifting of the needle, and after aspiration, 10 ml of anesthetic solution is injected. The needle is then advanced again as far as the first rib and another 10 ml of anesthetic is injected during the withdrawal of the needle as far as the fascia and not into the subcutaneous tissue. Immediately after this, the needle is inserted again 1 cm more medially and therefore closer to the subclavian artery, the pulsations of which can be seen or perceived on the needle. With the needle in contact once again with the first rib, as before, another 10 ml of anesthetic is injected during withdrawal of the needle. The last needle insertion is performed 1 cm posterolaterally to the first. If paraesthesias are registered during these reinsertions, the progress of the needle is arrested and 5 of the scheduled 10 ml of anesthetic are injected. If this technique is executed with all due care, the brachial plexus can be blocked with 40 ml of anesthetic solution.

If a haemostatic tourniquet is applied or if the surgery is to be performed on the arm or shoulder, a subcutaneous collar infiltration of the axillary and acromial areas is recommended in order to block the intercostobrachial nerve and the terminal branches of the cervical plexus, respectively.

6.4.5 Moore's Description

The patient is in the supine position, without a pillow under the head, which is turned to the opposite side.

The patient is asked to raise his head a few cm above the stretcher to show the clavicular head of the sternocleidomastoid muscle and, posterior to this, the anterior scalene muscle the position of which is marked X immediately above the clavicle. The X is 1.5–2 cm from the lateral border of the clavicular head of the sternocleidomastoid muscle. Laterally to the X lies the pulse of the subclavian artery which must be regarded as the main landmark. A skin wheal is produced at the point marked X. A 3–5 cm 22-G needle is connected to a 10 ml syringe filled with anesthetic solution. The needle is introduced via the skin wheal and directed caudad, slightly tilted posteriorly and medially. If paraesthesias are evoked, the progress of the needle is arrested, and after aspiration, 5 ml of anesthetic solution is injected and another 5 ml after rotating the needle through 180°. The needle is advanced, albeit with the syringe empty, as far as the first rib; the empty 10 ml syringe is replaced by a full one and its contents are delivered a little at a time during withdrawal as far as the fascia. It is important to observe carefully the depth at which the needle comes into contact with the first rib and to keep this as a reference point beyond which the needle should not be advanced in the subsequent insertions in attempts to elicit paraesthesia. To elicit paraesthesias, the needle may be directed in a slightly anterior direction or in a posterior direction. It must not be directed in a lateral or medial direction, because, in both cases, the pleura may be perforated, laterally between the first and second rib, and medially, perforating the dome. In an anterior direction, if the needle is advanced just a little at a time, the anesthetist can stop as soon as he feels the needle start to slip on the edge of the rib; in the posterior direction, in practice, there is no danger of perforation because the needle slips beyond the rib angle and ends up in the muscular territory outside the rib cage.

Five ml of anesthetic solution is injected whenever paraesthesia is elicited, and after rotating the needle through 180°, another 5 ml is injected. Once the block has been completed, vigorous massaging of the supraclavicular region will facilitate the spread of the anesthetic. If a haemostatic tourniquet needs to be applied to the upper part of the arm or surgery is to be performed on the medial or superomedial part of the forearm, a "bracelet" block of the axilla and anterior part of the arm (between the biceps and deltoid muscles) must be executed in order to anesthetize the medial cutaneous nerve of the arm, the medial nerve of the forearm and the intercostobrachial nerve.

Dosage: from 30 to 50 ml of 1 % lidocaine or mepivacaine.

Complications:
- pneumothorax, reported in 0.5–4 % of cases;
- block of the phrenic nerve in 40–60 % of cases;
- Bernard-Horner syndrome in 70–90 % of cases.

6.5 Winnie and Collins Subclavian Perivascular Technique (1964)

6.5.1 Patient Position

The patient lies supine with the head slightly turned to the opposite side. To lower the shoulder in this position, the patient is asked to stretch forward and touch the ipsilateral knee with the fingers of one hand. It would be better, if possible, to have another operator apply traction to the limb, otherwise the voluntary manoeuvre may subject the shoulder and neck muscles to traction with reduced palpability as a result.

6.5.2 Landmarks

In order to highlight the clavicular head of the sternocleidomastoid muscle, the patient is asked to raise his head. After using the dermatographic pencil to trace the transverse line of the neck starting from the cricoid cartilage, the anesthetist places his finger behind the lateral border of the sternocleidomastoid muscle at the point where the latter is crossed by the cricoid transverse line. This point corresponds to Chassaignac's tubercle, as the anterior tubercle of the transverse process of C6 is called. The finger thus positioned behind the lateral border of the sternocleidomastoid muscle touches the anterior scalene muscle. Maintaining slight pressure and sliding the finger posterolaterally, the finger will feel the interscalene groove between the anterior and middle scalene muscles. At this point, the finger is slid along the groove in a caudad direction. The step formed by the omohyoid muscle that crosses the interscalene groove at greatly variable levels is encountered (Fig. 1.4). After overcoming this obstacle, the interscalene groove can again be felt and in many cases the pulse of the subclavian artery can be palpated.

When the anesthetist's finger arrives at the end of the groove, both in the event that the groove is crossed by a particularly low omohyoid muscle which therefore makes it difficult or impossible to feel the pulse of the subclavian artery, and, in the event that the pulse is palpable, once this incomprehensible muscle step has been overcome, the exploratory movement of the finger is arrested, but the finger remains in position (Fig. 6.3).

6.5.3 Technique

A 35 mm 24-G needle is inserted immediately above the finger and is directed caudad, neither dorsally nor anteriorly nor medially. If the direction is correct, the needle cone must advance, remaining in contact with the skin (Fig. 6.3). It is important to bear in mind that the brachial plexus at this point is closer to the middle than to the anterior scalene muscle, which is closer to the subclavian artery. If, during the insertion of the needle, paraesthesia of the shoulder or a twitch attributable to the supraspinatus and/or infraspinatus muscle should occur, this means that the needle has come into contact with the suprascapular nerve arising from the primary superior trunk. This contact is not reliable because the suprascapular nerve, only a few mm from its origin, emerges from the sheath of the neurovascular bundle and it is impossible to establish whether it has been stimulated within or outside of the sheath. Paraesthesias evoked at a level below the shoulder (upper arm, forearm, hand) or twitches of the deltoid, biceps or triceps muscles, etc., are valid. If an electrical nerve stimulator is used, it is good policy to perform an extensive prior disinfection as far down as the middle of the arm. In this way, by resting the hand on the patient's shoulder one can clearly perceive the contraction of the deltoid muscle without mistaking it for a movement induced by contraction of other scapular muscles.

If the subclavian artery is punctured, it means that the needle has been inserted or directed anteriorly and therefore needs to be reinserted a little more dorsally.

Once the required twitch has been elicited, 1 ml of anesthetic is injected in order to test the tissue resistance to injection and establish that this is not intraneural (onset of shooting pain). This is followed by injecting another 2–3 ml which will result in a dull, troublesome pain, generally affecting the entire arm due either to pressure of the liquid or to cold stimulation caused by the fact that the temperature of the anesthetic on the nerve is generally room temperature.

After performing the injection of the entire amount of anesthetic scheduled, Winnie advises vigorous massaging in a cranio-clavicular direction to facilitate the spread of the anesthetic.

The complementary block of the intercostobrachial nerve and the medial cutaneous nerve of the arm is necessary when a haemostatic tourniquet needs to be applied. In this case, it is sufficient to inject a few ml of anesthetic into the subcutaneous tissue, medially to the axillary pulse, at a point corresponding to the teres major and to the aponeurosis of the latissimus dorsi muscle.

6.6 Moorthy's Block

In 1991, S.S. Moorthy of the Department of anesthesia, Indiana University School of Medicine, developed a technique apparently similar, but actually substantially different from the

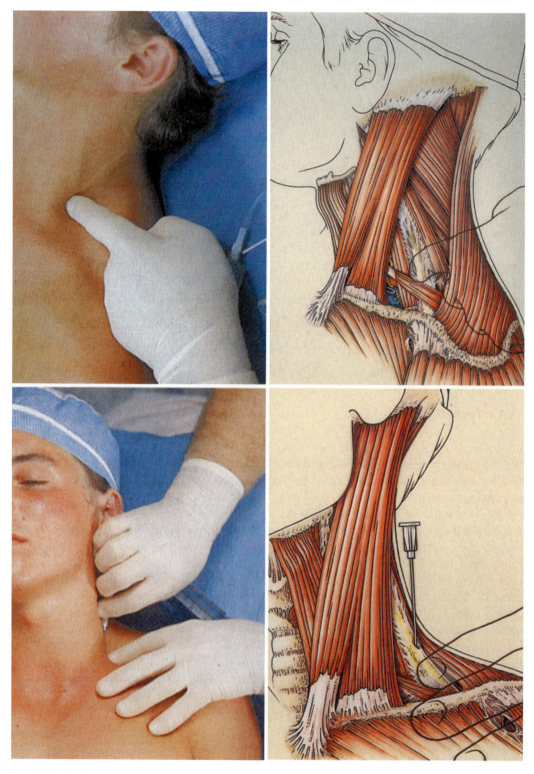

Fig. 6.3 In the four-panel page of this figure, we wish to present the original photos of Winnie's book with Buchoj's magnificent drawings, the clarity of which is inimitable (by courtesy of Winnie A.P.: *Tecniche Perivascolari di Blocco del Plesso Brachiale*, Verduci Editore, Roma 1984)

Winnie and Collins perivascular subclavian technique. Among other things, Moorthy seems to have been one of the first to use ultrasound to identify the vascular landmarks.

The author's intention was to modify the supraclavicular approach in order to avoid the most serious complication, that is to say pneumothorax.

6.6.1 Patient Position

The patient is placed in the supine position with the back raised 5–8 cm for the purposes of better exposing the clavicle and the sternocleidomastoid muscle. The arm is extended alongside the body and the head is turned 45° towards the opposite side to the one to be anesthetized.

6.6.2 Landmarks

An echo-Doppler probe is used to identify both the subclavian artery at the supraclavicular level and the axillary artery below the clavicle; the two points are marked and connected by a straight line segment that indicates the course of the subclavian artery which later becomes the axillary artery and which runs in the direction of the axilla with an inferolateral course. At supraclavicular level, the middle and upper trunks of the brachial plexus are in a superolateral position in relation to the artery (Fig. 2.5).

6.6.3 Technique

A skin wheal is induced with a small-calibre needle, 2 cm above the clavicle and 1 cm laterally to the straight line indicating the course of the subclavian artery. At the same point, an 18-G needle is introduced to a depth of a few mm, making a larger breach in the dermis for the purposes of facilitating the introduction and penetration of a stimulating needle. A Teflon-coated needle connected to an electrical nerve stimulator is introduced via the same hole produced by the 18-G needle. The stimulator is set at a current intensity of 0.5–0.2 mA and a frequency of 2 Hz.

The needle is advanced caudad, laterally and posteriorly to the course of the artery, and, in practice, towards the axilla. When the needle tip enters the neurovascular bundle, the motor stimulation of the upper limb begins; once stimulation of the deltoid or pectoralis muscles is provoked, the needle is advanced further in order to obtain, if necessary, muscle twitches at the level of the forearm, wrist and fingers. When appropriate twitches are elicited, the needle is fixed and, after aspiration, the anesthetic solution is injected.

With the Moorthy technique, the needle is directed laterally to the artery and does not come into contact with the first rib. Moreover, with this technique, the subclavian and axillary arteries are located with a Doppler probe. Any difficulties encountered in inducing a motor response are generally due to an excessively anterior position of the needle. In this case, the needle must be withdrawn and reintroduced with a more posterior path.

6.7 Parascalene Techniques

6.7.1 Posterior Approach

Kappis Technique
In April 1912, Kappis published his paravertebral block technique for all somatic nerves, including, as far as we are concerned, the cervical nerves. At this latter level, to avoid puncturing the vertebral vein or artery, the needle was directed laterally to the semicanals of the transverse processes.

The entry point of the needle was 3 cm laterally to the spinous process of C6.

After inducing a skin wheal, a 10 cm needle was advanced about 4 cm in a slightly medial direction in order to reach the articular process. Sliding the needle laterally to this process, it arrives at the transverse process of C6 which, if palpable from the outside, is indicated by the index or middle finger of the anesthetist's other hand. On coming into contact with the apophysis of the transverse process, 5 ml of anesthetic solution is injected after aspiration. The needle is then withdrawn as far as the subcutaneous tissue and reinserted, slightly changing its inclination, in the direction of another articular process and then of the corresponding transverse process, repeating the procedure.

If the patient is so muscular that palpation of the transverse processes proves impossible, once the articular process is reached, the needle is advanced laterally about a further 1.5 cm before injecting the anesthetic solution.

World War I, which afforded the opportunity to implement all the anesthetic techniques hitherto available, promoted the Kulenkampff technique in the field despite its defects, whereas the Kappis technique was little used because its execution was judged to be too painful for the patient.

6.7.2 Santoni Technique

In 1918, Santoni proposed a technique similar to the Kappis technique, which differed from the latter in that the needle was introduced via different cutaneous skin wheal metamere by metamere. At the level of T1, to overcome the obstacle of the first rib, the skin wheal was induced 3.5 cm laterally, but 2 cm above the level of the spinous process. On coming into contact with the first rib, the latter was overcome by directing the needle in a caudal direction and slightly medially. Santoni's technique failed to solve the problems, possibly multiplying them fivefold, by inserting the needle in five different points.

6.7.3 Posterior Approach According to Pippa *(written by Pippa himself)*

This technique, illustrated by Pippa in 1990, and originally employing the loss of resistance technique in order to locate the brachial plexus, today, thanks to the use of electrical nerve stimulation and more recently to the use of ultrasound in conjunction with regional anesthesia, has earned widespread approval on account of its success rate and safety profile.

6.7.4 Patient Position

The block is performed with the patient seated and with the neck bent slightly forward or with patient recumbent on one side. The anesthetist stands behind the patient when the latter is seated, or sits when the patient is recumbent. The patient is placed in the recumbent position on the side opposite to the side of the block, with the head positioned axially on a firm pillow, and the cervical region slightly flexed.

6.7.5 Landmarks

- The midpoint of the interspinous segment between C6 and C7 (Fig. 6.4).
- A transverse straight line is traced passing through this point.
- Another point 3 cm distal to the midpoint of the interspinous segment is marked on this line.
- This latter point marks the needle insertion point (Fig. 6.4).

6.7.6 Technique

The technique requires an 8–10 cm-long stimulating needle.

After inducing a skin wheal with local anesthetic, the needle is inserted according to a sagittal plane and directed first perpendicular to the skin and then in a caudocranial, oblique and lateral direction. The author recommends that the anesthetist should never abandon the sagittal introduction plane and should avoid any deviation of the needle in a medial direction (Fig. 6.5).

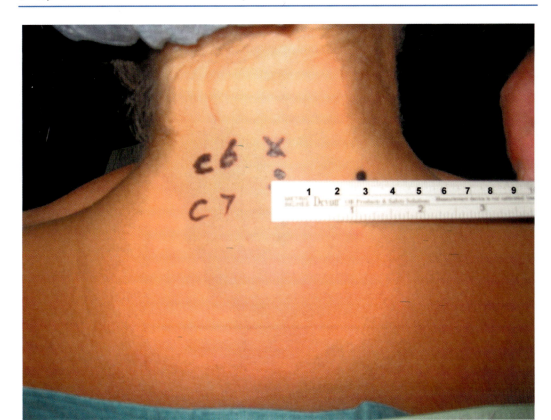

Fig. 6.4 Landmarks of the Pippa technique. At a distance of 3 cm from the *C6–C7* interspinous space the point where the skin wheal will be induced is marked

When the needle tip makes contact with the transverse process of the sixth or seventh cervical vertebra (this occurs at a depth of 4–5 cm), the upper edge of the transverse process is crossed and the needle is directed obliquely cephalad without deviating medially, but rather remaining fairly lateral. At a depth of 7–8 cm from the skin entry plane, at the onset of twitches of the biceps muscle or the muscles of the shoulder, after aspiration and after performing the Raj test, the anesthetic solution is injected at fractionated doses alternating with numerous aspirations.

Recently, to avoid the troublesome pain due to the needle penetrating into the trapezius muscle and the extensor muscles of the head, which occurs with the posterior approach, Boezaart has proposed a posterolateral approach, which, by entering in a position anterior to edge of the trapezius muscle, should enable anesthetist to direct the needle between lateral edge of the extensor muscles of the neck and the medial border of the levator scapulae muscle. This path, albeit via a virtual space, should be less painful, the needle being introduced in such a way as to skirt the external perimysium of the above-mentioned muscles.

With the advent of ultrasonography, the much feared risk of subarachnoid puncture attributed to this approach is no longer a credible hazard, inasmuch as, on proceeding with the ultrasound imaging, the passage of the needle at a safe distance from the spine is clearly visible (Fig. 6.5b).

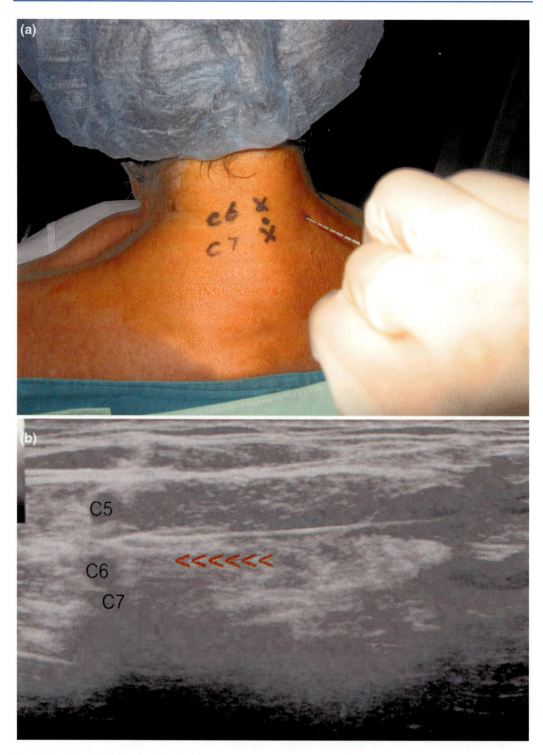

Fig. 6.5 a After inducing the skin wheal, the needle is introduced according to a sagittal plane in a direction perpendicular to the skin. In this photo, owing to an optical effect (parallax error), the needle appears erroneously to have a slightly medial direction. **b** Ultrasound image of the Pippa technique performed with an electric nerve stimulating needle

6.8 Anterior Approach

6.8.1 David L. Brown: Plumb-Bob Technique

If the article *Brachial Plexus Anesthesia: A Review*, published in the *International Monitor* No. 4, 1998—the journal edited by Narinder Rawal—had not been written by Brendan T. Finucane, I would probably not have read it with very much attention, and after a rapid glance to see whether anyone had by any chance noticed the technique I had published in *Minerva Anestesiologica* in 1992, I would have set it aside.

The first technique described was the "plumb-bob" technique proposed by David L. Brown et al. in *Anesthesia Analgesia* in 1993. The article was entitled "Supraclavicular nerve block: anatomical analysis to prevent pneumothorax". The description of the method by Finucane, albeit very short, as befits a review article, made it interesting and worth looking into. In addition to the article in *Anesthesia Analgesia*, it was also well described and illustrated in the *Atlas of Regional Anesthesia* by David L. Brown, edited in the Italian version by Antonio Delfino.

The concept on which this technique is based is simple, and the idea of the plumb line, as a guide to positioning the needle, is attractive.

6.8.2 Patient Position and Landmarks

The anesthetist performing the block stands alongside the patient at the level of the arm. The patient is placed in the supine position with his head turned to the side opposite to the block and with the arms extended beside the body. The patient is asked to raise his head a few cm in order to highlight the muscles of the neck, thus giving prominence to the clavicular head of the sternocleidomastoid muscle. The point where the latter encounters the clavicle is marked (Fig. 6.6a). The patient is asked to lower his head, while continuing to keep it turned to the opposite side to the block.

6.8.3 Technique

The needle is introduced at the point marked on the skin (Fig. 6.6b), close to the lateral edge of the clavicular head of the sternocleidomastoid muscle just above the clavicle. The direction is perpendicular to the floor, as though the needle were guided by a plumb line attached to its tip (Fig. 6.6c, d). It is precisely for this reason that it is useful to imagine a sagittal plane that passes through the point marked on the skin; the needle must remain on this plane without deviating either medially or laterally. If no paraesthesias or muscle twitches are elicited, the needle will be withdrawn as far as the subcutaneous tissue and reinserted gradually at an angle of no more than 30° in a cephalad direction; if, once again, no paraesthesias or twitches are elicited, the needle will be progressively orientated caudad at an angle of no more than 30°.

Once the needle comes into contact with brachial plexus, 30 ml of local anesthetic is injected, after fractionated aspiration, in a single injection. If, instead of the plexus, the needle comes into contact with the first rib, the author advises proceeding by shifting the needle laterally a little at a time, following the bony contact until it reaches the plexus. It is important never to orientate the needle medially so as not to increase the risk of pneumothorax.

6.8.4 Complications

The author reports pneumothorax as being the most feared complication. This occurs in 0.5–5 % of cases according to the amount of experience of the anesthetist.

Block of the phrenic nerve, again according to the author, occurs in 50 % of cases, which is in line with the results reported by Joseph Neal after supraclavicular block.

Another possible complication is puncture of the subclavian artery which, on the path of the needle, lies anterior to the plexus, but the only measures required are monitoring and compression, if a haematoma occurs.

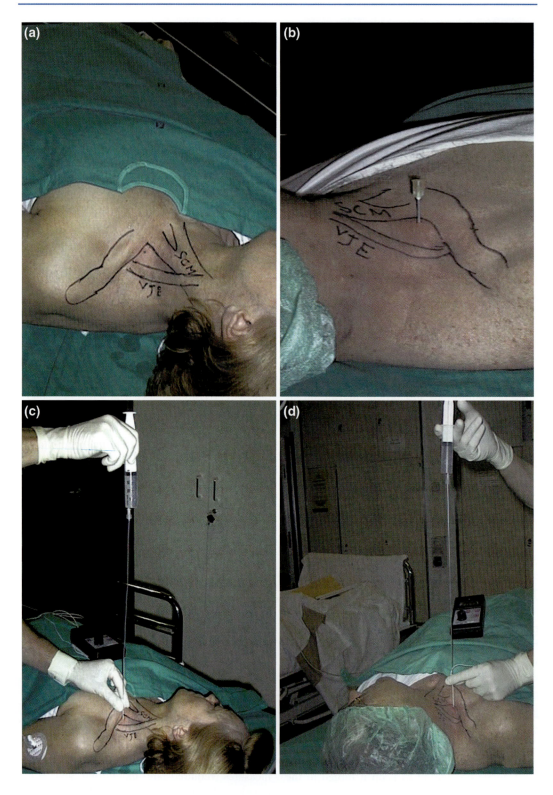

◀ **Fig. 6.6** This four-panel page illustrates the Brown technique. Panel **a** shows the landmarks marked on the skin and the point at which the needle is to be inserted; in panel **b**, the skin wheal has been produced and the 18-G needle, inserted immediately afterwards to enlarge the breach, has been left in place as a marker; in panels **c** and **d** to emphasize the plumb-bob concept the PVC tubing has been pulled upwards on the perpendicular of the needle

6.9 Lateral Approach (Lateral Paravertebral Techniques)

6.9.1 Mulley Technique

In 1919, Mulley described the first lateral paravertebral technique, basically for avoiding pneumothorax as well as puncture of the subclavian artery.

6.9.2 Patient Position and Landmarks

The patient lies in the supine position with his head turned to the side opposite the block.

In this way, the supraclavicular triangle is presented, formed by the anterior border of the trapezius muscle, the posterior border of the sternocleidomastoid muscle and the clavicle as the base. If the triangle is poorly delineated, an additional landmark is identified 3 cm above the clavicle and 0.5 cm posterior to the external jugular vein.

6.9.3 Technique

The needle is inserted at the centre of the triangle, perpendicularly to the skin, and, once paraesthesia of the first two fingers is obtained, 20 ml of anesthetic solution is injected, followed by another 10 ml in a slightly lateral position.

This technique has proved safe and efficacious, but has rarely been adopted.

6.9.4 Hilarowicz Technique

Six years later, in 1925, Hilarowicz, in an attempt to improve the Mulley technique and believing the centre of the triangle to be an imprecise landmark, described what in practice was a new technique.

As his main landmark, he adopted Chassaignac's tubercle on the transverse cricoid line (Fig. 6.7).

On reaching the tubercle with an 8 cm needle, at the onset of paraesthesias of the shoulder and first finger of the hand, 5 ml of anesthetic solution is injected (Fig. 6.8).

After subsequently identifying the transverse processes of C7, T1 and T2 and evoking paraesthesias of the other fingers of the hand, another 15 ml of anesthetic is injected, subdivided into boluses of 5 ml per metamere.

Winnie comments on this technique, describing it as a lateral version of the Kappis technique which hardly resembles the Mulley technique.

6.9.5 Etienne Technique

Defined by Winnie himself as the first true interscalene approach, the Etienne technique is based on the use of the same landmarks as in the Mulley technique, that is, the supraclavicular triangle (anterior border of the trapezius muscle, posterior border of the sternocleidomastoid muscle, clavicle). After drawing the triangle, the transverse cricoid line is traced passing through the two catheti of the triangle, formed by the posterior border of the sternocleidomastoid muscle and the anterior border of the trapezius muscle. The supraclavicular triangle is thus divided into a smaller triangle (superiorly) and a trapezium (inferiorly). At the midpoint of the straight line segment, identified by the points of intersection of the transverse cricoid line with the two catheti of the triangle, the needle is inserted and advanced in the direction of the opposite shoulder, slightly caudad, but on a plane parallel to that of the

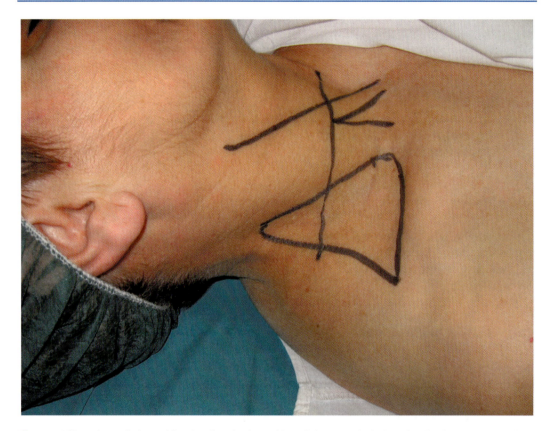

Fig. 6.7 Hilarowicz technique. After drawing the three sides of the supraclavicular triangle, the transverse cricoid line is traced which divides the triangle into another smaller triangle superiorly and a trapezium inferiorly

operating table. On making contact with the transverse process of the sixth or seventh cervical vertebra, without attempting to elicit paraesthesias, 20 ml of anesthetic solution is injected (Fig. 6.9).

6.9.6 Bonica's Lateral Paravertebral Approach

The author compares this block technique with that used for performing a deep cervical block.

A skin wheal is induced at the level of the transverse process of the fifth cervical vertebra.

An 8 cm-long needle is inserted as far as the transverse process, and as soon as the needle comes into contact with the latter, 5 ml of anesthetic solution is injected after aspiration. The needle, withdrawn as far as the subcutaneous tissue, is then directed towards Chassaignac's tubercle and, in succession, towards the transverse process of C7 and towards that of T1, injecting 5 ml of anesthetic each time.

The technique, though starting one metamere more cephalad, is similar to the Hilarowicz technique.

The indications for this type of block are limited to cases of infection of the supraclavicular fossa, cases of Pancoast syndrome due to tumours of the extreme apex of the lung and rare cases of fibrosis of the scalene muscles with distress due to compression of the brachial plexus.

6.10 Winnie's Interscalene Block

The interscalene brachial plexus block described by Alon P. Winnie is the most widely used technique in the world published in 1970. It definitively eliminates the risk of pneumothorax,

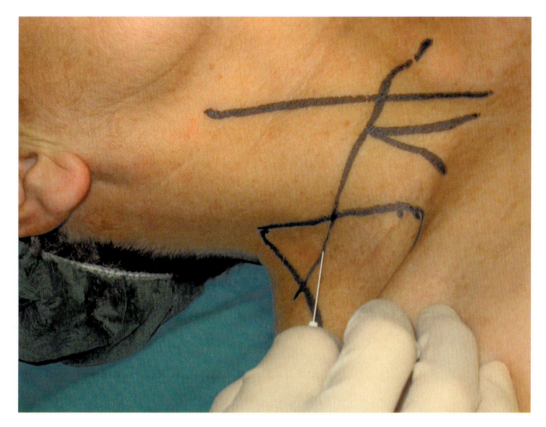

Fig. 6.8 Hilarowicz technique. Insertion of the needle at the level of Chassaignac's tubercle

and this, in our opinion, has been one of the most important reasons for its popularity.

We have to thank A. P. Winnie for developing the concept of the perivascular space and promoting its widespread application.

The first anesthesiologist to talk about the perivascular space was E. M. Livingston, whose technique had also been reported by Labat in the second edition of his textbook entitled *Regional Anesthesia* published by Saunders & Co in 1922. Labat had labelled Livingston's technique as "subfascial". Livingston wrote: "The plexus and the artery are separated from the surrounding structures by a fascial investment which represents two walls, the one in front belonging to the scalenus anticus muscle and the other belonging to the scalenus medius, These walls proceed laterally and slightly forward to meet the deep cervical fascia". Livingston's technique, which in terms of direction and landmarks resembles that of Kulenkampff, avoided contact with the nerve trunks and, as soon as the needle penetrated beyond the cervical fascia enveloping the plexus, 30 ml of anesthetic was injected without eliciting paraesthesias. But let's return to Winnie.

6.10.1 Patient Position

Supine with the head turned 45° to the opposite side to the one to be blocked.

6.10.2 Landmarks

The level at which the block is performed corresponds to that of the sixth cervical vertebra. What comes to mind immediately is that present at this level is Chassaignac's tubercle, as the transverse process of C6 is called, and that this might serve as an excellent landmark. The

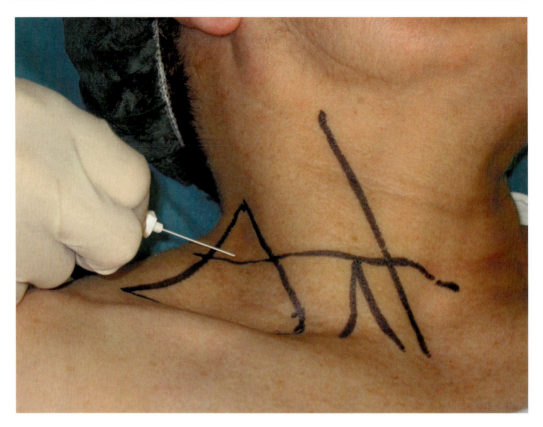

Fig. 6.9 Etienne technique. The needle is inserted at the midpoint of the base of the *small upper triangle* and directed towards the *opposite shoulder*, and therefore in a slightly caudal direction but parallel to the plane of the operating table

author, however, immediately plays down any initial enthusiasm in this sense, stating that this tubercle should not be used as a landmark because its palpation causes such discomfort as to undermine patient compliance.

A transverse line passing across the cricoid cartilage at the point where it crosses the lateral border of the sternocleidmastoid muscle is the most important landmark.

At this level, the external jugular vein is another important landmark that one should always seek to avoid. It is often evident or appears punctually during initial attempts at palpation (Fig. 6.10a).

To give prominence to the clavicular head of the sternocleidomastoid muscle, the patient is asked to raise his head. After tracing the transverse line of the neck departing from the cricoid cartilage (Fig. 6.10a, b), the anesthetist places his index finger behind the lateral border of the sternocleidomastoid muscle at the point where the latter is crossed by the transverse cricoid line. This point corresponds to Chassaignac's tubercle. The finger thus positioned behind the lateral border of the sternocleidomastoid muscle touches the anterior scalene muscle. Maintaining slight pressure and sliding the finger posterolaterally, the interscalene groove will be perceived between the anterior and middle scalene muscles. At this point, the anesthetist will also position his middle finger in the interscalene groove caudad to the index finger. It is good policy to bear in mind that, in the scalene triangle, the brachial plexus is closer to the middle than to the anterior scalene muscle, being distanced from the latter by the presence of the subclavian artery (Fig. 2.5).

6 Supraclavicular Brachial Plexus Block Techniques

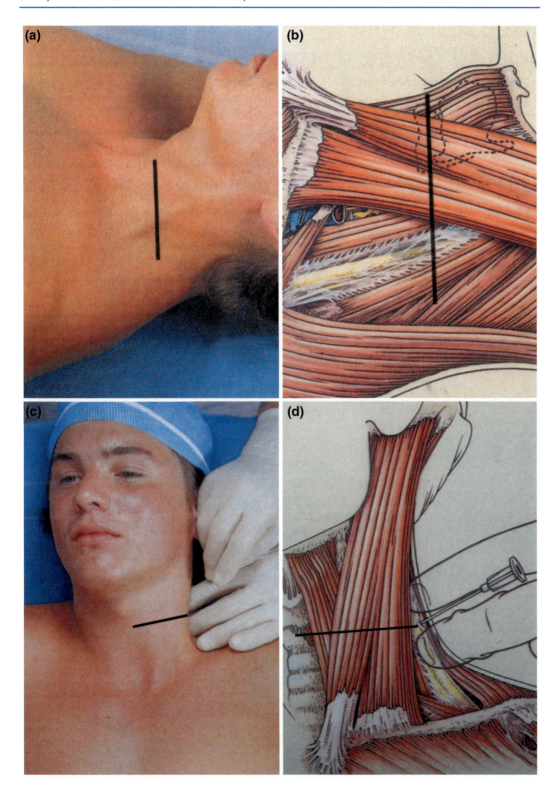

Fig. 6.10 a–d As in the case of the Winnie and Collins subclavian perivascular block, we have seen fit to group together the original photos of Winnie's book and Buchoj's magnificent drawings. A drawing is worth more than a thousand words. For an explanation see text. (By courtesy of Winnie A.P.: *Tecniche Perivascolari di Blocco del Plesso Brachiale*, Verducci Editore, Roma 1984)

6.10.3 Technique

The two fingers are slightly splayed, in the sense that whereas the index finger remains in position, the middle finger is moved approximately half a centimetre caudad, without exiting from the interscalene groove. A 35 mm short-bevel stimulating needle is inserted between the two fingers in a direction normal to the skin. The truncated cone shape of the neck must be borne in mind. Precisely for this reason, then, the needle will advance in a mostly medial but also in a caudal and posterior direction (Fig. 6.10c, d). If the external jugular vein is present, as it almost always is, it can be avoided by performing the needle entry puncture immediately above it. The needle is advanced until deltoid, biceps or triceps muscle twitches appear. Twitches of the supraspinatus and/or infraspinatus muscles, innervated by the suprascapular nerve, are not to be regarded as valid, because the suprascapular nerve abandons the neurovascular bundle of the brachial plexus at an early stage, and therefore, it is more likely that it is stimulated outside the brachial plexus. If the needle comes into contact with the bone without eliciting any twitches, it will be moved a little at a time, while remaining all the time in contact with the bone of the Chassaignac tubercle, until twitches occur. For the sake of safety, it is important that the needle be directed at least 30° caudad. A less inclined but more medial direction may result in the needle penetrating into the intervertebral conjugate foramen of C6 with stimulation of the root of C6 and the possibility of a peridural or, even worse, a subarachnoid block, if the presence of a valve mechanism of a small dural flap prevents the aspiration of cerebrospinal fluid.

When twitching of the deltoid, biceps or even the triceps muscles is registered, this should disappear if the current intensity is lowered below 0.2 mA, otherwise it would mean that the needle tip may be in an intraneural position. Once the twitch has been made to disappear, it can be reinduced by restoring the current intensity to a level above 0.2 mA. At this point, after aspiration, 2–3 ml of anesthetic is injected, which will cause a dull, troublesome but correct paraesthesia in the shoulder or along the arm, probably due to the relatively low temperature of the anesthetic liquid compared to that of the nerve, or to the pressure exerted by the anesthetic bolus directly on the nerve structures. The injection of the few ml of anesthetic will be sufficient to increase the impedance of the tissues, which will again abolish the twitch. Injection of the remaining anesthetic will be performed in 5 ml amounts with aspiration intervals in between. The author advises vigorous massaging in a caudal direction to facilitate the spread of the anesthetic. The amount of anesthetic recommended varies according to the patient's build from 20 ml, which often fails to reach the roots C8 and T1, to 40 ml, which usually allows a more complete anesthesia.

6.10.4 Complications

- Very rarely, pneumothorax; proper execution of the technique rules out this eventuality.
- Subarachnoid injection, injection into the vertebral artery and extension of the block to the peridural space are possible, again if the technique is not performed correctly.
- Block of the phrenic nerve, according to Urmey, occurs in 100 % of cases.
- Claude Bernard-Horner syndrome should not be considered a complication, but only a side effect, as should extension of the block to the inferior laryngeal nerve (recurrent nerve).
- The formation of a haematoma as a result of an arterial puncture requires only monitoring and compression.

6.11 Meier Technique

6.11.1 Patient Position

Supine with the head turned to the opposite side.

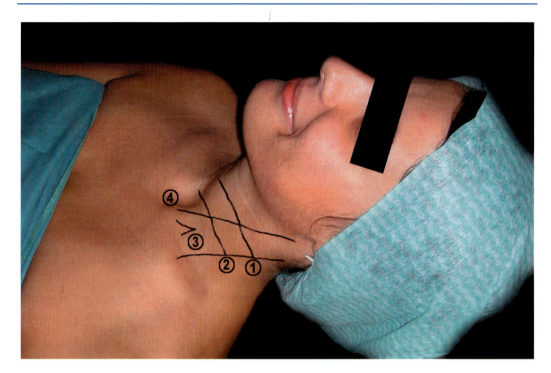

Fig. 6.11 Meier technique: *1* point of insertion with the Meier technique on the transverse thyroid line, behind the posterior border of the sternocleidomastoid muscle. *2* point of insertion with the Winnie technique on the transverse cricoid line, behind the posterior border of the sternocleidomastoid muscle; *3* clavicular head of the sternocleidomastoid muscle; *4* jugulum

6.11.2 Landmarks

The innovative aspect of this technique consists in the fact that the main landmark is the transverse line which rune from the superior margin of the thyroid cartilage and intersects with the posterior border of the sternocleidomastoid muscle. Thus, the point of insertion of the needle is about 2 cm above the insertion point with the Winnie interscalene technique, where the landmark is the intercricothyroid line (Fig. 6.11).

The external jugular vein lies in a slightly more anterior position than in the Winnie technique.

6.11.3 Technique

A skin wheal is induced at the point of intersection of the superior transverse thyroid line and the posterior border of the sternocleidomastoid muscle. The needle is directed caudad, tangential to the direction of the plexus, heading towards the midpoint of the clavicle. Normally, at a depth of 1 or 2 cm, the muscle twitch sets in. After performing the Raj test (injection of 2 ml of anesthetic which arrests the twitch), the planned volume of anesthetic is injected at fractionated doses in 5 ml boluses, each preceded by aspiration.

If shoulder movements are activated without contraction of the deltoid muscle, this means that the suprascapular nerve is being stimulated and therefore that the needle direction is too posterior. If, on the other hand, a diaphragmatic twitch occurs, it means that the needle has been directed too anteriorly and is stimulating the phrenic nerve, abutting upon the anterior scalene muscle, or that it has been directed medially, ending up by stimulating the anterior division of C4 which constitutes the main root of the nerve; in these cases, the needle must be withdrawn and directed with greater precision towards the midpoint of the clavicle.

The indications for this type of block, as in Bonica's lateral paravertebral approach, are cases of infection of the supraclavicular fossa, of Pancoast syndrome and cases of fibrosis of the scalene muscles with distress due to compression of the brachial plexus.

6.12 Dalens Parascalene Technique

This is a technique conceived and designed basically for paediatric patients, but which in any event can also be performed in adults.

6.12.1 Patient Position

Supine with the arm extended down alongside the body and the head turned to the opposite side to that where the block is to be performed. To hyperextend, the neck a small cushion is placed beneath the shoulders.

6.12.2 Landmarks

1. The midpoint of the clavicle.
2. Chassaignac's tubercle, localized by palpation, or better, to avoid a degree of discomfort that might jeopardize the compliance of a paediatric patient, localized at the point where the cricoid line intersects the posterior border of the sternocleidomastoid muscle.

A straight line segment joining the two landmarks is traced and subdivided into three-thirds.

6.12.3 Technique

A skin wheal is induced at the point between the upper two-thirds and the lower-third.

The needle is introduced in an antero-posterior direction. Once the muscular twitch required is elicited, the anesthetic solution is injected. If the direction is too lateral, the suprascapular nerve may be stimulated causing shoulder movements due to contraction of the supraspinatus muscle or the infraspinatus muscle but the deltoid muscle remains quiescent. If the needle is introduced too medially, the phrenic nerve may be stimulated with consequent twitching of the diaphragm. It should be borne in mind that, in children, the depth of the brachial plexus ranges from 7 to 30 mm according to the child's age and weight. The mepivacaine dose is 6–7 mg/kg.

Dalens reports that, as in all proximal techniques, the anesthesia may be unsatisfactory in the ulnar nerve territory.

6.13 Middle Interscalene Block (Alemanno Technique)

6.13.1 Why a New Technique? How This Technique Arose

In the late 'seventies, after two cases of pneumothorax in the space of just 1 week using the Kulenkampff technique as modified by Moore, I converted to Winnie's interscalene technique. Winnie's technique undoubtedly could be guaranteed to avoid any risk of this pulmonary complication and appeared to be efficacious above all for arm and shoulder surgery. During an orthopaedic surgical session in the mid 'eighties, I was using the interscalene block for what at the time was an open surgical operation on the shoulder. I had just elicited paraesthesia and, after fixing the needle, I was about to inject the anesthetic solution when, after aspiration, a thin trickle of blood appeared in the syringe, which, very optimistically, I gauged to be the result of a burst capillary; in actual fact, with the advantage of hindsight, the blood could only have come from the vertebral artery, puncture of which may result in spasm, especially in young subjects. Fortunately, I had cultivated the habit of initially injecting only 2 ml of anesthetic in order to be sure to avoid intraneural injection. However, the injection of a 2 ml bolus of 2 % mepivacaine was followed by a series of spectacular phenomena: the patient's eyes were glazed and rolled backwards and his tongue dropped back suddenly, obstructing his breathing; it was as if I had administered an intravenous injection of 300 mg of thiopentone sodium. I immediately extracted the needle, grabbed hold of the "to-and-fro" connected to an O_2 flowmeter which happened to be at hand behind me and proceeded to ventilate the patient, after inserting a Guedel oropharyngeal airway into his mouth. After a few minutes, the patient was intubated very easily without the aid of muscle relaxants. The patient, in fact, presented perfect muscle relaxation. By injecting the bolus of local anesthetic into the vertebral artery, via the basilar artery, I had probably anesthetized all 12 cranial nerves.

Once the patient was intubated, he was connected up to a Bird MK8 ventilator, a small, transparent, green plastic pressure-operated ventilator that permits the visualization of its mechanisms and circuits at high and low pressure. The patient showed signs of rearousal after about 20 min, and after another 10 min, he was completely awake and could be extubated. He remembered nothing, and the surgery was postponed and the patient sent back to the ward. He was operated on the next day under general anesthesia.

As always, when these misadventures occur, albeit with a happy ending, one is halted in one's tracks and for some time may feel reluctant to use a technique that has caused such a serious problem. I was no exception on that occasion and for a month or two, I almost always resorted to the use of general anesthesia.

One day, while looking at an anatomical drawing by Buchoj, upside down, on page 50 of Winnie's book *Plexus Anesthesia*, subtitled *Perivascular Techniques of Brachial Plexus Block*, published in the Italian version by Verduci in 1984, I came up with idea of using a needle to cannulate the neurovascular bundle along its main axis starting from near the midpoint of the clavicle (Fig. 6.12).

Above all, there could be no risk of pneumothorax owing to the direction of the needle tangential to the upper surface of the clavicle and not directed towards the pleura; in addition, unless the needle used was excessively long, it would have been difficult to reach the cervical spine and all the adjoining structures.

At the first attempt, the experiment was successful, but I did not realize I had found a new approach. It seemed impossible to me, in view of the simplicity of the technique, that it had not already been described.

Only a few years later, while lecturing at the Verona University Postgraduate School of Anesthesia and Resuscitation directed by Professor Stefano Ischia, I was explaining the various techniques (Kulenkampff, Kappis, Winnie, etc.) but concluded saying I no longer used any of these techniques, but rather a procedure of my own. One day, one of my brighter students asked me: "Excuse me, Professor, but have you already published this technique of yours?" Actually, "I haven't", was my answer, at which he said: "In that case, do it, otherwise we'll do it because, you know, we have tried it out in the operating theatre and it works very well". I then got a grip on the situation and reminded the students that in a few months time they would be sitting their examinations and that it would be wiser on their part if, in the meantime, they refrained from taking any untoward initiatives. I then rapidly consulted Winnie's textbook, doing some quick research with the aid of his most authoritative account of the historical evolution of the various brachial plexus block techniques, and I realized that my technique had, in fact, never been described. I therefore decided to publish the technique in *Minerva Anestesiologica* and it was included in the June 1992 issue of that journal. In the same year, I presented it at the S.I.A.A.R.T.I. National Congress held in Taormina. A few words of courteous congratulation, a few affectionate pats on the shoulder, but then no one took any further interest in it.

The acceptance and diffusion of a new technique are always something of a slow but sure process, also because the best technique to be used in routine practice in the operating theatre is the one you are most familiar with and best able to perform, and "it is always hard to break with old habits" as Thomas Stan wrote to me from Cleveland, Ohio.

At the E.S.R.A. Congress in 1999, which was held in Florence and organized by Paolo Busoni, I was sitting in the front row, listening to a lecture

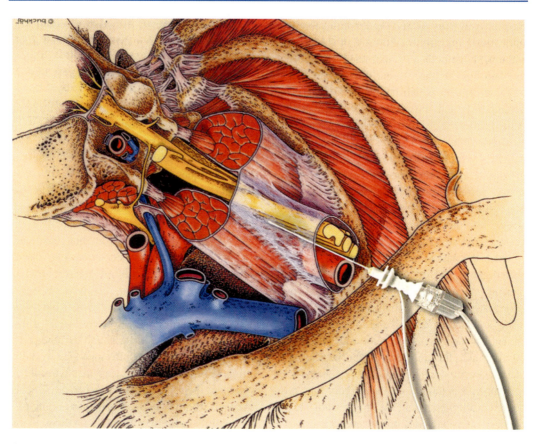

Fig. 6.12 The basic rationale of the middle interscalene block (MIB) is to cannulate the neurovascular bundle (by courtesy of Winnie A.P.: *Tecniche Perivascolari di Blocco del Plesso Brachiale*, Verduci Editore, Roma 1984, modified)

on the main brachial plexus block techniques. Sitting beside me was a distinguished-looking, unknown colleague, using a headset for the simultaneous translation, which enabled me to place him as a foreigner. The speaker, after presenting the various brachial plexus block techniques, went on to describe one last technique which he claimed to be "of his own devising", but which was incredibly identical to my technique! The lecture was followed by a lively discussion interrupted by the moderator who, to defuse this rather embarrassing situation, reminded everyone that it was time for a coffee break. The distinguished-looking foreign colleague sitting beside me received the translation of our discussion with a slight delay; when everyone had got up to leave the auditorium, he took off his headset and asked me: "Are you the real author of the last technique?" "Yes, sir. It was published 7 years ago in the June 1992 issue of *Minerva Anestesiologica*", I replied in my limited and consequently rather stilted English, at which he said: "Send me an abstract and I'll accept it for the International Symposium on Regional Anesthesia and Pain Medicine in Quebec City, Canada, in 2000". He then introduced himself as Professor Brendan Finucane, Chair of the Department of Anesthesiology and Pain Medicine of Alberta University, Edmonton, Canada.

In addition to the abstract, I sent him a poster which I would subsequently present at the Congress. He replied by sending me a fax in which he expressed a most flattering judgment which I am pleased to report.

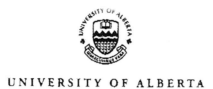

UNIVERSITY OF ALBERTA

April 19, 1999

Dr F Alemanno
Medico chirurgo
Specialista in Anestesia e Rianimazione
Facharzt für Anaesthesie und Wiederbelebung
Amb., Via del Vigneto 31, Weinbergstraße 31
39100 BOLZANO BOZEN

Dear Fernando:

Thank you for your communication about my publication on brachial plexus anaesthesia.

The information you sent me is very interesting and I intend to incorporate your technique in any future presentations or publications.

Thank you also for your excellent poster. Like Brown's method, yours is a very simple concept and appears much safer than the traditional approaches to brachial plexus anaesthesia.

Sincerely,

Brendan T Finucane, MBBCh, FRCPC
Professor and Chair
Department of Anesthesiology and Pain Medicine

BTF/ldb

Department of Anesthesiology and Pain Medicine
Office of the Chair

3B2.32 Walter C Mackenzie Health Sciences Centre • University of Alberta • Edmonton • Canada • T6G 2B7
Telephone: (780) 407-8887 • Fax: (780) 407-3200
E-mail: bfinucan@gpu.srv.ualberta.ca

6.13.2 Evolution of the Middle Interscalene Block

In the article published in *Minerva Anestesiologica* in June 1992, the technique was based on the eliciting of paraesthesias and was aimed at avoiding pneumothorax, which is possible with the techniques in which the needle is advanced in a caudal direction, and also at avoiding subarachnoid injection or injection into the vertebral artery, which is possible with the paravertebral techniques.

The patient was placed in the seated position with the feet off the bed, the back upright and the shoulders relaxed in order to make the brachial plexus more superficial.

The landmarks used were two: the pulse of the subclavian artery and the spinous process of C7.

The needle used was a normal 3 cm 23-G needle.

The technique was performed as follows:

A skin wheal was induced half a centimetre laterally to the pulse of the subclavian artery. The 3 cm G-23 needle, already attached to a 20ml syringe filled with anesthetic solution, was inserted laterally to the pulse of the subclavian artery. The needle was directed posterolaterally heading for the spinous process of C7. This first insertion rarely elicited paraesthesia, but was useful for identifying the transverse plane of C7 on which the needle was to operate. If, as was highly probable, no paraesthesia appeared, the needle was withdrawn as far as the subcutaneous tissue and reinserted, in succession, towards the vertebral arch, pedicle and body of C7. On eliciting paraesthesia, the needle was fixed and, after aspiration, 1 ml of anesthetic was injected to make sure that the needle tip was not in an intraneural position. It was also important that the injection should continue to cause a disagreeable sensation along the arm, not painful but paraesthetic, also during the subsequent first 5 ml fraction of anesthetic injected. If, however, the paraesthesia did not persist after the test injection and during the subsequent 5 ml fraction, it had to be re-elicited.

In 1999, after a certain delay, the electrical nerve stimulator was eventually used, which proved distinctly advantageous both for the patient and for the precision performance of the technique. In cases of fracture, however, we continued to use a normal needle for eliciting paraesthesia. Recently, it has proved possible to approach the nerve under ultrasound guidance.

More widespread knowledge and use of this technique have been facilitated by Professor Guido Fanelli's invitation to me to describe it in the volume entitled *Continuous Peripheral Nerve Block Techniques*, also coedited by Andrea Casati, Jacques Chelly and Laura Bertini and published in the United States in 2001 by Mosby International Limited, as well as by Battista Borghi's invitation to me to present the technique at the ESRA 2001 Congress held at the Rizzoli Institute in Bologna, and by Paolo Grossi's invitation to write a chapter on the middle interscalene block for the book entitled *I blocchi anestetici dell'arto superiore* published by Mattioli. Fidenza 2006.

A further contribution to the knowledge and diffusion of the technique came in the form of many invitations I have received to attend and speak at residential courses, and national and international congresses organized by Francesco Nicosia, Laura Bertini and Vincenzo Tagariello, Giuseppe Vairo and Aldo Barbati, Domenico Camaioni and Mario Bosco, Paolo Grossi, Alessandro D'Ambrosio and Michele Dambrosio, Silvio Colonna, Gerardo Martinelli, Gianfranco Di Nino and Nicolino Franceshelli, Paola Valentini Claudio Amodei and Claudio Lo Presti, Salvatore Montanini and Epifanio Mondello, Mohammad Saleh, Izdiad Badran and Hamdi Bader, Francesco Paoletti, Francesco Ambrosio, Gennaro Savoia, Yigal Leykin, Rui Sobral de Campos and Lucindo Ormonde, Giovanni Pinto, Giovanni Pittoni, Ezio Vincenti, Walter Mosaner, Stefano Brauneis, Consalvo Mattia and Flaminia Coluzzi.

All these initiatives and invitations, for which I will never be grateful enough to the organizers, have contributed considerably to augmenting the knowledge and more widespread use of the technique also at an international level.

In 2002, 10 years after the publication of the first paper, we proceeded to verify the indications and limitations of the technique. After 58 middle interscalene blocks, performed for shoulder surgery in the space of 3 months, we verified the extent of the anesthesia with the pinprick test applied to the entire surface of the upper limb, recording the following results referring to the involvement of the various nerves in their respective areas of competence:
- circumflex nerve 100 %;
- musculocutaneous nerve 100 %;
- radial nerve 100 %;
- median nerve 93 %;
- medial cutaneous nerve of the forearm 80 %;
- ulnar nerve 72.5 %;
- medial cutaneous nerve of the arm and intercostobrachial nerve (whose territories of competence are often imbricated or overlapping) 54 %.

We therefore concluded that the MIB technique, like all the other supraclavicular techniques, is indicated for shoulder and arm surgery, but its reliability progressively diminishes the more distal or peripheral the surgical field.

6.14 Middle Interscalene Block

6.14.1 Present State of the Art

The middle interscalene block is so-called in order to distinguish it from Winnie's technique which could be defined as a high interscalene block, since the scalene triangle is entered at its apex; nor could the block be called 'low' (apart from the negative semantic connotations of the adjective) because to reach the base of the triangle, except in the case of Kulenkampff's method and other similar caudad techniques, the only access route is the infraclavicular centripetal route.

6.14.2 Patient Position

The ideal position is the upright seated position with the head rest completely raised (deck chair position), with the legs extended and with the arm hanging limply outside the bed. In this manner, the shoulder is relaxed, the clavicle is rotated downwards, and the neurovascular bundle becomes more superficial. The head is turned 45° to the side opposite the one to be operated on. If the patient, for some reason, is unable to assume or maintain this position, the block can also be executed in the supine position (Fig. 6.13).

6.14.3 Landmarks

1. The pulse of the subclavian artery, marked **O**.
2. The midpoint of the clavicle, marked with a dot.
3. The spinous process of C7, marked **X** (Fig. 6.14).

A straight line segment is traced running from the midpoint of the clavicle tangential posterolaterally to the **O** marking the pulse of the subclavian artery (Fig. 6.15).

6.14.4 Technique

1. Thorough disinfection. It is important that the disinfection should be thorough, particularly for shoulder surgery, and this is for two reasons: in the first place, above all if one is working with a low current intensity, in order to be sure that the twitch is from the deltoid muscle, it may be useful to rest the hand not manoeuvring the needle on the skin investing the deltoid muscle so as to feel the muscle twitching; secondly, because, in the case of shoulder surgery, the operating field is disinfected twice rather than just once.
2. A skin wheal is induced with a 23-G needle 2 mm laterally to the pulse of the subclavian artery; the syringe is detached and the needle is left implanted in the skin as a marker; the 23-G needle is replaced by an 18-G needle (if possible in the same hole) so as to enlarge the breach in the dermis, thus facilitating the passage of the Teflon-coated needle and preventing invagination of the skin with the consequent unwanted microbial entrainment. The 18-G needle is also left in situ.

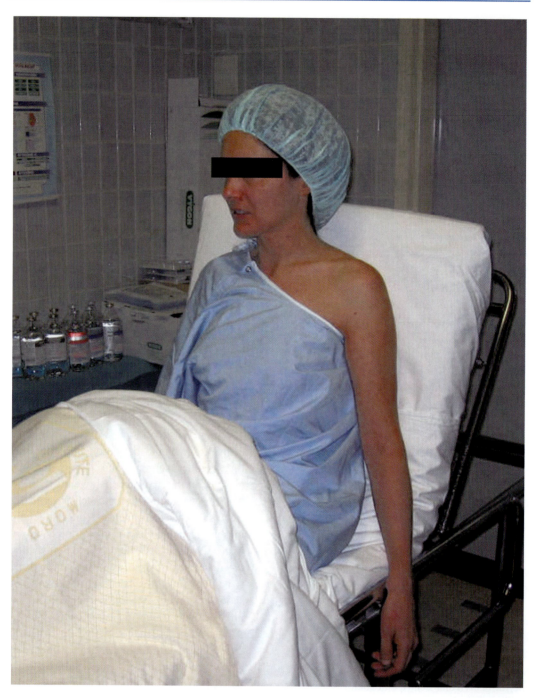

Fig. 6.13 Patient position. In a first description of the technique in 1992, the patient was placed in the seated position with the feet of the bed. This proved to be an uncomfortable position, the venous return of the lower limbs was not optimal, and in the case of lipothymia, it was necessary to make the patient change position completely in order to put him or her in the recumbent position. In the new position, on the other hand, with the legs resting on the bed and with the back propped up against the head rest, the patient will be in a much more comfortable position with a lower risk of lipothymia episodes

6 Supraclavicular Brachial Plexus Block Techniques

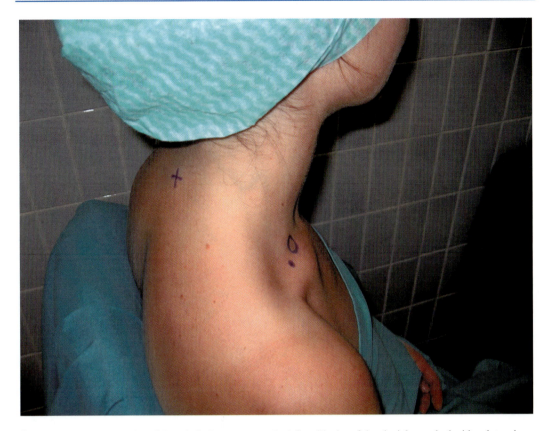

Fig. 6.14 Landmarks: pulse of the subclavian artery, marked **O**; midpoint of the clavicle, marked with a dot; spinous process of C7, marked **X**

3. Needle direction: the 18-G needle is replaced by a 35–40 mm Teflon-coated 24-G needle which is advanced along the straight line running from the midpoint of the clavicle and tangential posterolaterally to the **O** marking the pulse of the subclavian artery, but proceeding more deeply on the transverse plane of C7, indicated by the **X** denoting the spinous process of C7. The path of the needle, in practice, is parallel to the plane corresponding to the upper surface of the clavicle, or slightly rising in relation to the latter (Fig. 6.16 a, b). The direction of the needle must on no account ever be descending, otherwise we would be performing a different technique with a distinct risk of pneumothorax. The current intensity is set at 0.4 mA. On the basis of our experience, a current intensity greater than 0.5 mA may stimulate a nerve element which is in contact internally with the fascia enveloping the brachial plexus, even if the needle tip is positioned outside the fascia.

If, on the other hand, a nerve element is stimulated with the current intensity we suggest, the tip of the needle is sure to lie inside the neurovascular bundle. Once the desired twitch is induced, the current intensity is reduced below 0.2 mA; if the twitch persists, there is a risk that the needle tip may be intraneural, and therefore, the needle must be withdrawn, albeit only millimetrically; if, on the other hand, the twitch disappears, the previous stimulation values are restored and when the muscle contraction reappears 1 ml of anesthetic solution is injected.

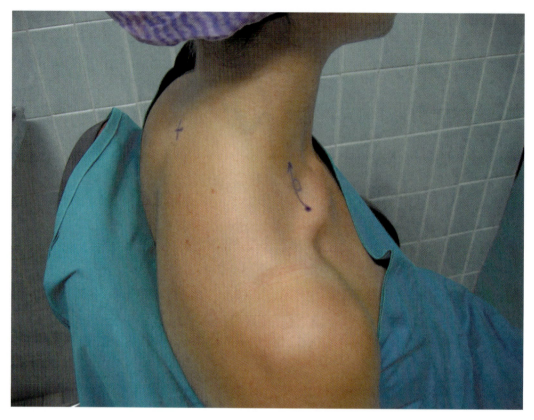

Fig. 6.15 A straight line segment is traced from the midpoint of the clavicle and runs at a posterolateral tangent to the O marking the pulse of the subclavian artery

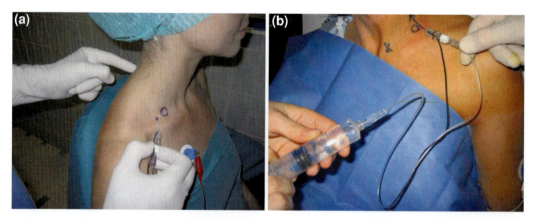

Fig. 6.16 *a-b* Technique. The direction of the needle is parallel to the upper surface of the clavicle or slightly rising in relation to it. In the first version of the technique (*Minerva Anestesiologica*, June, 1992) and also later, with the use of the electric nerve stimulator, the needle was directed first towards the spinous process of C7 and then, remaining on the transverse plane of C7, in succession towards the arch, pedicle and body of the same vertebra until paraesthesia was elicited or appropriate muscle twitches. The intention, however, praiseworthy, of finding the plane of C7 with the first needle insertion and not abandoning it with the successive insertions meant in practice that the first two insertions not only rarely led to the brachial plexus, but rather were capable of causing inappropriate paraesthesias or twitches due to stimulation of the supraclavicular nerve. These twitches could be misleadingly deceptive particularly for beginners who may sometimes mistake twitches of the supraspinatus muscle (with raising of the shoulder) for twitches of the deltoid muscle, thus risking injecting the anesthetic outside the neurovascular bundle

This small injection should not be followed by sharp pain, but only by a troublesome paraesthesia, and, moreover, the twitch should disappear completely (Raj test).

If no twitches appear at the first insertion, little adjustments are made to the path of the needle; the needle must be withdrawn as far as the subcutaneous tissue and reinserted in a direction slightly posterior or anterior to the straight line segment described above until the desired twitch appears.

On appearance of the deltoid, biceps or triceps muscle twitch, after aspiration and a Raj test, 0.4 ml/kg of anesthetic solution is injected. Like Silverstein, we prefer to inject all the anesthetic at the appearance of the first valid twitch rather than searching for others; in this case, in fact, we have to increase the current intensity after the first bolus of anesthetic which will alter the tissue impedance and, with that, our assessment of the distance between the needle tip and the nerve structure. The search for multiple twitches, moreover, may increase the complications associated with the blocks, without increasing their success rate.

Sometimes, however, the pulse of the subclavian artery is not present, and thus the main landmark for establishing the direction of the needle is lacking. In this case, we fall back on the use of three landmarks that are always present also in obese patients. These are as follows:

1. the midpoint of the clavicle (marked at the level of the posterior edge of the clavicle);
2. the spinous process of C7;
3. the sternoclavicular joint (marked at the level of the posterior edge of the clavicle).

By joining the first point to the other two, we obtain an angle whose bisector indicates the direction leading to the brachial plexus. It coincides with the straight line posterolaterally tangential to the **O** marking the pulse of the subclavian artery when the latter is present (Fig. 6.17).

A skin wheal is induced on the bisector at a distance of about 1.5 cm from the midpoint of the clavicle. The first insertion of the needle is performed following the bisector of the angle, but remaining on the transverse plane of C7, indicated by its spinous process. If no twitch appears at the first insertion, little adjustments are made to the path of the needle: the needle must be withdrawn as far as the subcutaneous tissue and reinserted in a direction slightly posterior or anterior to the above-mentioned bisector until the required twitch is elicited.

6.14.5 Indications

The most important indication for the supraclavicular techniques is unquestionably surgery of the shoulder and arm (the proximal half of the humerus). The potential efficacy of these techniques diminishes, the more distal or peripheral the surgical indication. As we have seen, in a study conducted in 58 patients, the median nerve was involved in 93 % of cases, the medial cutaneous nerve of the forearm in 80 % and the ulnar nerve only in 72.5 % of cases. The latter two are percentages, which are no longer acceptable in modern anesthesia and suggest the advisability of going over to the use of more peripheral techniques such as infraclavicular or axillary blocks. A number of exceptions can be made if the operative field lies in the territory of the radial nerve which is blocked by the middle interscalene technique in 100 % of cases, possibly supplementing the technique, if the extent of the anesthesia is incomplete, with peripheral blocks of the median or ulnar nerve or both at the elbow (e.g. for hand surgery). It is thus proves possible to exploit the possibility that the supraclavicular block affords of applying a haemostatic tourniquet at the level of the humerus.

As far as the continuous block is concerned, the indication for its use, other than for postoperative analgesia allowing the early application of physiokinetic therapy, consists in the prophylaxis of posttraumatic reflex sympathetic dystrophy (Sudeck's syndrome), it affords as a result of prolonged sympathetic block. In fact, the Claude Bernard-Horner syndrome in our single-shot case series is present in 93.5 % of cases, but the percentage is probably higher with the catheter because the latter protrudes for a

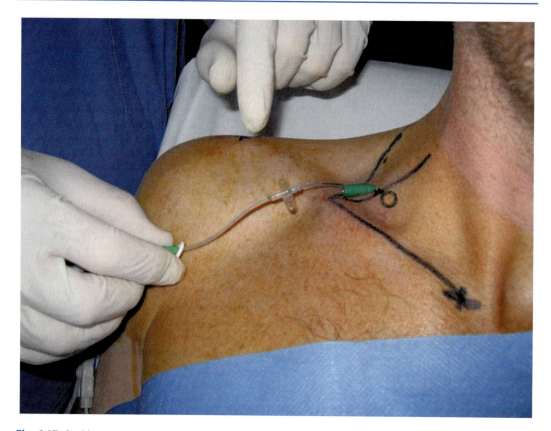

Fig. 6.17 In this case, the pulse of the subclavian artery was present, the bisector of the angle coincides with the posterolateral line tangential to the **O** marking the pulse

distance of 1–2 cm beyond the tip of the needle, thus approaching closer to the cervical spine and consequently to the paravertebral sympathetic chain.

6.14.6 Complications

In 692 cases published in *Regional Anesthesia and Pain Medicine*, Nov–Dec 2006, we registered the following complications:
- block of the phrenic nerve in 58 (60 %) of 97 cases monitored by chest X-rays on completion of surgery and therefore with the block certainly well established;
- block of the phrenic nerve with dyspnoea ($SaO_2 < 90$ %): 4 cases (0.6 %);
- arterial puncture with haematoma: 4 cases (0.6 %);
- dysphonia due to block of the lower laryngeal nerve: 6 cases (0.9 %);
- Claude Bernard-Horner Syndrome: 647 Cases (93.5 %):
- no cases of subarachnoid injection or injection into the vertebral artery;
- no cases of pneumothorax.

Pneumothorax should be very rare indeed. Proper execution of the technique should rule out any such eventuality.

In the course of more than 20 years, three anecdotal cases of pneumothorax have occurred, which, after thorough investigation, turned out to be due to technical errors, in the sense that the needle path presented a caudal inclination in the direction of the pleural dome.

In any event, we should always mistrust those patients presenting Stiller's characteristic asthenic habitus—tall, slim, flat-chested, drooping shoulders, chicken-wing shoulder blades—so well described by Bertold Stiller. In these cases, the lateral apophysis of the clavicle may be constitutionally rotated slightly downwards, superficializing the brachial plexus, admittedly, but also the first rib and therefore the pleural dome. Nor can ultrasonography, according to Brian D. Sites, be very much use in such cases because the reverberation caused by the first rib creates an acoustic shadow, which makes it impossible to establish the distance between the needle tip and the pleural dome.

In these cases, when performing the middle interscalene block, it is good policy to insert the needle half a centimetre higher than usual, but always on the straight line running from the midpoint of the clavicle posterolaterally tangential to the **O** marking the pulse of the subclavian artery, or, in the absence of the latter, on the bisector of the angle described above. In this case, the distance from the midpoint of the clavicle will no longer be 1.5 cm, but rather 2 cm, and it will be advisable to adopt a needle path which is slightly cephalad.

6.15 Anatomical Study

A cadaver has no subclavian artery pulse.

We therefore decided to verify the reliability of the bony landmarks on a cadaver. First of all, we reconstructed the angle and its bisector on a skeleton (Fig. 6.18).

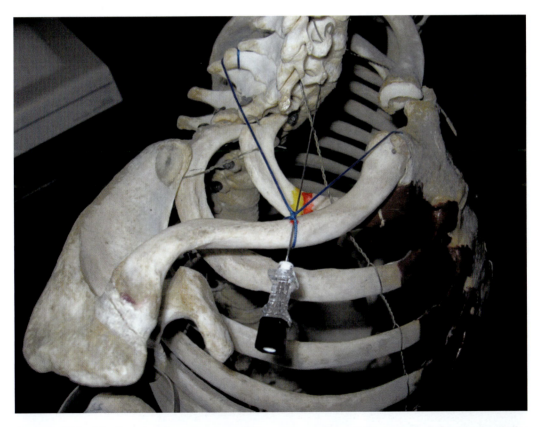

Fig. 6.18 With a Mersilene thread, we reconstructed the angle and its bisector on a skeleton. The bisector consisted in a 10-cm 22-G spinal needle, which reached the intervertebral conjugate foramen of *C7*. As can be seen, the needle passes above the yellow mark, on the upper surface of the first rib, indicating the shallow groove produced by the brachial plexus and just posterolateral to the red mark indicating the track of the subclavian artery

To this end, we knotted a blue Mersilene thread to the midpoint of the clavicle of a skeleton and then tied the two ends of the tautly strung thread, respectively, to the tip of the spinous process of C7 and to the sternoclavicular joint. The bisector consisted in a 10 cm-long 22-G spinal needle, which reached the intervertebral conjugate foramen of C7 (Fig. 6.18). As can be seen, the needle passes above the yellow mark, on the upper surface of the first rib, indicating the position of the brachial plexus, just posterolateral to the red mark indicating the track of the subclavian artery. We then drew the angle and its bisector on a cadaver (Fig. 6.19).

To better highlight the transverse plane of C7 during the anatomical dissection, we inserted a first 10 cm 22-G spinal needle following the straight line joining the midpoint of the clavicle to the spinous process of C7. A second needle was then introduced along the bisector of the angle (Fig. 6.20).

After introducing the two needles, it was the turn of the anatomical pathologist who removed the skin, the areolar subcutaneous tissue and the platysma in that order (Fig. 6.21). After removing the omohyoid muscle and the fascia enveloping the brachial plexus, it could be seen that the target had been reached: the needle inserted along the bisector of the angle had reached the brachial plexus (Fig. 6.22). In Fig. 6.23 the 2 needles have been removed and repositioned to indicate, respectively, the anterior and posterior limit of the insertions. We therefore were able to verify that as follows:

1. The line on the transverse plane of C7 joining the midpoint of the clavicle to the spinous process of C7 passes via the levator scapulae muscle.
2. This line, together with the middle half of the clavicle, forms an angle whose bisector passes through the brachial plexus. Thus, the

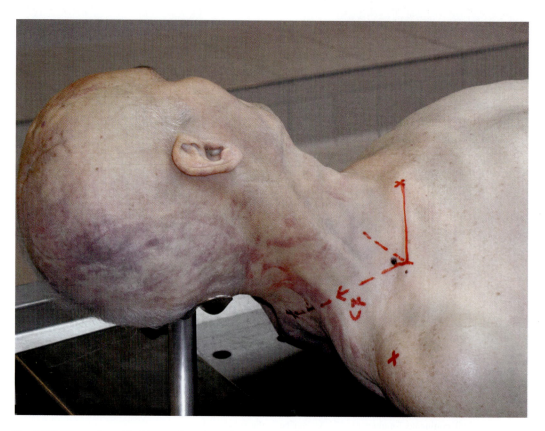

Fig. 6.19 The angle and its bisector have been drawn on a cadaver

6 Supraclavicular Brachial Plexus Block Techniques

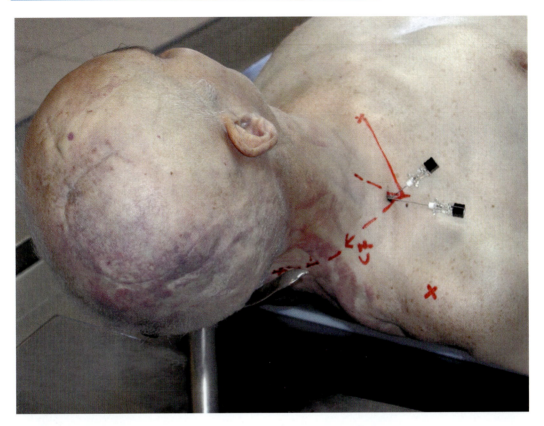

Fig. 6.20 To better highlight the transverse plane of C7 during the anatomical dissection, we inserted a first 10 cm 22-G spinal needle following the straight line that joins the midpoint of the clavicle to the spinous process of C7. A second needle was then introduced along the bisector of the angle

technique can also be performed in the absence of the subclavian artery pulse, which in cadavers, of course, is the rule.

To assess the safety of the manoeuvres of the technique in relation to the cervical spine, we measured the distance of the scalene triangle from the skin and, as regards the path we opted for, this distance was approximately 2.5–3 cm. We also measured the distance between the scalene triangle and the cervical spine at the level of the anterior scalene muscle, and the result was 3 cm (Fig. 6.24). Lombard and Cooper also measured the distance at the level of the middle scalene muscle, obtaining a value of 3.5 cm.

Doing the simple arithmetic, we find that the distance between the spinal column and the entry point of the needle ranges from 5.5 to 6.5 cm, which is a distance impossible to cover with a 3.5 or 4 cm needle.

6.16 Ultrasound-Guided Middle Interscalene Block

Another method, if the subclavian artery pulse is absent, is based on the use of ultrasonography. This method, which nowadays is very popular, can also be used when all the landmarks are present.

The procedure is as follows: after drawing on the skin the angle and its bisector (or, if the pulse is palpable, the straight line tangential to the pulse of the subclavian artery and passing from the midpoint of the clavicle), a linear probe is applied to the posterior edge of the medial half of the clavicle (Fig. 6.25) and is slid slowly in a lateral direction (Fig. 6.26a). At a certain point, the subclavian artery will appear on the screen as a pulsating "black hole" and just lateral to it we

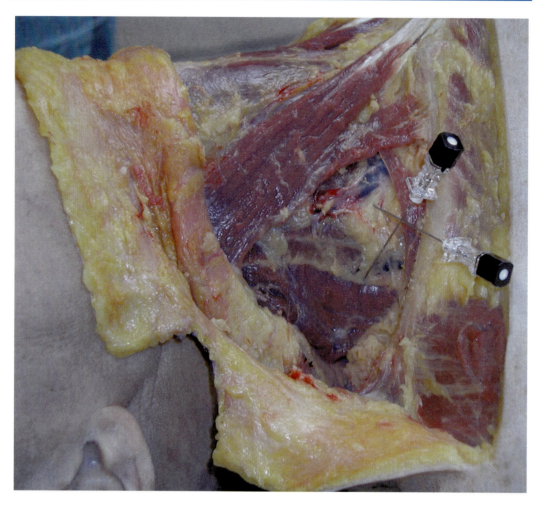

Fig. 6.21 The skin, the areolar subcutaneous tissue and the platysma have been removed. The omohyoid muscle in this case is fairly low down and partially hidden behind the clavicle

can see the "circular crowns" (hypoechogenic nerves surrounded by more echogenic epineurium) of the brachial plexus components severed transversely by the ultrasound beam (Fig. 6.26b).

Since the clavicle and the probe itself would tend to hamper the insertion of the needle along the characteristic path of this technique, the probe is rotated 45° (clockwise on the right and counterclockwise on the left), while keeping an eye all the time on the position of the artery on the screen (Fig. 6.26c).

The ultrasound image will remain substantially the same (Fig. 6.26d), but by rotating the probe, we are now able to see the bisector or straight line drawn on the skin and necessary for correctly directing the needle and having enough space to insert it "out of plane" (Fig. 6.26c).

To have an "in-plane" view of the needle, the probe must be applied along the bisector of the angle (Fig. 6.27a) or (when the subclavian artery pulse is present) along the straight line tangential to the **O**. In this way, the ultrasound image will change completely and the various elements of the brachial plexus, severed longitudinally by the probe, will appear on the screen in a very characteristic manner like a bundle of railway tracks between the anterior and middle scalene muscles. The siphon of the subclavian artery, cut longitudinally by the probe, will present an

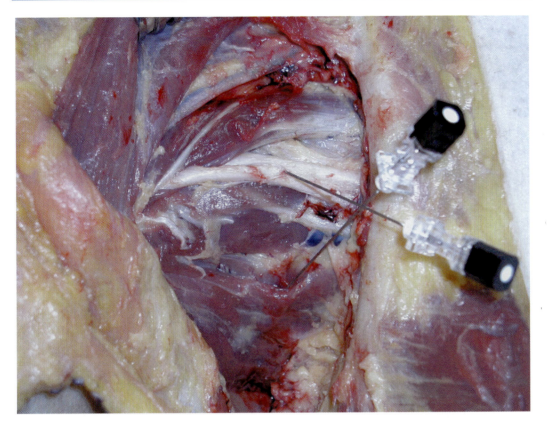

Fig. 6.22 After removing the omohyoid muscle and the fascia enveloping the brachial plexus, it can be seen that the target was reached: the needle inserted along the bisector of the angle has reached the brachial plexus. The large nerve that runs parallel to the brachial plexus is the suprascapular nerve, stimulation of which causes a false twitch; adhering to the anterior scalene muscle and clearly visible is the phrenic nerve, the stimulation of which causes visible twitching of the diaphragm

oblong, ovaloid appearance, like a hypoechogenic ellipse, surrounded by a wall whose echogenicity will be greater, the higher the degree of atherosclerosis (Fig. 6.27b).

In Fig. 6.28, we can see the application of the combined method—nerve stimulation plus ultrasound guidance. Figure 6.29 shows the "black hole" of the subclavian artery and close to it the components of the brachial plexus cut across transversely by the probe.

After eliciting the twitch required with a current intensity of 0.4 mA, we can see the typical spread of the anesthetic solution injected inside the neurovascular bundle which has the appearance of a hypoechogenic cloak wrapped around the artery and the brachial plexus (Fig. 6.30).

To conclude, then, we have to emphasize the importance of the following points when using this method:

- strictly maintain at all times the path prescribed by the technique, since this cannot fail to increase the safety of the ultrasound method as well. A casual insertion of the needle, that is, without following a safe, well tried and tested path, encouraged perhaps by the direct ultrasound view and lulled into a false sense of security, may lead to the reappearance of old complications which we thought we had put behind us;
- always use the electrical nerve stimulator as well simultaneously as Admir Hadzic says, "the two methods are complementary and not mutually exclusive".

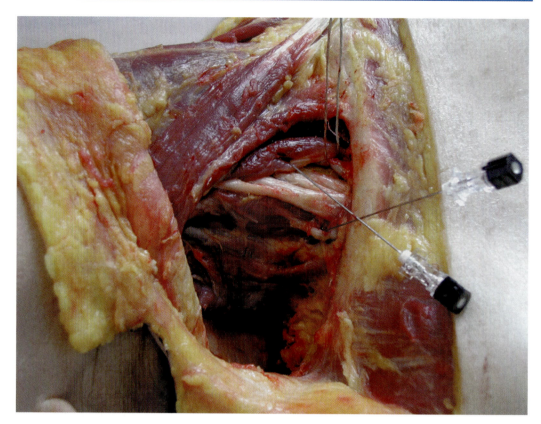

Fig. 6.23 The two needles have been removed and repositioned to indicate, respectively, the anterior and posterior limit of the insertions. The anterior limit is represented by the position of the needle at the level of the phrenic nerve (which crosses over the anterior scalene muscle obliquely lower down), while the posterior limit is represented by the suprascapular nerve, the stimulation of which causes false twitching of the supraspinatus muscle with raising of the shoulder. The subclavian artery has been isolated and raised with a thread

6.17 Continuous Middle Interscalene Block

More than 60 years have elapsed since Ansbro first described the possibility of executing a continuous brachial plexus block in 1946. He used a blunt-tipped needle inserted into the supraclavicular fossa as far as the first rib, according to Kulenkampff's classic technique. The needle was also inserted in a cork used as a rough and ready means of measuring depth acting as a brake to prevent further unwanted progression. The cork was attached to the skin with sticking plaster. The infusion of anesthetic (1 % lidocaine) was done with a syringe and a three-way faucet drawing the anesthetic solution directly from a tank. Five years later, Smirnov and Sarnoff described for the first time the use of a polyethylene catheter for performing a continuous peripheral block. It was probably a ureteral catheter whose metal mandrel was used for the first time for the electrical localization of a nerve.

6.17.1 Indications

The main indications for the insertion of an indwelling catheter for a brachial plexus block consist in the possibility of guaranteeing surgical anesthesia in operations that exceed the duration of action of ropivacaine or levobupivacaine

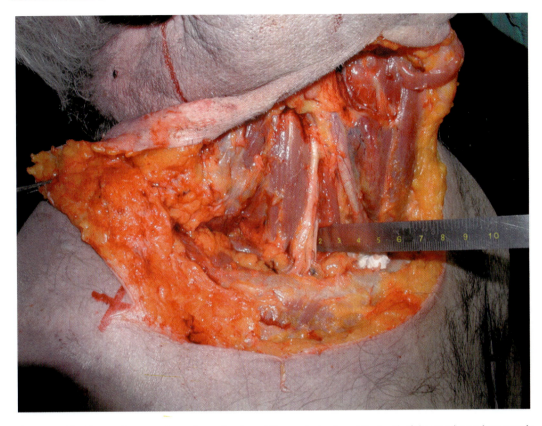

Fig. 6.24 The distance between the scalene triangle and the cervical spine at the level of the anterior scalene muscle has been measured: the value was 3 cm

(as in the reimplantation of limbs) and of guaranteeing good postoperative analgesia and an early initiation of physiokinetic therapy, as well as to ensure a continuous sympathetic block, superior in efficacy to the stellate ganglion block even when repeated. As we have already said, the sympathetic block affords the best prophylaxis for reflex sympathetic dystrophy (Sudeck's syndrome).

6.17.2 Patient Position

Seated upright, with the head rest raised (deck chair position) with the arm hanging limply outside the bed; in this way, with the shoulder relaxed, the clavicle is rotated slightly downwards and the brachial plexus becomes more superficial. The head is turned 45° to the opposite side. If the patient is unable to assume the seated position, the block can also be performed with the patient in the supine position.

6.17.3 Landmarks

1. Pulse of the subclavian artery.
2. Midpoint of the clavicle.
3. Spinous process of C7 indicating the transverse plane on which to operate.

6.17.4 Technique

The dermatographic pencil is used to mark the pulse of the subclavian artery with an **O**, the midpoint of the clavicle with a dot, and the spinous process of C7 with an **X**. Thorough

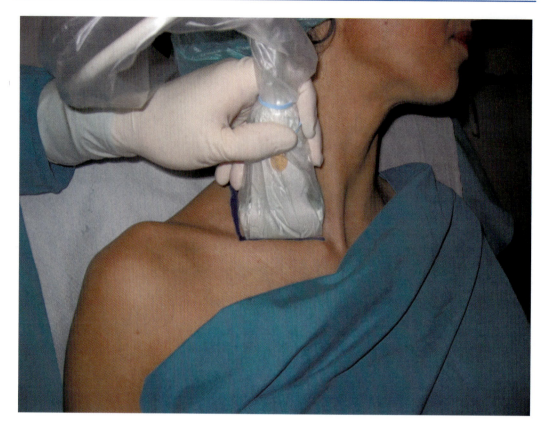

Fig. 6.25 A linear probe is applied to the posterior edge of the medial half of the clavicle

disinfection of the neck and the supraclavicular, pectoral and shoulder regions is mandatory. The operating field is delimited anteriorly by means of a sterile, self-adhesive drape, leaving the shoulder and arm visible, where the ground electrode is placed, in order to observe muscle twitches.

A skin wheal is induced with a 23-G needle laterally to the **O** marked on the skin, at 3 o'clock on the left and 9 o-clock on the right, injecting 1.5 ml of 1 % lidocaine. The syringe is detached, leaving the needle in situ. The 23-G needle is replaced by an 18-G needle, attempting to insert it in the same hole; in this way, via the enlarged breach produced in the dermis, the Teflon-coated needle will slide more easily and there will be no entrainment of cutaneous germs due to invagination of the skin in order to penetrate. The stimulating needle replacing the G-18 needle is inserted. The electrical nerve stimulator is set at a current intensity of 0.4 mA; the needle is directed towards C7 following the straight line connecting the midpoint of the clavicle to the entry point of the needle; when the twitch is obtained, the current intensity is progressively reduced to a value below 0.2 mA.

If the subclavian artery pulse is not present, we use three bony landmarks, namely:
1. the midpoint of the clavicle;
2. the spinous process of C7;
3. the sternoclavicular joint.

By connecting the first point to the other two, we obtain an angle whose bisector leads to the brachial plexus (see anatomical study). The skin wheal is induced on the bisector at a distance of 1.5 cm from the midpoint of the clavicle, whereupon one proceeds as described.

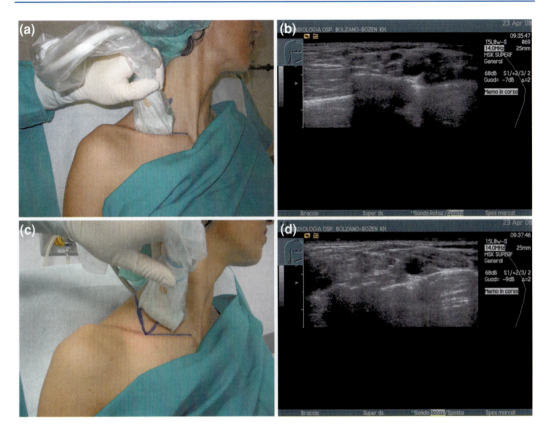

Fig. 6.26 a The probe is slid in a lateral direction. **b** Ultrasound view of the subclavian artery and brachial plexus with the probe adhering to the posterior edge of the clavicle. The cross section of the nerve elements is slightly ovaloid (like a slice of salami sausage) because the probe is not perpendicular to the plexus but slightly oblique. **c** The probe, rotated 45°, is now at 90° to the bisector of the angle (the long axis of the plexus). Its position now enables us to see the bisector of the angle and to introduce the stimulating needle "out of plane" according to a path already well tried and tested and therefore intrinsically safe. **d** As we have seen in Figure 6.25c, the probe is now at an angle of 90° to the plexus. The ultrasound image remains substantially unchanged, but the nerve elements transected at 90° have a more rounded appearance compared to the previous image (6.26b)

If no twitches are registered, minor adjustments are made withdrawing the needle to the level of the subcutaneous tissue and reinserting it in a slightly more posterior or a more anterior position. Generally speaking, it is not necessary to deviate more than 15 or 20° from the original line. If a movement of the scapula occurs, this means that the needle has been inserted too posteriorly and that we have stimulated the suprascapular nerve; if a diaphragmatic twitch occurs, it means that the position of the needle tip is too anterior, at the level of the anterior scalene muscle, where the phrenic nerve runs attached to the latter. After eliciting a twitch of the deltoid, biceps or triceps muscle, the current intensity is reduced progressively to a value below 0.2 mA; if the twitch disappears, the previous stimulation values are restored. After aspiration and a Raj test, the anesthetist then proceeds to inject 0.2 ml/kg of anesthetic, in order to pave the way for the catheter, with intermittent aspiration alternating with injections of 5 ml; the catheter must not be allowed to project more than 2 cm beyond the tip of the

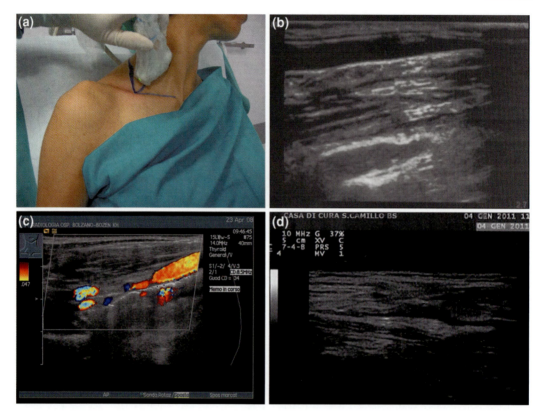

Fig. 6.27 *a* To perform an "in-plane" insertion of the needle in the plexus, the probe has been introduced along the bisector of the angle. *b* View of the brachial plexus cut longitudinally by the probe. The subclavian artery presents an oblong ovaloid appearance, like a hypoechogenic ellipse, surrounded by a wall whose echogenicity will be greater, the higher the degree of atherosclerosis. *c* The same longitudinal image of the plexus with the colour Doppler effect. *d* Longitudinal view of the brachial plexus after injection of the local anesthetic, which surrounds it like a sleeve

needle. The catheter is then fixed to the skin or tunnelled and another 0.2 ml/kg of anesthetic is injected, making 0.4 ml/kg in all. In the postoperative period, a continuous solution of 0.2 % ropivacaine or 0.125 % levobupivacaine is injected at the rate of 5–10 ml per hour, corresponding according to our calculations to 0.1 ml/kg/h.

The middle interscalene block lends itself particularly well to the placement of an indwelling catheter because the catheter is inserted into the neurovascular bundle along its main axis, because it enters the supraclavicular fossa at an extremely acute angle of incidence and therefore is not subject to untoward displacement, and because it is introduced close to the midpoint of the clavicle, which is not particularly responsive to movements of the body.

6.17.5 Complications

With the technique described above the most important complication is a block of the phrenic nerve, which is to be feared in the case of a patient suffering from respiratory insufficiency. As we have already mentioned, the frequency of involvement of the phrenic nerve in the single-shot middle interscalene block technique, in a study in which patients were monitored by means of X-ray investigations conducted in the immediate postoperative period in 97 patients, was 60 %.

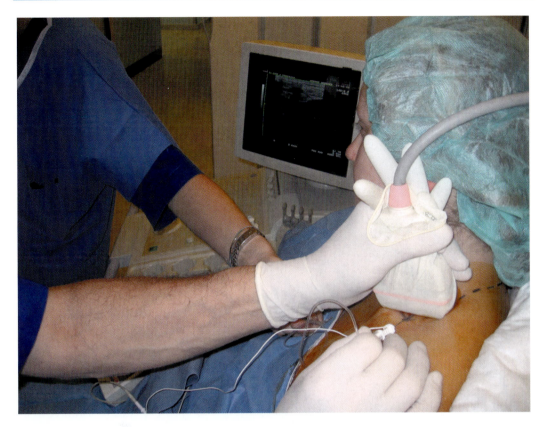

Fig. 6.28 Application of the combined method: ultrasound plus electrical nerve stimulation

At the end of the surgical operation, using fluoroscopy, the occurrence of a phrenic nerve block was verified in 80 patients. A substantial difference between the single-shot technique and the technique involving catheter placement was ascertained (Alemanno, unpublished observation). In the latter case, in fact, paresis of the diaphragm in 72 patients (90 %) as opposed to 60 % with the single-shot technique was observed.

We asked ourselves why there is this difference, and the only possible explanation we could come up with consisted in the fact that we had injected half the scheduled amount of anesthetic on appearance of the muscle twitch for the purposes of expanding the neurovascular space and paving the way for the catheter, and the other half after inserting the catheter. Our technique introduces the needle and therefore the catheter into the neurovascular bundle coaxially with the result that the tip of the catheter, projecting 2 cm beyond the tip of the needle is closer to the cervical column. In this way, the second half volume injected spreads more cephalad, involving the phrenic nerve and perhaps also it roots (Fig. 6.31a, b).

To verify the spread of the anesthetic along the paravertebral groove, we injected 30 ml of methylene blue into the cadaver using a needle introduced under direct vision beyond the cervical fascia in the central zone of the scalene triangle (Fig. 6.32a). The 30 ml of methylene blue did not rise beyond C6 (Fig. 6.32b). In a second case, using a normal 38 mm 20-G needle, placed in contact with the bone of the cervical column and then withdrawn 5 mm, we injected 40 ml into the upper part of the scalene triangle at the level of C6 and observed that the dye rose to the level of C4 (Fig. 6.33).

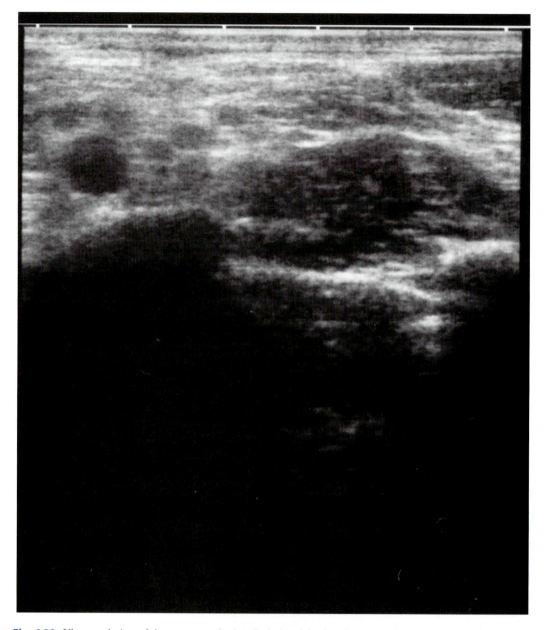

Fig. 6.29 Ultrasound view of the neurovascular bundle before injecting the anesthetic

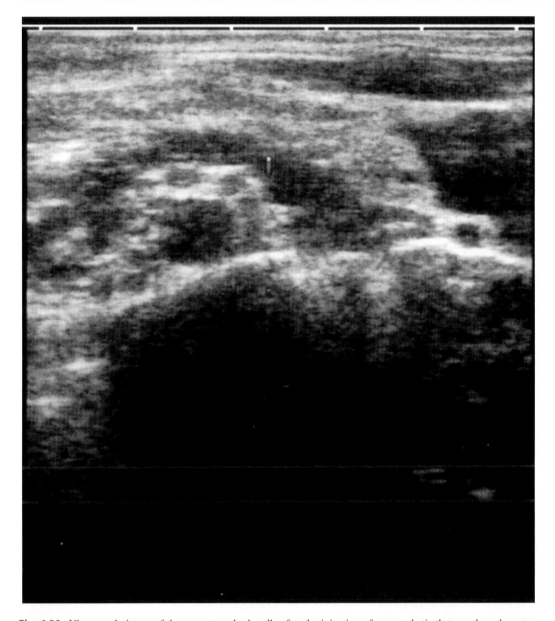

Fig. 6.30 Ultrasound picture of the neurovascular bundle after the injection of an anesthetic that envelops the artery and the brachial plexus like a cloak

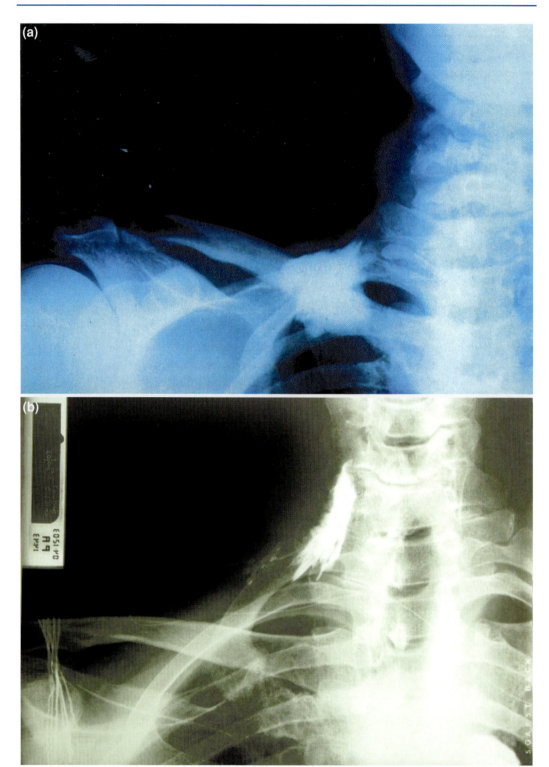

Fig. 6.31 a In this first case, 10 ml of iopamidol diluted with local anesthetic was injected, which spread in the neurovascular bundle in the paraclavicular area close to the middle third of the clavicle. **b** In this second case, after introducing the catheter 2 cm beyond the tip of the guide needle, 2 ml of iopamidol diluted with local anesthetic was injected. The spread of the contrast medium in the paracervical area is clearly visible

6 Supraclavicular Brachial Plexus Block Techniques

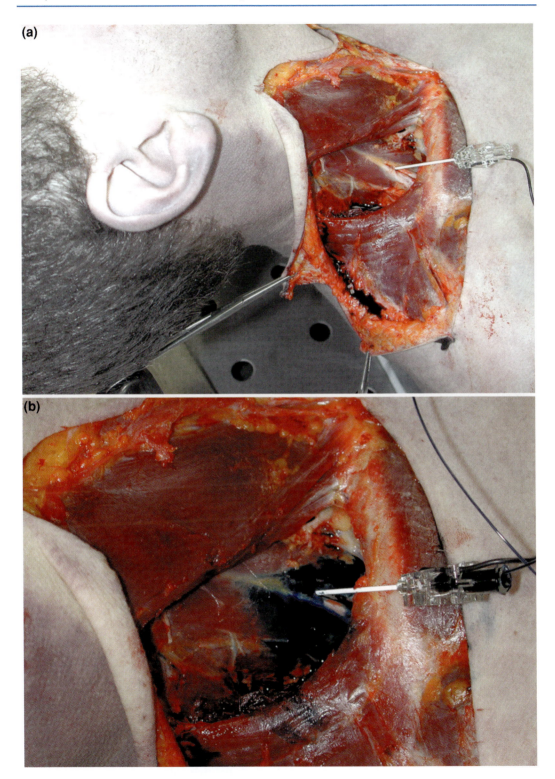

Fig. 6.32 **a** Introduction of a needle under direct vision into a cadaver, beyond the cervical fascia. **b** Injection of 30 ml of methylene blue. The spread did not rise beyond C6

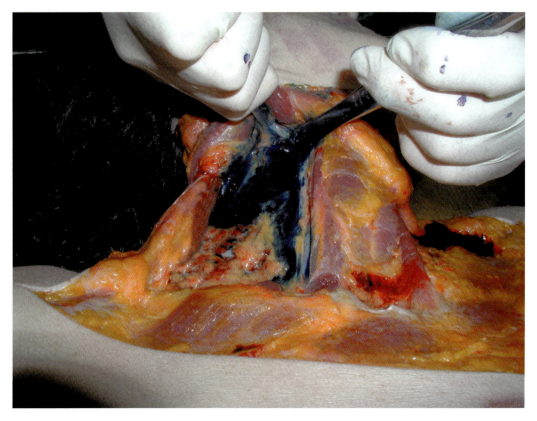

Fig. 6.33 Injection of 40 ml of methylene blue into the upper part of the scalene triangle, using a 38 mm-20 G needle, placed in contact with the bone of the cervical column and then withdrawn by 5 mm. The dye rose to the level of C4

Consequently, the phrenic nerve may be affected by the block because it crosses the neurovascular bundle at the level of the apex of the scalene triangle, especially if the injection is performed at this level, or, if the volume of anesthetic is substantial, the block may even extend to its roots.

In practice, with the catheter, the injection of a fair amount of anesthetic is effected 2 cm beyond the point at which the needle tip induces the muscle twitch, in a position therefore closer to the spine and with results similar to those reported by Urmey (100 %) using Winnie's interscalene block.

6.17.6 Tunnelling of the Catheter

If it is planned to leave the indwelling catheter in place in the neurovascular bundle for more than a few days, it is good policy to tunnel it in order to prevent it from being displaced. The tunnelling of the catheter must be done via a posterior path because an anterior path would be obstructed by the clavicle, while a lateral path would inevitably end up by invading the operating field in the case of shoulder surgery. What is recommended is that the tunnelling should take a subcutaneous path. In fact, the distance between the skin and the plexus is determined by the rectilinear course of the tunnelling needle. Once the catheter has been inserted, it is fixed to the skin, and therefore, the only mobile part is that close to the tip. As a result of the contraction of one or more muscles, the course of the needle is lengthened because what was initially a straight path becomes a sinusoidal or winding one. A transmuscular course thus tends to displace the tip of the catheter precisely on account of the muscular movements. These movements,

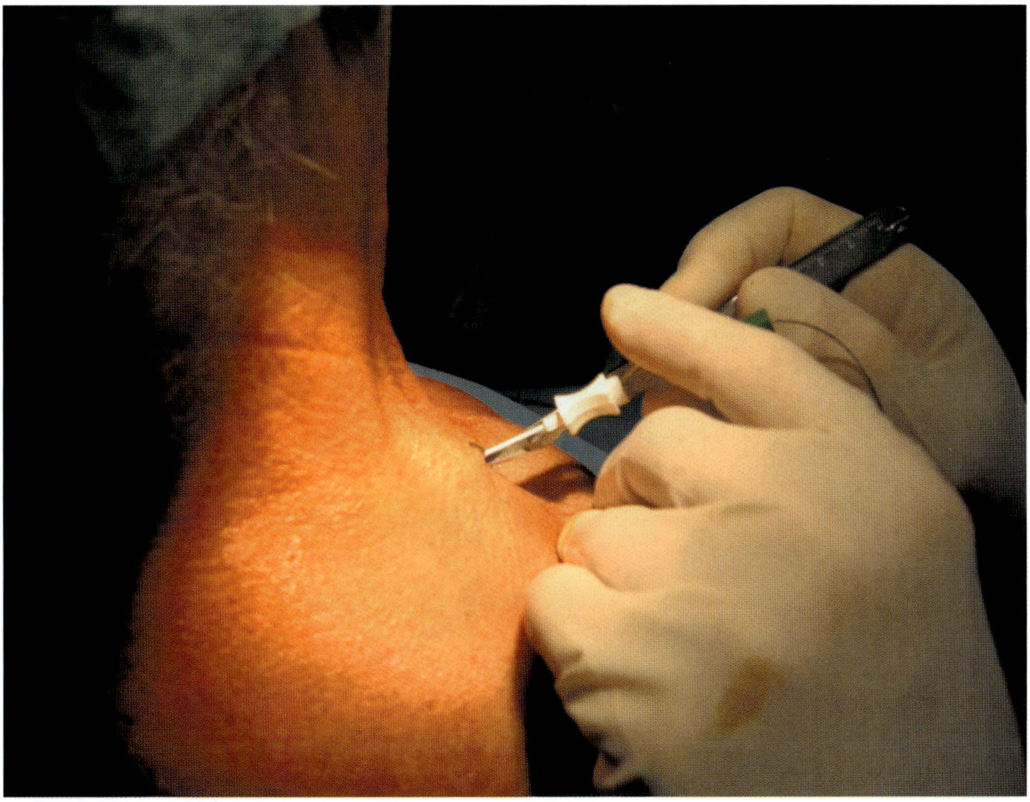

Fig. 6.34 Catheter tunneling. A triangular-bladed scalpel is used to make a small incision at the entry point of the stimulating needle. The stimulating needle was slightly raised

as we have said, tend to have an impact exclusively on the terminal part of the catheter which, if forced out of the neurovascular bundle, is obviously no longer capable of performing its function. This problem is minimized by our technique, where the catheter is inserted along the longitudinal axis of the brachial plexus and when going over from the direction of entry to the tunnel to a posterior direction, describes an angle of 90°; in any event, it is advisable to stick to the subcutaneous route so as not to expose the catheter to continual muscular stresses potentially capable of inducing its tip to deviate.

6.17.7 Tunnelling Technique

After inserting the catheter in the stimulating needle, making sure that it protrudes no more than 2 cm from the needle tip, the guide needle is left in situ in order to protect the catheter from possible damage as a result of the insertion manoeuvres of the tunnelling needle.

The technique uses a Tuohy 18-G needle or a spinal needle of the same calibre. We also use a G-22 spinal needle to perform the local anesthesia along the predetermined path. The local anesthetic we normally opt for is mepivacaine plus epinephrine. The procedure is as follows:

1. A subcutaneous skin wheal is induced at the stimulating needle entry point as reinforcement of the one already performed: 1 ml of mepivacaine plus epinephrine is injected at the apex of the acute angle that the skin forms with the needle;
2. using a triangular-bladed scalpel, a small incision is made at the entry point of the stimulating needle (Fig. 6.34). This small incision will facilitate the exit of the tunnelling needle and will make for a greater depth

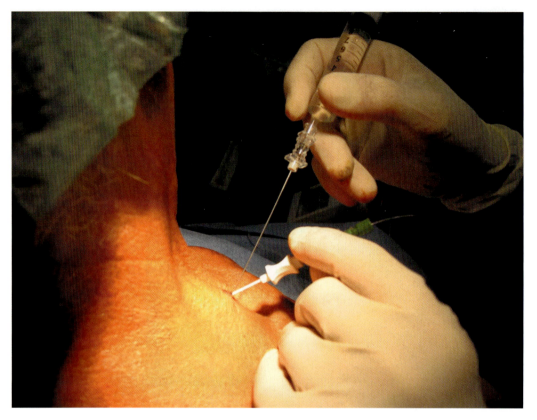

Fig. 6.35 Catheter tunnelling. Insertion of the 22-G spinal needle to a depth of 5 mm into the needle incision made by the scalpel

of the catheter at the point where it passes from the tunnel leading into the brachial plexus to the subcutaneous tunnel. To this end, the blade of the scalpel is pressed 5–6 mm deeper with the cutting edge turned towards the stimulating needle and making sure that the cutaneous and subcutaneous fringes between the cutting edge of the blade and the needle present a clean cut, otherwise the flexion angle of the catheter will become too superficial, preventing good healing of the small wound;

3. a 22-G spinal needle, already connected to the local anesthetic syringe, is inserted into the incision perpendicularly to the skin to a depth of 5 mm (Fig. 6.35) and then, after rotating it through 90°, it is pressed in a posterior direction, continuing to inject small boluses of anesthetic, while remaining at the subcutaneous level throughout, until it finally emerges from the skin at the level of the upper border of the trapezius muscle (Fig. 6.36);
4. at this point, the syringe is disconnected but the needle is left in situ;
5. a second small incision is made with the tip of the scalpel at the exit point of the 22-G needle to facilitate entry of the 18-G needle.

If the tunnelling needle is a Tuohy needle, we point it against the tip of the G-22 needle, exerting slight opposing pressure on the two needle cones in order to hold them point to point (Fig. 6.37) and pressing a little harder on the cone of the Tuohy needle. The tip of the latter will emerge from the skin exactly at the point where the other had entered, that is, at a depth of 5 mm. Its tip will be made to protrude from the small wound made by the scalpel in such a way as to cross over at least 3 mm beyond the stimulating needle which has been left in situ;

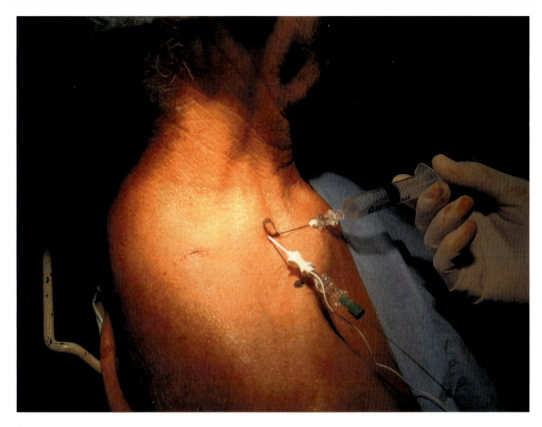

Fig. 6.36 Catheter tunnelling. Exit of the 22-G spinal needle at the level of the upper border of the trapezius muscle

the purpose of this is to avoid damage to the catheter by the tunnelling needle if the stimulating needle had been removed (Fig. 6.38).

If, instead of a Tuohy needle, we use an 18-G spinal needle as the tunnelling needle, the whole operation will be even easier: it will be inserted counter to the 22-G needle (which acts as a mandrel) as far as its cone and, after penetrating at least 3 mm beyond the stimulating needle, the G-22 needle will be withdrawn (Fig. 6.39).

6. That done, only now can the stimulating needle implanted in the neurovascular bundle be withdrawn; the free end of the catheter is then inserted in the bevel of the tunnelling needle (Fig. 6.40) and pushed delicately towards the cone until it protrudes just 1 cm (Fig. 6.41). At this point, taking hold of both the tip of the catheter and the cone of the needle, they are extracted together from the tunnel. Particular care must be taken to ensure that the catheter does not twist at the point of transition from one tunnel to the other. If this happens, it needs to be untwisted. The catheter is then settled into the angle of transition between the two tunnels by delicately pulling its end.

7. On exiting from the tunnel, the catheter is again fixed with a few strips of sterile sticking plaster or with any other form of adhesive bandage; the area is medicated with a single-layer sterile gauze dressing. As regards the small wound made by the scalpel, that will resolve rapidly, especially if the direction change angle of the catheter is 4–5 mm deep.

6.18 General Considerations Regarding Supraclavicular Techniques

We may consider the brachial plexus, with all its elements—roots, trunks, divisions and cords—as an anatomical complex which is enclosed by the

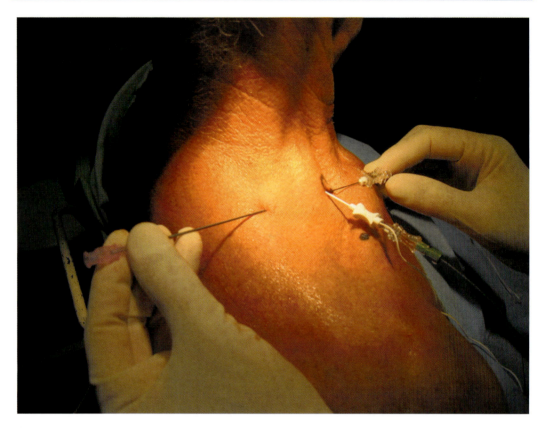

Fig. 6.37 Catheter tunnelling. Counter-insertion of the 18-G needle in the 22-G needle

investing layer of the deep cervical fascia fused with the vertebral extension of the superficial cervical fascia and develops in two directions:
- one vertical, paracervical segment that aligns all the points of origin of the roots (i.e. the anterior divisions of the spinal nerves) and extends laterally as far as the scalene triangle;
- another segment that changes direction at the level of the scalene triangle and appears to be largely horizontal, although, in actual fact, it is slightly inclined inferolaterally.

In short, these two segments constitute the longitudinal axes of the brachial plexus.

As we have seen in the anatomical description, the spatial configuration of the brachial plexus can be compared to that of a right-angled triangle (the classic set square) the height of which corresponds to the line joining the five conjugate foramina, from which its roots emerge, and the base of which rests on the first rib. At the supraclavicular level, then, it presents two longitudinal approach axes, one along the height of the triangle (i.e. interscalene technique) and the other parallel to the base, corresponding to the line passing at the level of the midpoint of the clavicle and directed towards the cervical column (i.e. middle interscalene block). As regards the antero-posterior thickness of the triangle, sandwiched between the anterior and middle scalene muscles, it ranges from a virtual thickness at the level of the apex of the scalene triangle to a thickness of 1–2 cm at the level of the first rib.

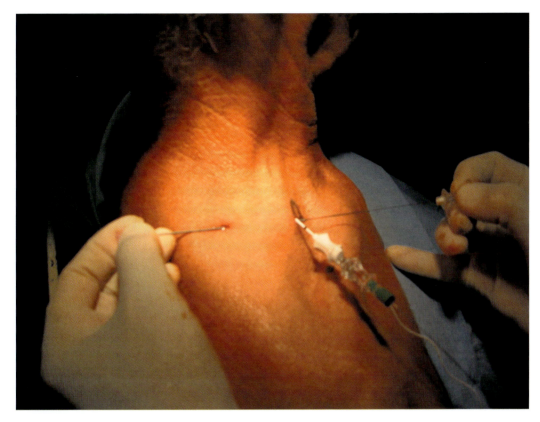

Fig. 6.38 Catheter tunnelling. The tip of the 18-G needle has penetrated beyond the stimulating needle and the 22-G needle is withdrawn

Winnie subdivides the supraclavicular brachial plexus block techniques into two groups, the parascalene techniques that reach the neurovascular bundle along its transverse axis, and the interscalene techniques that approach the plexus via the longitudinal axes.

One of these longitudinal axes, as we have said, is parallel to the height of the triangle corresponding to the line joining the intervertebral conjugate foramina from C5 to T1, while the other is parallel to its base which passes at the level of the midpoint of the clavicle.

The interscalene techniques include Winnie's two techniques (the subclavian perivascular technique and the interscalene technique) and Alemanno's middle interscalene block.

The parascalene techniques, on the other hand, include the antero-posterior techniques, for example, the Brown technique (plumb-bob method), the Dalens technique in children and the posterior-anterior techniques, that is, Kappis, Santoni and Pippa posterior approaches.

If there is a theoretical objection that can be brought against Alemanno's technique (MIB), it is that the needle is directed towards the intervertebral conjugate foramen of C7. In fact, if the needle fails to reach the upper primary trunk, it will probably stimulate the middle primary trunk from which basically the radial nerve originates with consequent twitching of the triceps muscle. If the path of the needle is prolonged further (another 3 cm), the tip of a fairly long needle

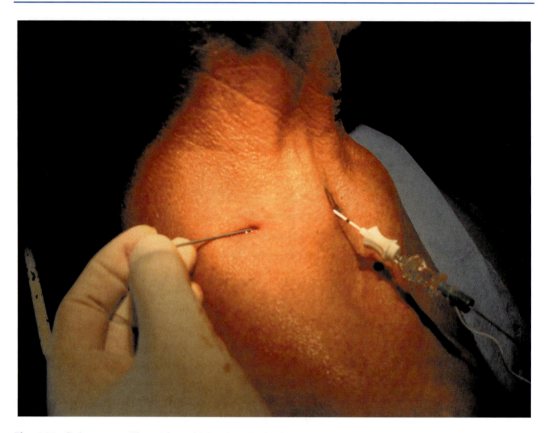

Fig. 6.39 Catheter tunnelling. After withdrawing the 22-G needle, the bevel of the 18-G needle projects a few millimetres beyond the stimulating needle. Only now can the latter be withdrawn

(>5 cm) might reach the conjugate foramen or come close to it. This is why it is important to use a 35–40 mm needle (less than 50 mm) which, in its path, starting from a point close to the midpoint of the clavicle (at a distance of 1–1.5 cm from the latter) at most is capable of reaching the centre of the scalene triangle. Therefore, when inserting an indwelling catheter into the neurovascular bundle, using the middle interscalene block, it is equally important not to let it advance more than 1–2 cm beyond the tip of the needle cannula. It is true that the end of the catheter is not the tip of a needle and consists of relatively soft material, but if the catheter is advanced excessively and comes into contact with, or inserts itself in the conjugate foramen, a peridural injection may occur.

6.19 Conclusions

A century has elapsed since Kulenkampff published the article describing his ground-breaking technique in 1911 and even today we are still debating as to which of the more than twenty techniques proposed over the years may be the most suitable. As regards the positive results they yield, these techniques are more or less

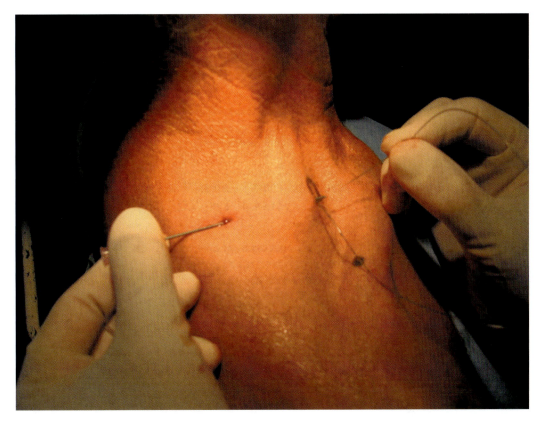

Fig. 6.40 Catheter tunneling. Insertion of the end of the catheter into the bevel of the tunneling needle

equivalent, but what makes the difference in their respective evolutions is the continuous attempt by the various authors to reduce the complications by proposing various different approach routes. It is true to say that, for practical purposes, the best technique is the one the anesthetist is most familiar with and best able to perform, and that it is difficult to change old habits, but this should not prevent us from trying out the latest proposals with all due caution.

In any event, we go along with the opinion that it is more appropriate to employ supraclavicular techniques for surgery of the shoulder and upper arm, while more peripheral techniques are advisable for forearm and hand surgery.

We do not re-read our old text books often enough:

> "The supraclavicular compartment is shielded on the outside by a thin layer of soft tissue parts comprising the middle cervical aponeurosis along with the omohyoid muscle, the superficial cervical aponeurosis, the subcutaneous connective tissue and the skin.
>
> These various planes are successively and methodically crossed by the surgeon in order to gain access to the compartment and its contents. To this end one can follow either the posterior

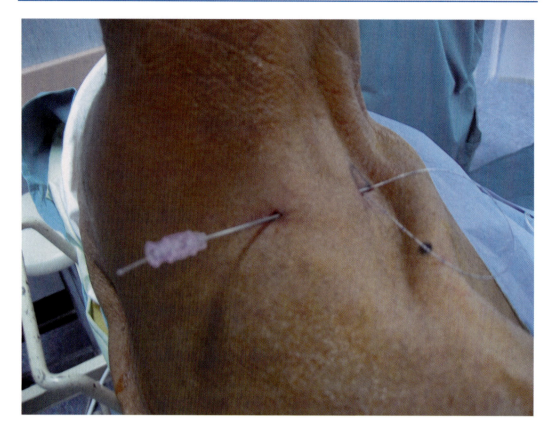

Fig. 6.41 Catheter tunnelling. The end of the catheter now projects from the cone of the tunnelling needle; and that's it

border of the sternocleidomastoid muscle or the superior edge of the clavicle, or both together, or even a line joining the midpoint of the sternocleidomastoid muscle and the midpoint of the clavicle. Of these various routes, the first two lead more often than not to the vessels and the last one to the brachial plexus".

Theodore Tuffier 1897

Bibliography

Alemanno F, Accinelli G, Pfaender M (1985) Una semplice metodica di tunnelizzazione e fissaggio del catetere peridurale. Acta Anaesth Italica 36:143–146

Alemanno F, Bertini L, Casati A, Di Benedetto P (2001) Plesso brachiale. In: Fanelli G, Casati A, Chelly JE, Bertini L (eds) Blocchi periferici continui. Milano, Mosby Italia, pp 47–58

Alemanno F, Capozzoli G, Egarter-Vigl E, Gottin L, Bartoloni A (2006) The middle interscalene block: cadaver study and clinical assessment. Reg Anesth Pain Med 31(6):563–568

Alemanno F, Capozzoli G, Egarter-Vigl E (2004) A new approach to the supraclavicular block. Reg Anesth Pain Med 29(1):72–73

Alemanno F, Graziano G, Maccabruni F, Pinali R (2000) Brachial plexus block for shoulder surgery: our experience with Alemanno's technique. ALR 9(3):122–126

Alemanno F, Gretter R, Di Leo Y, Bellini L (2003) Alemanno's brachial plexus block ten years later: topographic study of anesthetized areas. Minerva Anest 69(6):575–581

Alemanno F (2000) Brachial plexus block. International Symposium on Regional Anesthesia & Pain Medicine. Quebec, Canada, May 31–June 3 2000, SYLLABUS, page 20

Alemanno F (1992) Un nuovo approccio al plesso brachiale. Minerva Anestesiol 58:403–406

Ansbro FP (1946) A method of continuous brachial plexus block. Am J Surg 71:716–722

Barutel C, Vidal F, Raich M, Montero A (1980) A neurological complication following brachial plexus block. Anesthesia 35:365–367

Bellucci G (1982) Storia della anestesiologia. Piccin Editore, Padova

Benumof JL (2000) Permanent loss of cervical spinal cord function associated with interscalene block performed under general anesthesia. Anesthesiology 93:1541–1544

Boezaart AP, Koorn R, Rosenquist RW (2003) Paravertebral approach to the brachial plexus: an anatomic improvement in technique. Reg Anesth Pain Med 28:241–244

Bonica JJ (1959) Il dolore. Francesco Vallardi Editore, Milano

Borgeat A, Blumenthal S (2007) Unintended destination of local anesthetics. In: Neal JM, Rathmell JP (eds) Complications in regional anesthesia & pain medicine. Saunders Elsevier, Philadelphia

Brandt L (1997) Illustrierte Geschichte der Anästhesie. Wissenschaftliche Verlagsgesellschaft mbh, Stuttgart

Brown DL, Cahill DR, Bridenbaugh LD (1993) Supraclavicular nerve block: anatomic analysis of a method to prevent pneumothorax. Anesth Analg 76:530–534

Brown DL (1995) Atlante di anestesia regionale. Antonio Delfino Editore, Roma

Chelly JE, Casati A, Fanelli G (2001) Continuous perpheral nerve block techniques. Mosby International Limited

Dalens B, Vanneuville G, Tanguy A (1987) A new parascalene approach to the brachial plexus in children: comparison with supraclavicular approach. Anesth Analg 66:1264–1271

Dalens B (1995) Anestesia loco-regionale dalla nascita all'età adulta. Fogliazza Editore, Milano

Finco G, Alemanno F et al (1999) Ropivacaina 1 % vs Bupivacaina 0, 5 % nel blocco del plesso brachiale secondo Alemanno nella chirurgia dell'arto superiore. Minerva Anestesiol 65(Suppl. 2):53

Finco G, Capozzoli G et al (2000) Ropivacaina 1 % vs Ropivacaina 0, 75 % nel blocco del plesso brachiale secondo Alemanno nella chirurgia della spalla. ALR 3:122–126

Finucane BT (1998) Brachial plexus anaesthesia: a review. The International Monitor. Medicom International. IMRAPT 10(4):3–8

Finucane BT (1999) Complications of Brachial Plexus Anesthesia. In: Brendan T (ed) Finucane: complications of regional anesthesia. Churchill Livingstone, New York

Gauthier-Lafaye P (1986) Manuale di anestesia locoregionale. Masson Italia, Milano

Hadzic A (2007) Nerve stimulation should be used in conjunction with ultrasound-guided nerve blocks. ASRA NEWS, pp 7–9

Harrop-Griffiths AW, Denny MB (2006) Eponymicity and the age of ultrasound: how should new blocks be introduced into clinical practice? Reg Anesth Pain Med 31(6):492–495

Kappis M (1912) Über Leitungsanästhesie an Bauch, Brust, Arm und Hals durch Injektion ins Foramen Intervertebrale. München Med Wochenschr 59:794–796

Kulenkampff D (1911) Die Anästhesierung des Plexus brachialis. Zentralblatt für Chirurgie, Sonnabend den 7 Oktober 1911; 40: 1337–1340

Labat G (1922) Regional Anesthesia. Saunders & Co., Philadelphia

Labat G (1927) Brachial plexus block: details of technique. Anesth Analg 6:81–82

Labat G (1927) Brachial plexus block. Br J Anaesth 4:174–176

Livingston EM, Wertheim H (1927) Brachial plexus block: its clinical application. Anesth Analg 6:149–154

Lombard TP, Couper JL (1983) Bilateral spread of analgesia following interscalene brachial plexus block. Anesthesiology 58:472–473

Meier G, Bauereis C, Maurer H, Meier T (2001) Interscalenäre Plexusblockade. Anatomische Voraussetzungen-anästhesiologishe und operative Aspekte. Der Anaesthesist 50(5): 333–341 © Springer-Verlag 2001

Moore DC (1969) Anestesia regionale. Piccin Editore, Padova

Moorthy SS, Schmidt SI, Dierdorf SF, Rosenfeld SH, Anagnostou JM (1991) A supraclavicular lateral paravascular approach for brachial plexus regional anesthesia. Anesth Analg 72:241–244

Murano L, Accinelli G, Alemanno F (2002) Supraclavear technique of Alemanno with a nerve stimulator. ALR 11:125–129

Neal JM, Moore JM, Kopacz DJ, Liu SS, Kramer DJ, Plorde JJ (1998) Quantitative analysis of respiratory, motor and sensory function after supraclavicular block. Anesth Analg 86:1239–1244

Niesel HC, Panhans C, Zenz M (1981) Regionalanaesthesie. Gustav Fisher Verlag, Stuttgart

Partridge BL, Katz J, Benirschke K (1987) Functional anatomy of the brachial plexus sheath: implications for anesthesia. Anesthesiology 66:743–747

Pippa P, Busoni P (2010) Anestesia locoregionale. Verduci Editore, Roma

Pippa P, Cominelli E, Marinelli C, Aito S (1990) Brachial plexus block using the posterior approach. Eur J Anaesth 7:411–420

Scott DB (1996) Tecniche di anestesia regionale. Verduci Editore, Roma

Silverstein WB, Saiyed MU, Brown AR (2000) Interscalene block with a nerve stimulator: a deltoid motor response is a satisfactory endpoint for successful block. Reg Anesth Pain Med 25:356–359

Sites BD, Brull R, Chan VW, Spence BC et al (2007) Artifacts and pitfall errors associated with U.S. guided regional anesthesia. Part II: a pictorial approach to understanding and avoidance. Reg Anesth Pain Med 32(5):419–433

Sites BD, Brull R, Chan VW, Spence BC, Gallagher J, Beach ML, Sites VR, Abbas S, Hartman GS (2010) Artifacts and pitfall errors associated with ultrasound-guided regional anesthesia: part II: a pictorial approach to understanding and avoidance. Reg Anesth Pain Med 35(2)Suppl 1:S81–S92

Stiller B (1907) Die asthenische Konstitutionskrankheit. Enke, Stuttgart

Smirnov SJ, Sarnoff LC (1951) Prolonged peripheral nerve block by means of indwelling plastic catheter. Treatment of hiccup. (Note on the electrical localization of peripheral nerve). Anesthesiology 12:270–275

Testut L, Jacob O (1977) Trattato di anatomia topografica. UTET, Torino

Testut L (1943) Anatomia umana. Libro Ottavo. UTET, Torino

Thompson GE, Rorie DK (1983) Functional anatomy of the brachial plexus sheaths. Anesthesiology 59:117–122

Tuffier T (1977) Vie d'accesso alla loggia sopraclavicolare. In: Testut L, Jacob O: Trattato di anatomia topografica, vol II. UTET, Torino, pp 159

Urmey W, Talts KH, Sharrock NE (1991) One hundred percent incidence of hemidiaphragmatic paresis associated with interscalene brachial plexus anesthesia as diagnosed by ultrasonography. Anesth Analg 72(4):498–503

Vongvises P, Panijayanond T (1979) A parascalene technique of brachial plexus anesthesia. Anesth Analg 58(4):267–273

Winnie AP, Collins VJ (1964) The subclavian perivascular technique of brachial plexus anestesia. Anesthesiology 25:353–363

Winnie AP, Franco CD (2000) L'approccio sopraclavicolare al plesso brachiale. In: Urmey W (ed) Tecniche di anestesia loco-regionale e di terapia antalgica, nuovi concetti e tecniche del blocco del plesso brachiale, a cura di Brendan T. Finucane: pp 5–18. Traduzione italiana di Paolo Busoni. Promo Leader Service, Firenze

Winnie AP (1984) Anestesia plessica. Tecniche perivascolari di blocco del plesso brachiale. Verduci Editore, Roma

Winnie AP (1970) Interscalene brachial plexus block. Anesth Analg 49:455–466

Ultrasound-Guided Interscalene and Supraclavicular Blocks

Astrid U. Behr

The ultrasound-guided nerve block technique has been in use now for about 15 years, and its diffusion is steadily growing with optimal clinical results. The main advantage in comparison with the other techniques consists in the direct visualization of the local anesthetic spreading around the nervous structures to be blocked. The ultrasound guidance also allows us to follow in real time what happens under the skin layer, with a close control on the needle approaching its target, thus reducing the risk of damage to any sensitive anatomical structures, such as blood vessels or the pleura.

The desirable clinical consequences are as follows: a reduction in the number of necessary attempts, a faster performance, a reduced risk of iatrogenic damage due to vascular and/or nerve puncture and a shorter block onset time. All the former lead to higher block quality and greater comfort for the patient, which allow to consider a reduction in the volume of required local anesthetic.

Numerous clinical studies have been conducted in order to evaluate the superiority of one technique over the others. In the editorial introducing Casati's important clinical paper on the axillary block, which compared the multiple nerve stimulation technique with the ultrasound-guided technique, Borgeat and Capdevila commented that it is extremely difficult to find statistical differences between the two techniques in terms of qualitiy of regional anesthesia, onset time, incidence of complications and patient comfort, considering that these clinical studies are often based on the work of anesthesiologists well experienced in nerve blocks. The number of patients needed to make these minor differences statistically significant should be so high as to make them a largely non-feasible proposition. The authors conclude that a combination of the two techniques may help us to better understand the scientific basis of regional anesthesia.

In 2010, the Cochrane group published a review article, where the ultrasound-guided technique and the traditional one were compared, analyzing 18 studies with a total of 1,344 patients, to the conclusion that, when performed by experts, the success rates of the two approaches are similar.

Individual studies have demonstrated that the ultrasound-guided technique is associated with a reduced complication rate, an improved quality of the block, a faster execution time and a reduced onset time.

There are also numerous case reports showing that ultrasound guidance reduces the complication rate, but cannot completely eliminate complications, inasmuch as it is an operator-dependent technique with given limitations. Hadzic comments on the publication of a series of case reports describing complications under

A. U. Behr (✉)
Department of Medicine DiMed Anaesthesiology and Intensive Care Unit, University of Padua, Padua, Italy
e-mail: astridursula.behr@gmail.com

ultrasound guidance pointing out that the US-guided technique is undoubtedly one of the most important developments in the field of regional anesthesia, but that it would be a mistake to consider it such a safe technique that it should replace all the previous strategies. The most suitable approach for improving the safety of our patients would be to employ ultrasound guidance as an important supplementary procedure in the context of the already existing and future protocols for raising standards in the execution and monitoring of regional anesthesia. It should not be forgotten, however, that there are clinical or patient situations in which nerve stimulation would be impossible: ultrasound guidance in such situations proves indispensable as in the case of amputated patients or patients with neurological or neuromuscular diseases.

7.1 Exploration of the Anatomical Site

As first step in the execution of an ultrasound-guided block, it is advisable to explore the anatomical site in order to visualize and recognize the structures in the 'target area'. The brachial plexus is explored in the supraclavicular sites, from the interscalene area -at the level of the cricoid cartilage (C6)- to the base of the neck, using a linear ultrasound probe at a medium-high frequency (6–15MHz).

The patient should be supine and/or semi-seated, with the head turned 45° contralaterally. The position of the arms is indifferent. In these patients, above all, an attempt must be made to avoid any contractions or tension of the sternocleidomastoid muscle in order to allow good adhesion of the probe to the skin. To improve the adhesion between probe and skin, it is advisable to apply an abundant amount of gel.

The operator should then disinfect the skin, covering the probe with a sterile cover or tegaderm and applying sterile gel on the skin.

The operator must place himself in an ergonomic position allowing a direct visualization. A seated position should be considered.

The dominance of the operator's right or left hand conditions the position of the anesthetist in relation to the patient. The operator can place himself behind the patient's head or in front of the patient. As a rule, the probe is held in the non-dominant hand in order to use the dominant hand to handle the needle.

7.2 Ultrasound Anatomy of the Supraclavicular Region

A sound knowledge of topographical and functional anatomy is necessary to recognize the structures under ultrasound guidance. Since we can only recognize what we know, a good knowledge of both topographical anatomy and basic elements of sonoanatomy is advisable.

Generally speaking, the nerves are visualized in cross-section (short axis). The nerve presents itself ultrasonographically exactly as it is described histologically. The pure nerve tissue appears hypoechoic and/or anechoic, whereas the connective structures surrounding the nerve (epineurium, perineurium, etc.) appear as hyperechoic images. The composition of the nerve changes according to its anatomical site, and, therefore, the nerve changes its ultrasonographic appearance according to its connective component. In a central site, a mono- or oligofasciculated nerve can be seen, with a prevalent component of pure nerve tissue and a very modest connective component, often with only a hyperechoic connective outline, a pattern often called "dark bubbles" (Fig. 7.1).

While moving towards the peripheral sites, far from the neuraxis, the nerve changes its structure and assumes a honeycomb appearance, typical of the peripheral nerve (Fig. 7.2). The hypoechoic nerve fascicles are surrounded and interposed by hyperechoic connective structures, which present precisely the histological appearance of the peripheral nerve. The nerve can be seen in longitudinal section (long axis), rotating the probe through 90°, in its filamentous appearance with multiple parallel hyperechoic bands and interposed hypoechoic fascicles (Fig. 7.3).

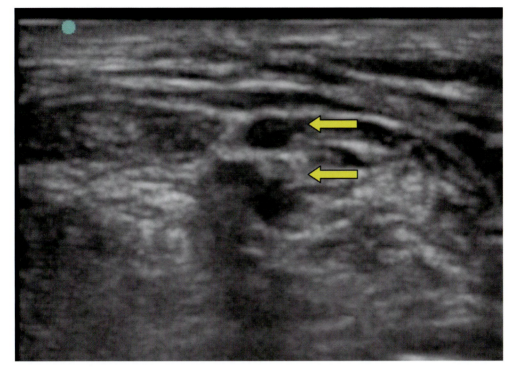

Fig. 7.1 Central nerve (nerve root and/or trunk) in short axis

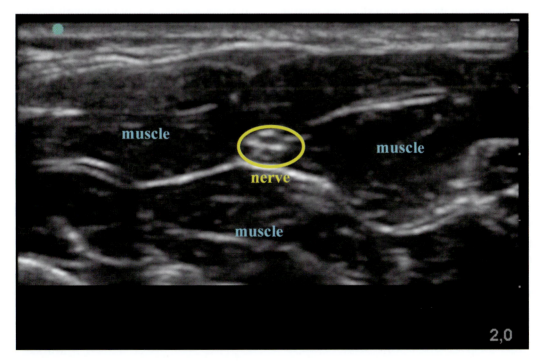

Fig. 7.2 Median nerve; example of polyfasciculated peripheral nerve presenting a honeycomb appearance, surrounded by the flexor muscles of the hand and fingers

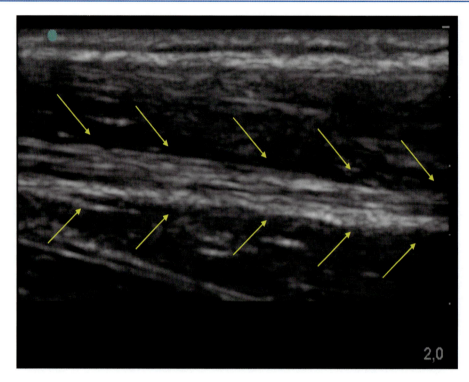

Fig. 7.3 *Yellow arrows* indicate the median nerve in long axis (longitudinal projection)

The brachial plexus is formed by the anterior divisions of the spinal nerves from C5 to T1 and crosses the interscalene groove between the anterior and middle scalene muscles. The nerve roots descend at various angles and join to form the trunks at various distances from the intervertebral foramina.

The angle between the spinal axis and the nerve roots decreases while moving downwards, and, therefore, an optimal image of each nerve root can only be obtained varying the angulation of the probe (tilting continuously), in an attempt to capture the roots and the trunks with a perpendicular angulation. In this way, it proves practically impossible to capture all the nerve roots in a single image with a single angulation of the probe. The typical appearance of the three bubbles in a row is obtainable only when trunks run parallel as happens more easily in distal part of the neck, just before reaching the supraclavicular site.

It is not always easy to distinguish between roots and trunks, and this depends above all on the position of the probe in relation to the course of the nerve structures.

During the exploratory phase, it is useful to adjust the pressure of the probe, tilting it to change the angulation, in order to optimize the image and recognize the anatomical structures with certainty, and continuously aligning it so as to follow the course of the structures and rotating it in an attempt to render the anatomical structures more easily recognizable.

The interscalene groove in the supraclavicular site can be identified in two ways: starting from the medial zone at the level of the cricoid cartilage (C6) and moving laterally with the probe, the following structures are recognizable: the trachea, the thyroid gland and the vessels of the neck (Fig. 7.4), the carotid artery, a round, anechoic, pulsatile structure and, anterolaterally, the internal jugular vein, a compressible, more oval-shaped,

7 Ultrasound-Guided Interscalene and Supraclavicular Blocks   121

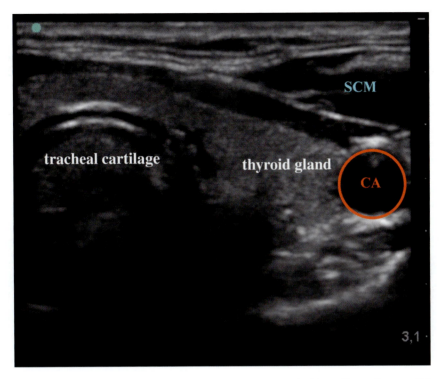

Fig. 7.4 Approach to the interscalene groove at the level of the cricoid cartilage, from medial to lateral; sternocleidomastoid muscle (*SCM*); carotid artery (*CA*)

anechoic structure (Fig. 7.5). Moving laterally, we can see -close to the surface- the sternocleidomastoid muscle, which progressively flattens, and the external jugular vein, which often disappears with the pressure exerted by the ultrasound probe. Below, the anterior scalene muscle and, more laterally, the middle scalene muscle, can be recognized. The roots and/or the trunks are detectable between the two scalene muscles by tilting the probe appropriately in relation to the nerve structures and their course (Fig. 7.6). The image presented is comparable to that of a butterfly with the body represented by the chain of hypoechoic bubbles in the interscalene groove and the two wings by the bellies of the anterior and middle scalene muscles. It is not easy to distinguish ultrasonographically between roots and trunks, or at what level the roots become trunks. Descending from top to bottom, the roots of C5 and C6 merge to form the upper trunk, C7 forms the middle trunk, and the roots of C7 and C8 form the upper trunk, located deeper down. The anterior scalene muscle appears very small in the cranial part of the neck, whereas in the caudal neck area its size is comparable to that of the middle scalene muscle. The vertebral artery can be located below the level of C6 and it is found deeper down and more medially in relation to the nerve structures (C7–C8). Moving further down with the probe, the divisions are shaped from the trunks and the brachial plexus in the supraclavicular site takes on a bunch-of-grapes appearance, that is, a mass of several hypoechoic bubbles. Here, the subclavian artery serves as a vascular landmark, and the brachial plexus lies in a site posterolateral to the vessel, surrounded medially by the distal part of the anterior scalene muscle and laterally by the middle scalene muscle (Fig. 7.7).

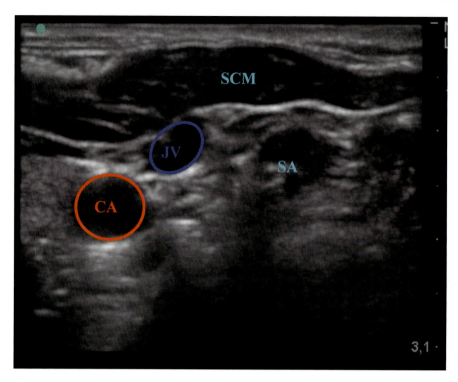

Fig. 7.5 The sternocleidomastoid muscle (*SCM*) at the surface, thinning as one proceeds laterally; carotid artery (*CA*); internal jugular vein (*JV*); anterior scalene muscle (*SA*)

The second method for locating the interscalene groove is particularly useful in more difficult anatomical situations. In these cases, it is advisable to start from lower down with a scan on the oblique coronal plane with the probe positioned parallel to the clavicle (Fig. 7.7). In the supraclavicular cavity, the subclavian artery is identified as a round, pulsatile, anechoic structure, which constantly serves as a landmark at this level. Colour Doppler may be used for verification. Below the subclavian artery, the hyperechoic and hyperreflecting pleura is recognizable as, more laterally, is the hyperechoic edge of the first rib with the underlying acoustic shadow. The brachial plexus lies laterally and dorsally to the subclavian artery, sandwiched between the anterior scalene muscle -medially-and the middle scalene muscle -laterally. It is triangular in shape with the apex towards the external aspect. Here, the trunks have already given rise to the divisions, and the nerve plexus consists of a mass of hypoechoic rings in a fairly superficial site (hardly deeper than 2.5 cm).

Following the structures of the plexus in a cranial direction towards the interscalene site, the three trunks are detectable as hypoechoic bubbles with a hyperechoic border, between the anterior scalene muscle –medially- and the middle scalene muscle -laterally. The image of the trunks is lost when ascending further (above C6), and the nerve roots become visible while passing in front of the hyperechoic image of the transverse processes.

7.3 Ultrasound-Guided Block Technique

In the early phases of the learning curve, it is advisable to take advantage of the dual guidance technique for a safer execution of ultrasound-guided blocks. This means that the ultrasound

7 Ultrasound-Guided Interscalene and Supraclavicular Blocks

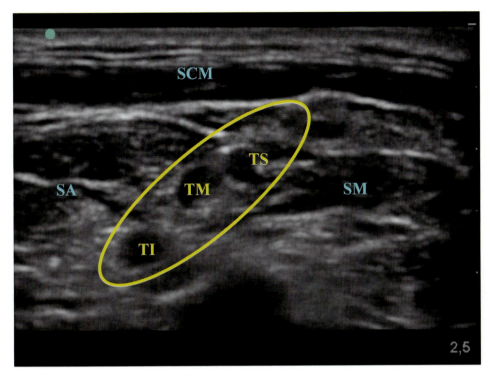

Fig. 7.6 Between the anterior scalene muscle (*SA*) and, more laterally, the middle scalene muscle (*SM*), we see the roots and/or trunks of the brachial plexus; the *upper* trunk (*TS*), the *middle* trunk (*TM*) and the *lower* trunk (*TI*). Close below the surface we see the sternocleidomastoid muscle (*SCM*)

guidance is combined with electrical nerve stimulation, thus availing oneself of an important aid in identifying the nerve structure in the proximity to the needle. It is advisable to maintain the nerve stimulator at a fixed setting of 0.6 mA in order to obtain confirmation of the correct twitch without causing muscle contractions that could be painful to the patient.

It should be noted that direct contact with the needle does not always prompt a neuromuscular response. Perlas, in a paper published in 2006, describes a 38.7 % nerve sensitivity for paresthesias and a 74.5 % neuromuscular response, when ultrasonographically monitoring the correct position of the needle in contact with the nerve. These results confirm the possibility of false negatives in roughly one-third of cases.

On the basis of the position of the needle in relation to the ultrasound probe, we can distinguish between two approach methods: the 'in-plane' technique, with the needle parallel to the long axis of the probe, and the 'out-of-plane' technique, with the needle orthogonal to the probe. The 'in-plane' technique allows the continuous monitoring of the needle along its entire length and, above all, enables the operator to precisely locate the needle tip. Nevertheless, the alignment of needle and probe is by no means easy and requires considerable practice. With the 'out-of-plane' technique, the route is often more direct and similar to the traditional approaches. As the needle is orthogonal to the probe, only a cross-section of the needle can be seen and it is difficult to precisely know the depth of the needle tip. With the aid of the tissue movements due to the passage of the needle and with hydrolocalization, the correct position of the needle tip can be confirmed. The hydrolocalization is achieved by injecting small amounts of non-conductive solution (5 % glucose) in order to check the hypoechoic halo produced by the liquid, without interfering with the nerve stimulation.

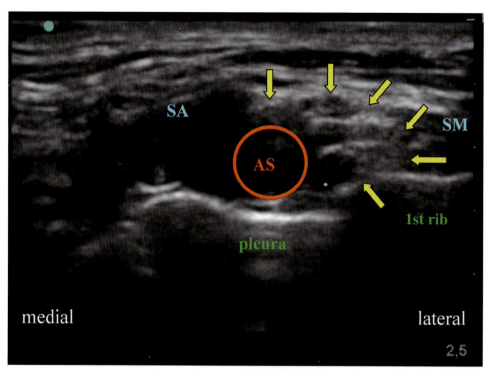

Fig. 7.7 *Left* supraclavicular site: *yellow arrows* indicate the brachial plexus; *SA* anterior scalene muscle; *SM* middle scalene muscle; *SA* subclavian artery; below is the hyperreflecting image of the pleura and, more laterally, the first rib

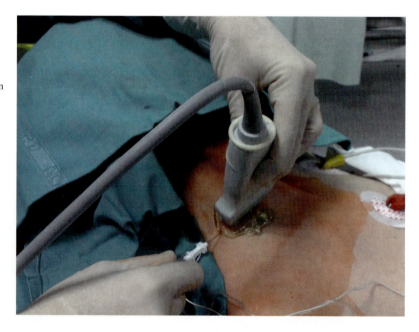

Fig. 7.8 *Left* lateral-to-medial interscalene 'in-plane' approach. The position of the operator will depend upon the dominance of the hand; in this case the position is behind of the patient

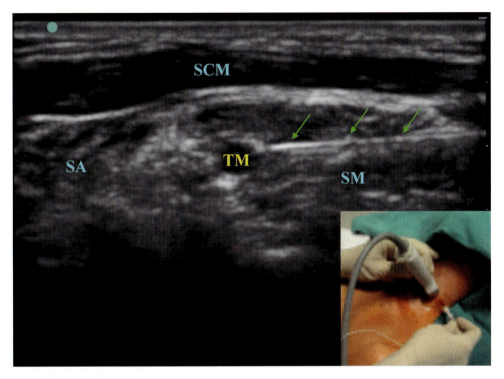

Fig. 7.9 *Right* interscalene block with the 'in-plane' approach: needle direction lateral to medial; the needle tip is close to the middle trunk (*TM*) of the brachial plexus between the anterior scalene muscle (*SA*) and the middle scalene muscle (*SM*); at the surface the sternocleidomastoid muscle (*SCM*)

7.4 Performing the Block at the Interscalene Level

7.4.1 'In-plane' Procedure

Before performing the block, it is advisable to find an appropriate position for the operator, the ultrasound appliance and the probe. According to the dominant hand and the side to be blocked, the operator decides whether to place himself behind (Fig. 7.8) or in front of the patient's head. The patient is in the supine or semi-seated position with the head turned slightly towards the contralateral side. After identifying the interscalene groove with the roots and trunks, an attempt is made to position the target, that is, the roots of C5–C6 and/or the middle trunk (C7), in a central position on the monitor. Normally, we find ourselves 1–2 cm below the level of the cricoid cartilage. The needle is inserted approximately 1–2 cm laterally to the probe in an attempt to penetrate the skin with an acute entry angle (angle between needle and skin). With an acute entry angle (possibly ≤45°), a greater incidence angle (angle between needle and ultrasound beam) can be obtained, which allows better visualization of the needle beneath the ultrasound beam. The frequent presence of the external jugular vein in this site may require to move the needle entry site laterally. After perforating the skin, an attempt is made to align the probe and needle, advancing in a lateromedial direction until the interscalene groove is reached (Fig. 7.9). It is important to move only one hand, keeping the other still, in order to align the probe and the needle; either the needle or the probe must be moved. The syringe containing the local anesthetic must be kept in aspiration by a second operator or by a nurse.

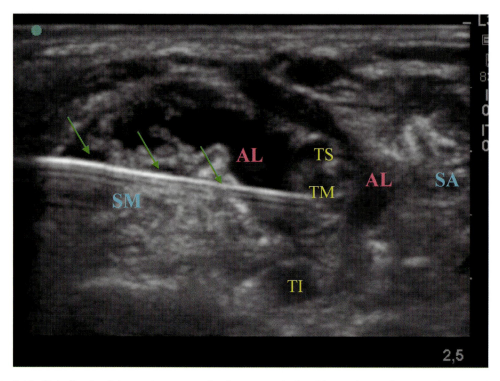

Fig. 7.10 *Right* 'in-plane' interscalene approach after the spread of the anesthetic around the nerve trunks: *TS* upper trunk; *TM* middle trunk; *TI* lower trunk; *AL* local anesthesia; *SA* anterior scalene muscle; *SM* middle scalene muscle; *green arrows* indicate the needle, the tip of which is close to the middle trunk

The correct position of the needle tip can be confirmed by the neuromuscular response desired at 0.6 mA (best twitch). A test injection of liquid may be performed in order to rule out maldistribution, as may occur in the eventuality of an intramuscular or extrafascial injection. To maintain the help that nerve stimulation can provide, it is advisable to use a non-conductive solution such as 5 % glucose for the hydrolocalization. After confirming the correct position of the needle, the anesthetic is injected slowly, avoiding turbulence or the presence of air bubbles, which may impair good visual monitoring of the procedure (Fig. 7.10). On the basis of the spread of the local anesthetic, the operator may decide to reposition the needle to improve the area of distribution of the drug. With a good infiltration of the plexus, the nerve structures become more visible due to the presence of the hypoechoic anesthetic solution around the hyperechoic contours of the roots and trunks.

7.4.2 'Out-of-plane' Procedure

The 'out-of-plane' technique, that is, with the needle orthogonal to the long axis of the probe, does not allow the continuous monitoring of the needle and, above all, does not allow recognition of the needle tip (Fig. 7.11).

The advantages of the 'out-of-plane' technique are a more anatomical approach to the interscalene groove, with a shorter needle path (less than 1 cm in depth) and a more direct access to the nerve structures. The interscalene groove is reached without having to cross the middle interscalene muscle. The execution of the technique is similar to the approach used for the classic interscalene block techniques such as the Winnie's or Meier's technique.

According to the dominant hand and the side to be blocked, the operator decides whether to place himself behind or in front of the patient's head. The patient is in the supine or semi-seated

7 Ultrasound-Guided Interscalene and Supraclavicular Blocks

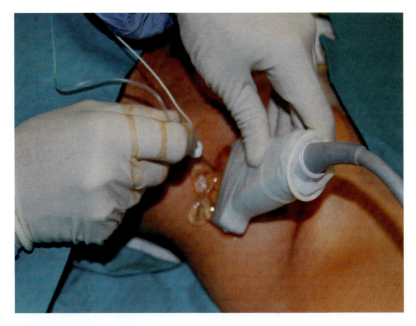

Fig. 7.11 *Right* interscalene approach with 'out-of-plane' technique

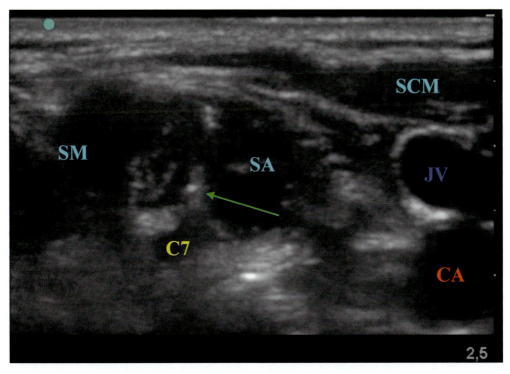

Fig. 7.12 *Right* 'out-of-plane' interscalene approach: the *green arrow* indicates a cross-section (tip?) of the needle, which is directed towards C7 or the middle trunk (*TM*); *SCM* sternocleidomastoid muscle; *SM* middle scalene muscle; *SA* anterior scalene muscle; *JV* internal jugular vein; *CA* carotid artery

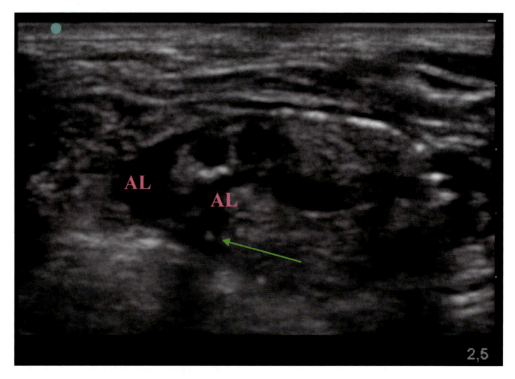

Fig. 7.13 'Out-of-plane' interscalene block: the *green arrow* indicates a cross-section of the needle (tip?); the spread of local anesthesia (*AL*) can be seen in the interscalene groove

position with the head turned slightly towards the contralateral side. After locating the interscalene groove containing the roots and trunks, an attempt is made to move the target, that is, the roots of C5–C6 and/or the middle trunk (C7) into a central site on the monitor. The needle is introduced close to the probe at a point corresponding to the centre of the probe and, in this way, the target is made to coincide with the penetration point at the centre of the image. The needle is introduced, observing the tissue movements in an attempt to identify the needle tip (Fig. 7.12). With the 'out-of-plane' technique, the acoustic shadow cone that forms beneath the probe in cross-section is an artefact that helps us to locate the needle.

The needle tip has to be positioned in proximity to the root of C7, confirming the position of the needle by nerve stimulation with a fixed voltage of 0.6 mA or the injection of 5 % dextrose as a pilot injection. After confirmation of the correct positioning of the needle, the local anesthetic is injected, monitoring the spread for any corrections of the needle position (Fig. 7.13).

7.4.3 'In-plane' Procedure Posterior Approach

The posterior approach is an old access route to the brachial plexus, which, with the advent of the ultrasound-guided technique, has been rediscovered and re-evaluated.

The patient is in the lateral decubitus position lying on the sound shoulder. The operator is to the rear of the patient with the ultrasound device positioned in front of him. The probe is positioned on the neck in short axis in relation to the brachial plexus (Fig. 7.14). The sonoanatomy recognition procedure (Fig. 7.15) is mainly the same as that described above. Once the interscalene groove has been identified, the needle is inserted in the posterior part of the neck, and the

Fig. 7.14 Posterior 'in-plane' interscalene approach; the patient is lying in the lateral decubitus position

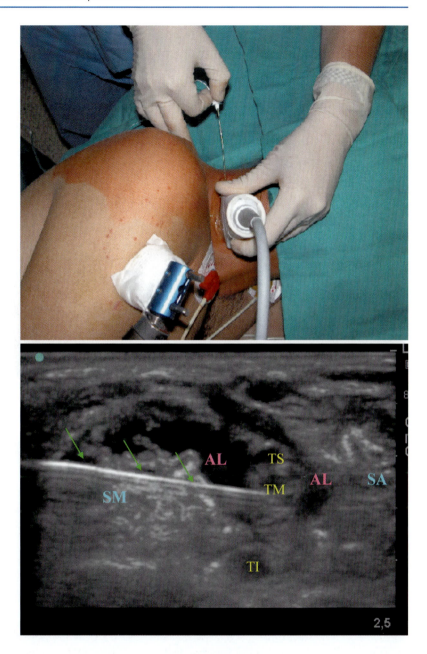

junction between the levator scapulae muscle and the trapezius muscle is marked as the ideal penetration point. The needle is directed on the anteroposterior plane with the 'in-plane' technique, crossing the trapezius muscle and the paraspinal extensor muscles in an anterior direction. The needle is advanced leaving the posterior scalene muscle medially and crossing the middle scalene muscle (Fig. 7.16). When the needle tip arrives close to the roots or, more laterally, to the trunks, the contraction of deltoid muscle or the biceps muscle is elicited by nerve stimulation at 0.6 mA and the operator proceeds to inject the local anesthetic, monitoring the spread of the liquid to make sure that the distribution around the nerve structures is correct

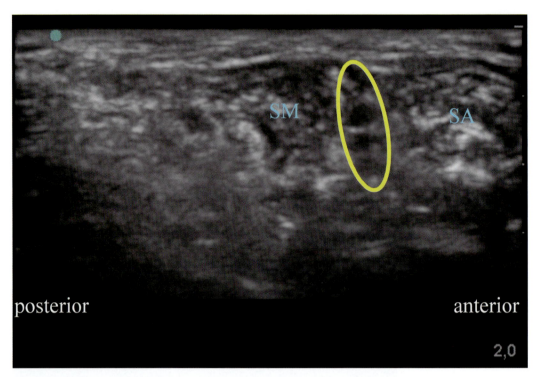

Fig. 7.15 Posterior interscalene approach; middle scalene muscle (*SM*); anterior scalene muscle (*SA*); the brachial plexus is outlined in *yellow*

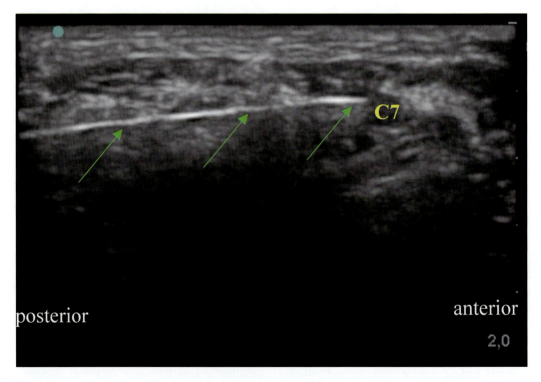

Fig. 7.16 Posterior 'in-plane' approach from posterior to anterior; *green arrows* indicate the 100 mm needle, which is directed towards the root of C7 or the middle trunk

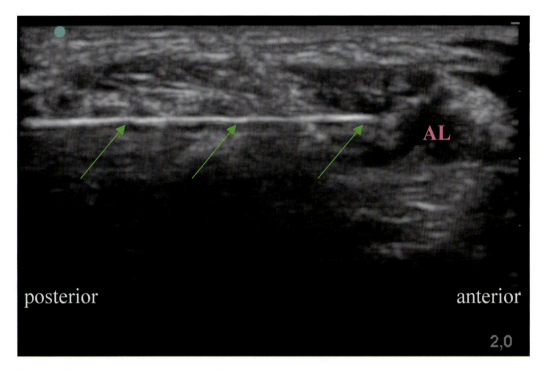

Fig. 7.17 Spread of the local anesthetic (AL) in the interscalene groove; *green arrows* indicate the needle in plane

and avoiding intramuscular and/or intravascular injections (Fig. 7.17).

This technique is particularly indicated in the case of surgical procedures with medium-to-intense postoperative pain that may require the placement of a continuous perineural catheter for the antalgic treatment.

The main advantage is that the catheter crosses a substantial layer of muscles, measuring from 4 to 6 cm in depth and is thus held more firmly in situ in the postoperative period. The interscalene catheter positioned with an anterolateral approach is much more superficial, thus with a higher incidence of displacement.

Other advantages of the posterior approach for catheter introduction are that the entry point is far from the surgical field and that there is no risk of entering into conflict with the external jugular vein which often passes in that site.

It has been reported that, despite the technological efforts made to improve ultrasound visibility, the ultrasonographic imaging of perineural catheters often proves difficult (Fig. 7.18): it is necessary to use indirect indicators such as hydrolocalization in order to ensure they are correctly positioned.

7.5 Performing the Block at the Supraclavicular Level

The supraclavicular site is anatomically and functionally an ideal site for performing anesthesia for the distal part of the humerus, elbow, forearm and hand. In this site, the components of the brachial plexus are closely packed together and therefore are all easy to be blocked by a single injection, with a reduced dose of local anesthetic and with very rapid anesthesia onset times. For these reasons, the technique was considered 'the spinal anesthesia' of the upper limb.

Despite these positive characteristics, the technique has not been widely adopted in clinical practice on account of the substantial risk of serious complications, particularly pneumothorax. With the advent of ultrasound guidance, it

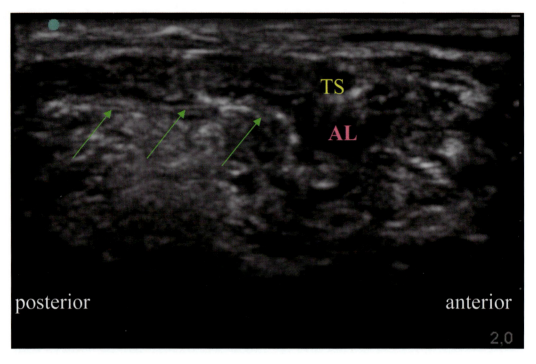

Fig. 7.18 Posteriorly positioned perineural catheter in an interscalene site. It is by no means easy to trace the course of the catheter, which is indicated by the *green arrows*. It is useful to perform a pilot injection in order to verify correct deposition of the local anesthetic (*AL*)

has proved possible to reduce the incidence of this complication. The possibility of seeing and localizing the structures to be avoided and of monitoring the needle in real time during the execution of the procedure make unwanted contact with the pleura unlikely.

In the supraclavicular site, the nerve structures of the brachial plexus are very superficial and close to the subclavian artery, which is useful as a landmark for a rapid ultrasound identification. For the above described reasons, it is necessary to perform the brachial plexus block at the supraclavicular level using the 'in-plane' technique, which allows continuous monitoring of the needle tip, in order to effectively reduce the risk of iatrogenic lesions such as pneumothorax or intravascular injection.

The patient position is supine with the head turned to the contralateral side. It may be helpful to have the patient sat in a 'beach-chair' position in order to effectively lower the shoulders.

The operator places himself behind or in front of the patient's head depending upon the side to be blocked and the operator's dominant hand (Fig. 7.19). It is always advisable for the operator to assume an ergonomic position with easy view of the images on the ultrasound monitor.

Once the anatomical site is identified, with the probe parallel to the clavicle, it is advisable to perform a colour Doppler check (Fig. 7.20) in order to rule out the presence of vascular structures within the mass of hypoechoic structures belonging to the nerve plexus. The ultrasonographic appearance of vascular and nervous structures is similar (both are hypoechoic), and it is important to detect the presence, if any, of vessels in this site with the aid of colour Doppler. In this way, it is possible to choose a safe path avoiding contact with vessels and/or an intravascular injection. The vessels most often present in this site are the transverse cervical artery and the suprascapular artery.

Fig. 7.19 *Right* 'in-plane' lateral-to-medial subclavian approach: the anesthetist places himself behind the patient and uses the dominant hand to perform the block; *green arrows* indicate the needle, which is directed towards the angle formed by the subclavian artery (*AS*), pleura and first rib

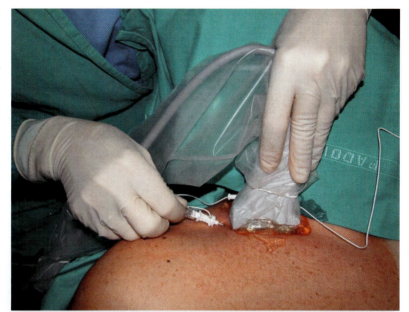

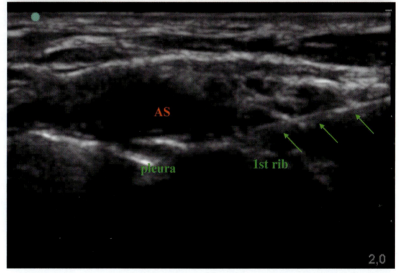

7.5.1 Lateromedial 'In-plane' Approach

With the probe positioned parallel to the clavicle, the needle is introduced lateral to the probe and advanced in a lateromedial direction. In order to have a good view of the needle under ultrasound guidance, an attempt is made to optimize the angle of incidence by moving the needle 1–2 cm lateral to the edge of the probe. The ideal end position of the needle tip for the local anesthetic injection is the angle formed by the subclavian artery, the first rib and the pleura, which anatomically corresponds to the site of the lower trunk. It is important to monitor the spread of local anesthetic during the injection in order to withdraw and reposition the needle, as and when such correction is necessary (Fig. 7.21). The spread should ideally be distributed laterally and caudad in relation to the subclavian artery and should then infiltrate completely the plexus. By avoiding the spread of local anesthetic towards

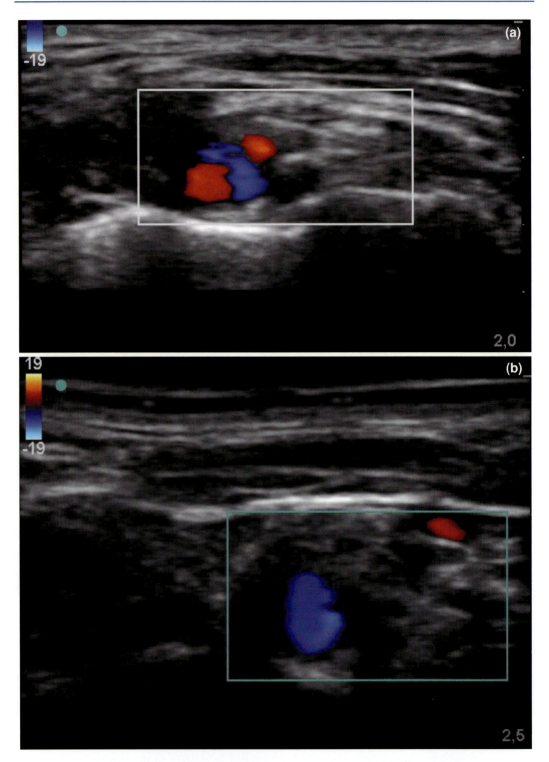

Fig. 7.20 Supraclavicular site. Colour Doppler has been employed in order to verify the position of the subclavian artery **a** and to detect the presence, if any, of vascular structures in the vicinity of the brachial plexus **b**, which could interfere with the path of the needle

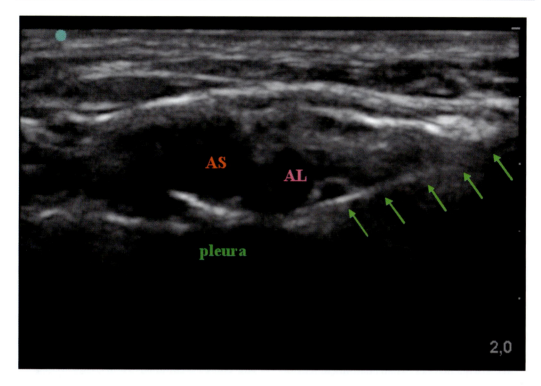

Fig. 7.21 Supraclavicular site: beginning of injection of local anesthetic and monitoring of its correct spread. *AS* subclavian artery; *AL* local anesthetic; the *green arrows* indicate the needle in plane

C4, it is possible to limit the incidence of a phrenic nerve block, which is a present consequence of the block in the supraclavicular site.

7.5.2 Medial-to-Lateral 'In-plane' Approach

This approach is a valid alternative to the foregoing technique. In this case, the entry point of the needle is medial to the probe. Some may consider this approach the safest one, since it aims the needle laterally, far from the pleura and thorax. The subclavian artery, however, may be an obstacle.

The introduction of a catheter in this site is proposed for any surgical procedure on the elbow, forearm and hand, that may be associated with medium-to-intense postoperative pain. The technique is widely similar to that described for the single-shot procedure. With this approach, the catheter is situated in a superficial site and, given an equal distribution of local anesthetic, the infraclavicular site is to be preferred.

A parasagittal approach has recently been described for a supraclavicular continuous catheter positioning. The entry point of the needle is at the level of the trapezius muscle, the techniques requires a posterior-to-anterior 'in-plane' approach. In this way, a more conspicuous layer of musculature is crossed, which may be useful for keeping the catheter firmly in situ.

The ultrasound location of the course of the catheter and particularly of the tip of the catheter is very difficult and often impossible. Apart from the visual identification of the course of the catheter, it is however possible to verify the site of the tip by monitoring the correct distribution of local anesthetic after injection.

7.5.3 Ultrasound-Guided Middle Interscalene Block (Alemanno Technique)

For a description of the ultrasound-guided procedure when using Alemanno's technique, the reader is referred to Chap. 6, Ultrasound-guided Block.

7.6 Final Considerations

Unfortunately, anatomy is not always predictable, and anatomical variations at the level of the interscalene site are fairly frequent. At present, ultrasonography is the only instrumental examination at the patient's bedside that enables us to discover and document this variability. One possible anatomical variant is the presence of the root of C5 or the upper trunk (C5–C6) superficially or within the belly of the anterior scalene muscle, which consequently acts as an anatomical barrier to the correct spread of the local anesthetic. The presence of the roots of C5 and C6 medially to the anterior scalene muscle, and outside the interscalene groove, has also been described. These situations may lead to an incomplete interscalene block, above all in concomitance with a reduced volume of local anesthetic. Ultrasound monitoring of the correct distribution of the drug around the nerve structures and correction, where necessary, of the position of the needle tip may spare us from achieving only partial success of the perineural block.

Anatomical variants are also identified in the supraclavicular site, such as, for instance, a brachial plexus more than 1.5 cm far from the subclavian artery.

The ultrasound-guided techniques are known to be subject to the complications or -better- the known consequences of blocks using traditional techniques, such as block of the stellate ganglion with Claude Bernard-Horner syndrome, block of the phrenic nerve and paresis of the recurrent nerve. It has been demonstrated in clinical studies that injecting a smaller amount of local anesthetic may reduce the risk of these sequelae.

During the execution of the interscalene block, by orientating the needle towards the middle trunk (C7) and reducing the volumes of local anesthetic to 10 ml, an optimal analgesic block can be obtained in shoulder surgery without involving the phrenic nerve. This may be a necessity and/or a very precise and useful indication in patients with respiratory insufficiency who would hardly bear a block of the phrenic nerve.

Similarly, the supraclavicular block has also been studied, and it has been found that the incidence of phrenic nerve block can be reduced by carefully monitoring the spread of local anesthetic and avoiding a rostral and medial distribution in relation to the subclavian artery.

As regards the reduction in the volumes of local anesthetic, there are numerous clinical studies that report data in favour of the ultrasound-guided techniques. In my view, reduction in the amounts of drug injected is becoming a natural process, because the visual monitoring of the precise and optimal distribution of LA around the nerve structures will spontaneously lead us to reducing our habitual volumes.

I would like to conclude with a few considerations regarding the learning of the ultrasound-guided technique.

The use of an ultrasound appliance is in no way a substitute for knowledge of anatomy. Indeed, it should be a stimulus for going back to the study of anatomy and of the relationships between the various anatomical structures themselves.

It is important to study the characteristics and limitations of the ultrasound technique and equipment in order to correctly interpret images and recognize artefacts, thus avoiding misinterpretations. There are 'good' ones that can help us to recognize the anatomical structures and 'bad' artefacts (Fig. 7.22) that can induce us to deviate from the correct diagnosis. It is important to know them in order to avoid the so-called pitfalls.

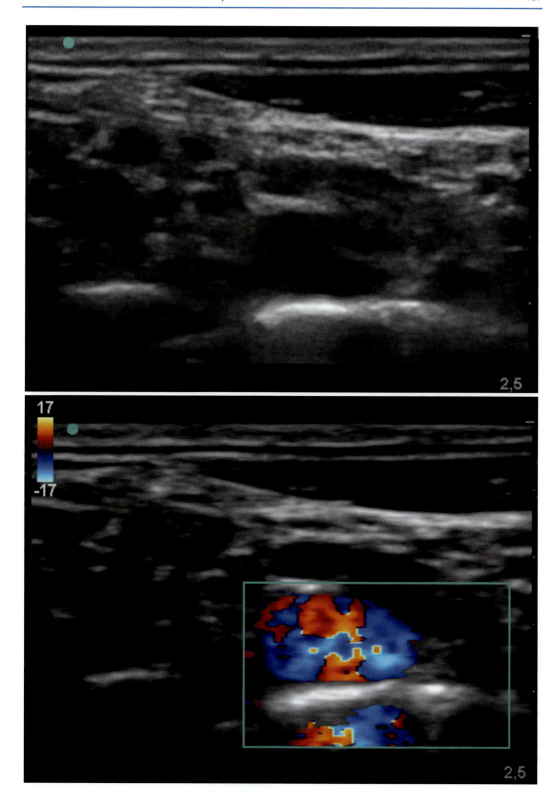

Fig. 7.22 Reverberation artefact in a supraclavicular site: the hyperreflecting pleura creates the artefact that gives a double mirror image of the subclavian artery. This artefact is also produced with the colour Doppler effect

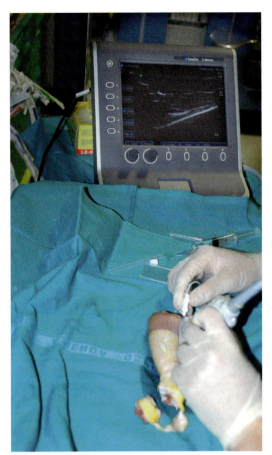

Fig. 7.23 An exercise useful for needle–probe coordination on a phantom

which initially allows us to operate safely and helps us in difficult situations.

To achieve valid clinical results with the ultrasound technique, unquestionably one must invest heavily in terms of time, patience and a great deal of practice.

A third important factor is manual practice in exploring with the probe, applying the four movements described above (pressure, alignment, rotation and tilting), and practice in coordinating the probe and needle, which can be done initially on a phantom (Fig. 7.23), only later carrying out the practised manoeuvres on the patients. There can be no doubt that the 'in-plane' technique is more difficult, with a less steep learning curve compared to the 'out-of-plane' technique, but, as we mentioned above, with the great advantage of affording the possibility of continuous visual monitoring of the needle and needle tip.

One absolutely fundamental piece of advice is to start with the dual guidance technique involving the simultaneous use of US and ENS,

Bibliography

Abrahams MS, Panzer O, Atchabahian A, Horn JL, Brown AR (2008) Case report: limitation of local anesthetic spread during ultrasound-guided interscalene block. Description of an anatomic variant with clinical correlation. Reg Anesth Pain Med 33(4):357–359

Aguirre J, Ekatodramis G, Ruland P, Borgeat A (2009) Ultrasound-guided supraclavicular block: is it really safer? Reg Anesth Pain Med 34(6):622

Antonakakis JG, Sites BD, Shiffrin J (2009) Ultrasound-guided posterior approach for the placement of a continuous interscalene catheter. Reg Anesth Pain Med 34(1):64–68

Bohannon DS (2009) Ultrasound guidance: posterior approach to brachial plexus nerve roots, trunks. Reg Anesth Pain Med 34(6):609

Brull R, Chan VW, McCartney CJ, Perlas A, Xu D (2007) Ultrasound detects intraneural injection. Anesthesiology 106(6):1244

Brull R, Perlas A, Cheng PH, Chan VW (2008) Minimizing the risk of intravascular injection during ultrasound-guided peripheral nerve blockade. Anesthesiology 109(6):1142

Borgeat A, Capdevila X (2007) Neurostimulation/ultrasonography: the Trojan war will not take place. Anesthesiology 106(5):896–898

Casati A, Danelli G, Baciarello M, Corradi M, Leone S, Di Cianni S, Fanelli G (2007) A prospective, randomized comparison between ultrasound and nerve stimulation guidance for multiple injection axillary brachial plexus block. Anesthesiology 106(5):992–996

Chan VW (2003) Applying ultrasound imaging to interscalene brachial plexus block. Reg Anesth Pain Med 28(4):340–343

Chin KJ, Niazi A, Chan V (2008) Anomalous brachial plexus anatomy in the supraclavicular region detected by ultrasound. Anesth Analg 107(2):729–731

Cornish PB, Leaper CJ, Nelson G, Anstis F, McQuillan C, Stienstra R (2007) Avoidance of phrenic nerve paresis during continuous supraclavicular regional anaesthesia. Anaesthesia 62(4):354–358

Cornish P (2009) Supraclavicular block–new perspectives. Reg Anesth Pain Med 34(6):607–608

Duggan E, El Beheiry H, Perlas A, Lupu M, Nuica A, Chan VW, Brull R (2009) Minimum effective volume of local anesthetic for ultrasound-guided supraclavicular brachial plexus block. Reg Anesth Pain Med 34(3):215–218

Fredrickson MJ, Kilfoyle DH (2009) Neurological complication analysis of 1,000 ultrasound guided peripheral nerve blocks for elective orthopaedic surgery: a prospective study. Anaesthesia 64(8):836–844

Ganesh A (2009) Interscalene brachial plexus block-anatomic considerations. Reg Anesth Pain Med 34(5):525

Hadzic A, Sala-Blanch X, Xu D (2008) Ultrasound guidance may reduce but not eliminate complications of peripheral nerve blocks. Anesthesiology 108(4):557–558

Kapral S, Greher M, Huber G, Willschke H, Kettner S, Kdolsky R, Marhofer P (2008) Ultrasonographic guidance improves the success rate of interscalene brachial plexus blockade. Reg Anesth Pain Med 33(3):253–258

Kessler J, Gray AT (2007) Sonography of scalene muscle anomalies for brachial plexus block. Reg Anesth Pain Med 32(2):172–173

Klaastad O, Sauter AR, Dodgson MS (2009) Brachial plexus block with or without ultrasound guidance. Curr Opin Anaesthesiol 22(5):655–660

Mariano ER, Afra R, Loland VJ, Sandhu NS, Bellars RH, Bishop ML, Cheng GS, Choy LP, Maldonado RC, Ilfeld BM (2009) Continuous interscalene brachial plexus block via an ultrasound-guided posterior approach: a randomized, triple-masked, placebo-controlled study. Anesth Analg 108(5):1688–1694

Perlas A, Lobo G, Lo N, Brull R, Chan VW, Karkhanis R (2009) Ultrasound-guided supraclavicular block: outcome of 510 consecutive cases. Reg Anesth Pain Med 34(2):171–176

Perlas A, Chan VW, Simons M (2003) Brachial plexus examination and localization using ultrasound and electrical stimulation: a volunteer study. Anesthesiology 99(2):429–435

Perlas A, Niazi A, McCartney C, Chan V, Xu D, Abbas S (2006) The sensitivity of motor response to nerve stimulation and paresthesia for nerve localization as evaluated by ultrasound. Reg Anesth Pain Med 31(5):440–445

Plunkett AR, Brown DS, Rogers JM, Buckenmaier CC 3rd (2006) Supraclavicular continuous peripheral nerve block in a wounded soldier: when ultrasound is the only option. Br J Anaesth 97(5):715–717

Renes SH, Rettig HC, Gielen MJ, Wilder-Smith OH, van Geffen GJ (2009) Ultrasound-guided low-dose interscalene brachial plexus block reduces the incidence of hemidiaphragmatic paresis. Reg Anesth Pain Med 34(5):498–502

Renes SH, Spoormans HH, Gielen MJ, Rettig HC, van Geffen GJ (2009) Hemidiaphragmatic paresis can be avoided in ultrasound-guided supraclavicular brachial plexus block. Reg Anesth Pain Med 34(6):595–599

Sites BD, Chan VW, Neal JM, Weller R, Grau T, Koscielniak-Nielsen ZJ, Ivani G (2009) American society of regional anesthesia and pain medicine; european society of regional anaesthesia and pain therapy joint committee. The American society of regional anesthesia and pain medicine and the European society of regional anaesthesia and pain therapy joint committee recommendations for education and training in ultrasound-guided regional anesthesia. Reg Anesth Pain Med 34(1):40–46

Sites BD, Spence BC, Gallagher J, Beach ML, Antonakakis JG, Sites VR, Hartman GS (2008) Regional anesthesia meets ultrasound: a specialty in transition. Acta Anaesthesiol Scand 52(4):456–466

Soares LG, Brull R, Lai J, Chan VW (2007) Eight ball, corner pocket: the optimal needle position for ultrasound-guided supraclavicular block. Reg Anesth Pain Med 32(1):94–95

Soffer RJ, Rosenblatt MA (2007) Teaching ultrasound-guided interscalene blocks: description of a simple and effective technique. J Clin Anesth 19(3):241–242

Tsui B (2007) Ultrasound-guidance and nerve stimulation: implications for the future practice of regional anesthesia. Can J Anaesth 54(3):165–170

van Geffen GJ, Rettig HC, Koornwinder T, Renes S, Gielen MJ (2007) Ultrasound-guided training in the performance of brachial plexus block by the posterior approach: an observational study. Anaesthesia 62(10):1024–1048

Walker KJ, McGrattan K, Aas-Eng K, Smith AF (2009) Ultrasound guidance for peripheral nerve blockade. Cochrane Database Syst Rev 4:CD006459

Complications of Supraclavicular Techniques

8

F. Alemanno

Danger is such a complex and very special fact that only rarely can its existence be asserted or denied with certainty. And yet this is what is demanded of the physician, it is as if, in states of severe disease, between danger and non-danger, there was the Great Wall of China.

Dr. De Carolis
General Practitioner, Porto Recanati 1905

8.1 Failed Block

Although it is not the most serious complication, it is undoubtedly the most embarrassing because of the protests of the patients and the complaints of the surgeon; moreover, it induces depression in the anesthetist as a result of reduced self-esteem.

Failure of the block may be considered to all intents and purposes a complication, which in general is associated with a high incidence in brachial plexus block techniques owing to a series of factors. First and foremost of these is an inadequate time period elapsing between injection of the anesthetic and the start of the operation. In this connection, we cannot emphasize too strongly the need to make sure that the patient arrives in the operating unit well in advance. With the long-lasting anesthetics available today, there is no risk that excessively early administration of the anesthesia will result in the effect wearing off too soon. In addition, the anesthesia technique must be performed in the preoperating room, because if it is done in the operating room while the surgeon is sharpening his instruments, it may be difficult to stop him and expect him to hold fire patiently before operating.

One of the reasons for a slow induction is a particular anatomical disposition of the septa described by Thompson and Rorie, with the relative lack of communication pathways between one compartment and another. In this case, the time the anesthetic takes to spread to the other compartments of the plexus from the point where it was injected may be considerable. The various expedients or adjuvants aimed at speeding up the induction of anesthesia have not proved particularly useful. Also the idea of using as the first bolus an anesthetic with a shorter induction time (as mepivacaine is generally reputed to be) or a mixture of two different anesthetics fails to yield any effective benefit. If the anesthetic has come into contact with the nerve, there is no appreciable difference between the various anesthetics, the difference between induction times not being more than just a few minutes. The duration of action, on the other hand, will differ as a function of the chemical characteristics of the molecule.

The completeness of the block is related to the spread of the anesthetic to all the compartments of the brachial plexus. At the supraclavicular level, the spread is facilitated by a greater measure of communication between the various compartments as compared to the axillary level.

In any case, however, in the eventuality of failure of the block, it can be repeated if there is enough time available. As Moore suggests, most

F. Alemanno (✉)
Institute of Anesthesiology, Resuscitation and Pain Therapy, University of Verona, Verona, Italy
e-mail: fernando@alemannobpb.it

patients do not realize that they have had a second block if this second block is preceded by a phrase of the type such as '… well, now I'm going to inject a bit more anesthetic to block this zone'.

Clearly, if there is a risk of exceeding the maximum permitted dose of anesthetic or there is not enough time available, it is advisable to administer general anesthesia without further delay.

8.2 Pneumothorax

Pneumothorax, though not the most serious, is the most feared complication of the supraclavicular techniques. It constitutes a risk that may occur even in the most expert hands or when using techniques that seem to be the safest possible. The percentage incidence of this complication varies considerably as a function of the technique and the anesthetist's experience. A simple cough during the plexus location manoeuvres should immediately alert the anesthetist to the risk of an unwanted needle tip placement. Nor can the use of ultrasound protect against this risk, because with the supraclavicular techniques, as suggested by Brian Sites, the first rib acts as a reflecting mirror, thus creating an acoustic shadow that makes it impossible to gauge the distance between the needle tip and the dome of the pleura, which may exceed the upper surface of the rib by some 2–3 cm.

One should always mistrust those, mainly female, patients with the asthenic habitus—drooping shoulders and winged scapulae—so well described by Berthold Stiller as long ago as 1907. In these patients, the lateral apophysis of the clavicle may present as constitutionally rotated downwards, thus superficializing the brachial plexus, but also the first rib and the pleural dome.

Nor can ultrasonography be of much help in this case, because as we have already said, the reverberation caused by the first rib creates an acoustic shadow that makes it impossible to gauge the distance between the needle and the pleural dome and this may be 2–3 cm higher than the upper surface of the rib. Despite being convinced that something is visible, one cannot avoid puncturing what, in actual fact, cannot be seen.

One should always beware of the supraclavicular techniques, even the ultrasound-guided ones, in which the needle is directed caudad! As George Santayana wrote: 'Those who cannot remember the past are condemned to repeat it'.

It may happen that the air bleb produced may be minimal and may thus go undiagnosed clinically, but if the portion of collapsed lung exceeds 25 %, it is necessary to put a thoracic drain in place.

Any anesthetist should be capable of performing this simple procedure without having to involve the surgeon who, being used to placing the drain under direct vision with the chest open, generally tends to put it in the same position (7th to 8th intercostal space on the anterior axillary line and in the same direction) also with the chest closed. At this level, to avoid a hepatic lesion, the surgeon, as is his wont, tends to insert a blunt-tipped catheter in a cranial direction and thus with a very acute angle in relation to the chest wall. In this way, the risk of inserting it between the parietal pleura and the internal thoracic fascia exists. This intervention may show up well at an X-ray check-up but affords no drainage efficacy. The scenario may be further complicated if the anesthetist, lacking experience and expertise in the placement of thoracic drains, tries to imitate the surgeon.

The procedure for the placement of a drain for the treatment for pneumothorax is simple and consists in three easy manoeuvres:

1. The first manoeuvre consists in administering the local anesthetic at the point at which the thoracic drain is to be inserted—the third intercostal space on the hemiclavicular line. With a 5-ml syringe filled with anesthetic, a skin wheal is induced. The needle is inserted on the hemiclavicular line at the level of the third intercostal space in a direction normal to the skin and taking care to skirt the upper border of the fourth rib so as to keep some distance away from the neurovascular bundle of the third. Proceeding gradually step by

step and injecting small boluses of anesthetic, preceded by frequent aspirations, one penetrates into the thoracic cavity without any risk of damaging any of the underlying structures. At a certain point, in fact, the aspiration will be followed by abundant influx of air into the syringe, which means that the needle has reached the cavity. The syringe is disconnected, and the needle is left in the chest both as a marker and, above all, to allow the efflux of air in the case of hypertensive pneumothorax.

2. In the same hole, the needle is replaced by a triangular-bladed scalpel, which is introduced down to the handle.
3. The triangular-bladed scalpel is replaced by a drain fitted with a sharp-edged mandrel that is gripped in the left hand which, resting against the thoracic wall, acts as a brake (as in the peridural procedure), whereas the right hand grips the tail knob of the mandrel and imparts the force. We proceed with a series of light taps on the mandrel until a dull click indicates that the drain tip has penetrated beyond the parietal pleura and has entered the thoracic cavity. As we have already said, it is good policy not to use blunt-tipped drains because they easily create false paths, insinuating themselves between the parietal pleura and the internal thoracic fascia. The latter can be used in the eventuality of a subsequent replacement of the drain. Lastly, a fairly large thread (No. 0) is used to construct a tobacco-pouch suture on the skin at a distance of half a centimetre from, and around, the entry point of the drain so as to guarantee the sealing. After tightening the thread, though not so much as to render the tissues ischaemic, a string is constructed, measuring a few centimetres in length, with a series of simple knots in succession, which is finally tied around the drain. To make sure that this last knot, which must secure the drain in place, does not slip along the drain, we have to tie a three-turn knot (one turn is a simple knot, two turns a surgical knot and therefore one turn more than the surgical knot). This latter three-turn knot guarantees that it does not loosen while we are tying the second simple holding knot. Not only this, but if when tightening it, we slightly squeeze the drain, forming a kind of collar, it will not be subject to slackening, thus guaranteeing the absolute stability and fixity of the system. Finally, the drainage tube will be connected to a large bottle equipped with a water valve.

8.3 Nerve Injuries

The possibility of causing a serious nerve injury is relatively rare, but should be borne in mind whenever approaching a nerve with a needle. The use of electrical nerve stimulation or of ultrasound should not make us feel safe from this complication which, even in its least severe manifestations, may cause the patient troublesome paraesthesias as well as even more troublesome forensic sequelae for the anesthetist, associated with lawsuits for damages as a result of symptoms, which are hard to quantitate and which, once they set in, one is never able to establish objectively when they will finish.

The first measure that needs to be adopted in order to avoid puncturing the target nerve to be identified is not to be in a hurry. For this reason, too, it is necessary to bring the patient to the operating unit in good time. The insertion of the needle must be slow. If it is not inserted slowly, there is a risk that it will reach the target before one realizes that the stimulation has taken effect. This is also valid even if the block is simultaneously ultrasound-guided.

Another problem has to do with the cutting angle of the needle bevel. This is a problem that dates back to the time when the injection of the anesthetic necessarily followed an initial paraesthesia induced by contact of the needle with the nerve structure. 'No paraesthesia, no anesthesia' declared Daniel Moore.

It may seem obvious, as maintained by Selander, that when you have to elicit a paraesthesia by contact, a sharper-tipped needle may cause greater damage to the nerve by penetrating more deeply and that, at first sight, a blunt-tipped needle may seem less damaging, but there are other arguments that counterbalance this assumption.

The first is that a sharper needle proceeds in the tissue with a uniform movement, whereas a more blunt-tipped needle, endowed with poorer penetration, undergoes sudden, though minor, accelerations related to the resistance which it encounters and then overcomes, albeit thanks to a small increase in '*vis a tergo*' ('force from behind'). In this case, the needle risks reaching the target with an accelerated movement and therefore without sufficient control and with the possibility of causing a lesion; there is consequently not enough time to induce a visible muscle contraction useful for arresting the course of the needle in good time.

A second consideration is that a needle with a long bevel has a much more oval exit hole than a short-bevel needle, with the result that, in the case of partial insertion in the nerve, the long-bevel needle presents the possibility of discharging the anesthetic via the part of the lumen that has not penetrated into the nerve, whereas the short-bevel needle is more likely to have all its lumen embedded in the nerve structure with the result that the anesthetic will be injected more easily at the intraneural level. Lastly, studies by Rice and McMahon have demonstrated that short-bevel needles are effectively more damaging.

On the other hand, however, the long-bevel needle tip, if it impacts against a bony structure, may be bent into the form of a kind of microscopic hook, which may snag on, and damage a nerve structure during needle withdrawal or direction-changing movements.

Be that as it may, regardless of the type of needle tip, if, regrettably, an intraneural injection were to occur, the consequences would be more severe, because in addition to the mechanical damage caused by the needle tip (nerve lesion plus haemorrhage due to rupture of the *vasa nervorum*), there would also be ischaemic damage related to the increased pressure and/or the presence of adrenaline in the anesthetic mixture.

Sunderland has classified nerve injuries as belonging to five different degrees of severity.

A first-degree injury occurs when moderate pressure is applied to a nerve for a brief period. Belonging to this degree of severity is compression of the sciatic nerve due to an incorrect posture followed by the classic paraesthesia of the lower limb or compression of the ulnar nerve due to an incorrect position of the forearm on the armrest of the operating table for surgery of brief duration. Another cause may be an excessively inflated haemostatic tourniquet applied to a limb with reduced muscle mass. In all these cases, the mechanism of action consists in compression of axonal fluids but, above all, in ischaemic compression of the *vasa nervorum* followed by anoxia proportional to the compression time. The pathogenic mechanism is that of a transient ischaemic attack. The nerve function recovery time will be proportional to the intensity of the pressure applied and its duration, but also to the presence of concomitant diseases such as diabetes or other degenerative diseases. In normal conditions it should not exceed about a fortnight; otherwise, we have to suspect a second-degree injury.

Classified as second-degree nerve injuries are those in which, as a result of the death of the nerve segment concerned, the distal part of the axons no longer receives the axoplasm from the respective neurons with consequent Wallerian degeneration also involving the myelin sheaths.

What remains, as the only important traces for future regeneration, are the endoneurial tubules, which are scavenged of debris by the macrophages and Schwann cells. New axoplasm, from the respective neuron, then revitalizes the tubules, regenerating their contents; this regeneration takes place at the rate of 2–3 mm per day. The Schwann cells simultaneously envelop and myelinate the tubules.

Sunderland's third-degree injury is a nerve fibre interruption. In third-degree injury, there is a lesion of the endoneurium, but the epineurium and perineurium remain intact. The third-degree injury is a lesion of the endoneurial tubules, but the structure of the fascicles is substantially preserved. This occurs in lesions caused by needles, but not followed by injection.

A fourth-degree injury is defined as a lesion in which the fascicles and tubules, in addition to being damaged, are disorganized as in the case of intraneural injection.

In third- and fourth-degree lesions, both the axons and the myelin sheaths degenerate, but not the Schwann cells which, in conjunction with the macrophages, proceed to clear away the degeneration debris. Immediately after the injury, the Schwann cells proliferate, thus restoring an anatomical continuity, which is extremely important for the regeneration of the nerve. This regeneration comes about fortunately in a shorter time period than the proliferation of the fibroblasts, which therefore do not have time to cause cicatricial obstacles. The Schwann cells of the segment proximal to the nerve also proliferate, thus reconnecting to those of the distal segment. The proliferation of these cells takes place longitudinally, leaving spaces that will be reoccupied in the regeneration process by the interrupted axons at the rate of 2 mm per day.

If the axons are severed transversely, the myelin sheath is also interrupted; in this case, the proximal stump degenerates over a brief segment in a retrograde sense; after a few days, axonal sprouts begin to form which, emerging from the severed stump, start to progress. Normally, this regeneration reaches the peripheral stump, the tubules are reoccupied by axons, and eventually the function of the respective peripheral receptors is restored. Even in the best of aseptic conditions or normal mesenchymal reactivity, however, a certain number of fibres regenerate successfully, but others are trapped in the fracture line and their sprouts therefore form a 'neuroma-in-continuity'. Even after only partial lesions, the growth of small fascicles of axons or even of single axons may give rise to the formation of microneuromas.

The regeneration does not always reoccupy the right tubule, and therefore, it may occur that motor fibres may restore sensory fibres and vice versa with an unsuccessful outcome or that a sensory fibre may reoccupy another with a different function, but in this latter case, the sensory function is remodulated at central level.

In normal conditions, once the endoneurial tubules have been regenerated, the Schwann cells reenvelop the tubules completely and then deposit myelin around them.

The situation is complicated if the needle tip has carried with it germs or other substances (undried disinfectant or ultrasonography gel) or if the patient has a hyperergic mesenchymal habitus; in these cases, the progression of the axonal sprouts is obstructed first by inflammatory processes and then by cicatricial processes, tending to form a tangled mass.

One can never overemphasize the importance of asepsis and the need to wait until the disinfectant has dried out (also in order to give it time to act!) and to take care not to drag ultrasonography gel in with the movements of the needle. The needle must first be inserted in the subcutaneous tissue, and then, the gel and the probe are applied, in such a way that the needle tip, which is the part that may finish up intraneurally, does not draw in gel and its additives, particularly into the bevel, not to mention the bad habit of using the disinfectant liquid in the place of gel with the risk of drawing the liquid in when manoeuvring the needle, or, worse still, beyond the perineurium in the case of nerve puncture. We should not forget that iodine is an extremely aggressive disinfectant. Free iodine captures electrons to form iodine ions which combine with various organic substrates, oxidizing lipids, amino acids and proteins, hence its action against bacteria, fungi and mycobacteria, but also viruses and protozoans. Before suturing a wound, surgeons generally disinfect tissues and viscera rather carelessly, preferring a slight degree of tissue mortification to a hypothetical bacterial contamination. It is quite another matter to carry active iodine into the perineurium, or, even worse, into the axon!

If the anesthetist suspects that he or she has caused a nerve injury, the use of antibiotic prophylaxis and cortisone is justified in order to block any possible fibroblast proliferation.

In the paravertebral approaches, the needle may come into contact with the spinal nerve both in the intervertebral conjugate foramen and immediately outside it. If the conjugate foramen is stenotic for various reasons such as scoliosis, arthrosis (present in 10 % of the adult population) with the presence or otherwise of osteophytic spurs, the nerve has less freedom of movement when in contact with the needle and therefore is more likely to be injured.

8.4 Phrenic Nerve Palsy

The phrenic nerve is formed by the spinal nerves C3, C4 and C5. As we have already said in the chapter on the anatomy of the cervical plexus, the main root of the phrenic nerve consists in the anterior division of C4 with a contribution from the anterior divisions of C3 and C5. The nerve, thus formed, emerges from the neurovascular space at the level of the apex of the scalene triangle and runs, adhering to the anterior surface of the anterior scalene muscle, in an inferomedial direction until it reaches the medial angle that the scalene muscle forms with the first rib where it passes into the thorax.

Its involvement in brachial plexus block techniques is all the more probable, the more closely the techniques approach the cervical column and the greater the volume of anesthetic injected.

The incidence ranges from 100 % in the high interscalene block, as reported by Urmey, to 67 % reported by Knoblanche, and 50 % reported by Neal. In our experience (middle interscalene block) in a radiographic study of 97 patients subjected to arthroscopy of the shoulder, anesthetized with 0.4 ml/kg of 0.75 % levobupivacaine, we registered 60 % diaphragmatic paresis at the end of the intervention (approximately two hours after induction and therefore with the block well stabilized).

Obviously, numerous diseases and conditions contraindicate the use of supraclavicular plexus anesthesia precisely on account of the risk of blocking the phrenic nerve. These include a previous pneumonectomy or even a simple contralateral lobectomy, a lesion of the contralateral phrenic nerve, chronic obstructive lung disease, asthmatic disease, even if quiescent at the time, myasthenia and all the neuromuscular degenerative diseases.

In any event, even in a healthy subject, in view of the fact that we have to consider that at least 50 % of cases present this complication, albeit in asymptomatic form, we must pay particular attention to the saturation measurements, especially in those cases where more or less heavy sedation is required. The intubation of the patient in the seated position 'is likely to prove so awkward and inelegant as to be formally inadvisable' (Gasparetto); the patient needs to be rapidly placed in the supine position, upsetting the entire operating field and the mental stability of the surgeon. Nor would it be much easier in the seated position to insert a laryngeal mask airway, even if with a bit of practice and tempting fortune.

All in all, in certain situations which it would be wise to prevent as early as the time of the preoperative visit, one should not regard giving up the idea of administering regional anesthesia right from the outset and resorting instead to the use of general anesthesia as a sort of *'diminutio capitis'* (a diminishing of personal status).

8.5 Vascular Lesions

The arterial circulation of the cervical spinal cord occurs via an extraspinal network, to the formation of which three different types of arteries contribute—the anterior spinal arteries, the posterior spinal arteries and the lateral spinal arteries, all branches of the vertebral and/or ascending cervical artery.

The two anterior spinal arteries, right and left, originate, respectively, from the two vertebral arteries at a level lower than the point where the two vertebral arteries unite to form the basilar artery. From their point of origin, the two arteries converge and merge into the anterior spinal trunk, which, following the anterior median fissure of the spinal cord, terminates at the level of C5. This path is not always so regular, but often forms rhombi and ellipses, where the two arteries, separating once again, spread out only to reunite medially to continue the anterior spinal trunk. This apparently curious behaviour always occurs at the origin of the pairs of spinal nerves.

In the same way as the anterior spinal arteries, the right and left posterior spinal arteries also originate from the vertebral arteries, posterior to the latter, and then travel to the posterior surface of the spinal cord without merging, running laterally to the posterior median sulcus. At the level of C2, they divide into two branches, one of which runs medially to the posterior roots, practically following Burdach's fascicle, while the other runs laterally to the roots. Their course remains parallel to the posterior median sulcus and terminates at the level of C5. Caudally, their function, like that of the anterior spinal arteries, will be taken over by the lateral spinal arteries.

The cervical lateral spinal arteries originate from the vertebral artery and from the ascending cervical artery, a branch of the thyrocervical trunk. This arises from the arch of the subclavian artery between the vertebral artery and the common carotid artery and soon divides into four branches: the inferior thyroid artery, the transverse scapular artery, the superficial cervical artery and, last but not least, the above-mentioned ascending cervical artery. The latter also supplies branches to the levator scapulae muscle and to the anterior scalene muscle, on whose surface it runs parallel to the phrenic nerve.

Once the lateral spinal arteries separate from the vertebral artery or the ascending cervical artery, they penetrate into the intervertebral foramen together with the spinal nerves and, at the bifurcation of the latter into the anterior and posterior roots, also divide into two branches which, following the respective roots, terminate one in the anterior median fissure and the other in the posterolateral groove.

The anterior branch, on reaching the internal midline of the spinal cord, divides into an ascending branch, which anastomoses with the descending branch of the upper metamere, and a descending branch which merges with the ascending branch of the lower metamere.

The posterior branch, on reaching the posterolateral groove of the spinal cord, likewise divides into an ascending branch and a descending branch, which merge with the respective descending and ascending branches of the neighbouring metameres.

The anterior branches of the lateral spinal arteries, anastomosing with those of the overlying and underlying metameres, thus form a middle trunk that is a continuation of the anterior spinal trunk originating from the vertebral arteries and terminating at the level of C5.

In the same way, the posterior branches of the lateral spinal arteries continue, at a level below C5, to assure the presence and function of the posterior spinal arteries that originate, in the upper cervical region, from the vertebral arteries.

To conclude, then, the spinal cord is coaxial, from top to bottom, with five arterial systems: one anterior, two right posterior that follow the right posterolateral groove and two left posterior that follow the left posterolateral groove. The two posterior systems on each side anastomose not only with each other but also with the two systems on the opposite side via transverse anastomoses.

The spinal cord, then, is surrounded by a cylindrical arterial network, the perimedullary circuitry, from which stem the arteries that supply it in depth. These are as follows: the anterior and posterior spinal arteries that penetrate along the anterior median fissure and along the posterior median septum; the anterior and posterior radicular arteries that enter the spinal cord along the radicular grooves; and the peripheral arteries which generally number eight to ten do not enter the spinal cord from precise reference points and are mainly destined to supply the white matter.

It is precisely the vertebral artery, the ascending cervical artery and the lateral spinal arteries that are exposed to the risk of mechanical injury. In general, however, an arterial lesion rarely indexes a spinal ischaemia thanks to the numerous anastomoses present in the perimedullary circuitry. There can be no doubt, however, that the intra-arterial injection even of small amounts of anesthetic can lead to an unwanted segmental spinal anesthesia. Other contributory causes are necessary to bring about the occurrence of an ischaemic syndrome; these include a concomitant hypotension that occurs as a result of the often tardy onset of Bezold–Jarisch syndrome.

Another adverse event might be a multifragmented fracture of an atheromatous plaque caused by the needle with microembolization of the spinal arteries.

Haematomas are relatively rare when using supraclavicular techniques. They may be caused not so much by puncture of the subclavian artery as by puncture of the transverse artery of the neck or of the vertebral artery. Normally, this complication requires only compression and observation. The anesthetist may have doubts as to whether the block may be less efficacious due to dilution of the anesthetic with a non-easily estimated amount of blood and/or as a result of plasma protein binding which might retard the effect.

8.6 High Spinal Block

This is one of the most serious complications that can occur. The signs and symptoms take very little time to set in, and therefore, they need to be recognized early so as to be able to treat them in time. Generally speaking, the patient manifests an early bilateral block of the brachial plexus and dyspnoea, becomes agitated and experiences first tachycardia and then bradycardia; cyanosis and convulsions set in rapidly, and the patient may stop breathing altogether. The respiratory arrest is due to bilateral block of the phrenic nerve and the accessory respiratory muscles (scalene muscles, intercostal muscles, etc.) and/or to cerebral anoxia due to severe hypotension. The first remedial measure consists in the administration of O_2 in a mask with a to-and-fro, immediately followed, if necessary, by intubation of the patient and connection to an automatic respirator, amongst other things in order to have the hands free in case cardiac arrest occurs. The hypotension is corrected by administering ephedrine or ethylephrine (Effortil-R) in addition to an adequate infusion of fluids and plasma expander with the flow restrictor fully open. In the eventuality of cardiac arrest, after an adequate heart massage has failed to yield a result, one should proceed with an intravenous injection of one or two ampoules of adrenaline followed immediately by heart massage. If the ampoules of adrenaline and the subsequent heart massage fail to yield the desired results, the anesthetist should not hesitate to inject a third ampoule. If high-voltage ventricular fibrillation follows, electrical defibrillation must be performed. I believe it is useful to implement ECG monitoring of the patient right from the start of the anesthetic procedures, in addition to the monitoring of SpO_2 and arterial blood pressure. Unfortunately, a substantially lax, 'economic' monitoring is often practised using only the oxygen saturation meter and forgetting that, in the case of cardiac arrest, the timing of the therapy for such arrest or for ventricular fibrillation (apart from heart massage) is very different.

If cardiac arrest occurs, even when treated with an effective heart massage, one should always suspect the onset of cerebral acidosis, particularly if the patient shows no immediate sign of rearousal. In this case, an infusion of tromethamine (THAM) would be useful. Bicarbonate, in fact, takes approximately 30 min to cross the blood–brain barrier! We should not forget, however, that THAM is so potent and has such an immediate action also on cells of the respiratory centre, which are known to function on the basis of H^+ ions, as to give rise to respiratory failure, if the latter are neutralized. This, however, should not be a major concern for the anesthetist–resuscitator who possesses all the means necessary to guarantee the patient's breathing.

8.7 Toxic Reactions

Toxic reactions due to absorption are somewhat rare, even though substantial amounts of anesthetic are used for brachial plexus blocks. The neurovascular bundle is a relatively closed, poorly capillarized system, despite the fact that vessels of fairly large calibre run within it, but these are practically impermeable to the anesthetic. The tissue consists of adipose and loose cellular connective tissue in addition to a few lymph nodes. The absorption is distinctly slower compared to that of an intramuscular injection. A number of muscles, such as the scalene muscles, seem to be in close contact, but the anesthetic would have to penetrate not only the deep cervical fascia that constitutes the actual sheath of the neurovascular bundle, but also the external perimysium of said muscles before coming into contact with the rich muscular capillary system.

The toxic reaction, on the contrary, will be very rapid even if only a few millilitres are injected into a vessel, particularly the vertebral artery. As we have already stated in a previous chapter, while performing an interscalene block, I had the misfortune of narcotizing a patient by injecting 2 ml of 2 % mepivacaine into the vertebral artery. The effect was similar to that of an intravenous injection of 300 mg of sodium thiopental: the patient's eyes glazed over and the tongue dropped back suddenly. Manual ventilation with a face mask and orotracheal intubation were easily performed without the aid of muscle relaxants; the muscles of the head and neck were completely relaxed. It is likely that local anesthesia of all twelve cranial nerves was induced via the basilar artery. The narcosis did not last more than fifteen minutes; the patient was extubated, fortunately remembering nothing, and was taken back to the ward and, after a thorough neurological examination, was operated on the next day under genuine general anesthesia.

The intravascular injection of local anesthetic, especially if intravenous, may lead to cardiac disorders, because, precisely on account of its mechanism of action, it induces repolarization alterations. This occurs above all with the use of racemic anesthetic solutions because the dextrorotatory form tends also to occupy the potassium channels.

According to Finucane et al., the administration of anesthetic should not be based only on the patient's weight, which certainly, if low, must limit the amount injected, but in the case of higher weights, one should also take account of the patient's height, as suggested by Winnie, or the length of the patient's arm, which would make for a better calculation of the capacity of the neurovascular bundle.

In anesthesiological practice with the middle interscalene block, the volume of anesthetic is normally calculated as 0.4 ml/kg. In patients weighing more than 80 kg, our calculation is no longer based on body weight in kg, but on height in cm exceeding one metre (0.4 ml/cm). If, however, the height in cm above one metre exceeds the weight in kg, we revert to calculating the volume of anesthetic in ml/kg (0.4 ml/kg).

There has recently been considerable interest in the disintoxicating action of 20 % lipid emulsions in cases of acute intoxication due to local anesthetics. The first study published on this subject was a report by Weinberg et al. in 1998, demonstrating that the toxic dose of bupivacaine that induced asystole in rats was altered by a lipid infusion. Five years later, the same author published a second article in which he demonstrated that the lipid infusion, administered to dogs in which bupivacaine toxicity was induced, was capable of improving hemodynamics and survival. The first reports on the use of lipid infusion in human subjects as an antidote to the systemic toxicity of local anesthetics were those published by Rosenblatt who used it immediately after resuscitation manoeuvres applied as a result of cardiac arrest, presumably due to bupivacaine and by Litz et al. after ropivacaine-induced cardiac arrest following axillary plexus block. These instances were followed by a report by Zetlaoui et al. who employed lipid infusion as a remedy for intravascular injection of local anesthetic in an ultrasound-guided axillary plexus block and by an article by Stephen Markowitz and Joseph Neal who reported a case of convulsions followed by cardiac arrest at the end of a block of the femoral nerve performed with the aid of electrical nerve stimulation. Another article by David H. Sonsino and Marc Fischler described a case of convulsions followed by cardiac arrest after the injection of 20 ml of 0.75 % ropivacaine in the course of an infraclavicular brachial plexus block, immediately treated (within 2 min of the cardiac arrest) with 50 ml of lipid emulsion. Yet another case was that reported by Hélène Charbonneau who described the rapid and successful treatment with a lipid emulsion of a 19-year-old patient intoxicated by 2 % mepivacaine administered for an axillary block performed under ultrasound guidance together with electrical nerve stimulation.

All these reports of acute intoxication due to intravascular injection in blocks mostly ultrasound-guided demonstrate, as reported by Alexander Gnaho et al., not only the efficacy of the lipid solution, but also the fact that ultrasound guidance does not prevent intravascular injection, because the ultrasound probe may compress the vascular structures, particularly venous structures, making it difficult or impossible to see whether the needle has finished up in a blood vessel or not. These authors even attribute the possible responsibility for the accident to unwanted shifting of the needle off course due to the muscle twitches caused by the electrical nerve stimulator. In this connection, we feel it is appropriate to stress once again that the use of a current intensity—even initial—above 0.5 mA in brachial plexus block is never justifiable because it may stimulate the nerve structures even if the needle tip is just outside the neurovascular bundle. A high current intensity is even less justifiable with the simultaneous use of ultrasound guidance because it is this that enables us to see the progression of the needle towards the nerve. Our job is to stimulate the nerve, and not to subject it to an electroshock!

Lastly, worthy of interest is the report by Marco Baciarello, Giorgio Danelli and Guido Fanelli, who describe the real-time ultrasound visualization of injection of local anesthetic into the femoral artery, interrupted after 4 ml, on observing a hyperechoic variation in the vessel lumen.

8.8 Bezold–Jarisch Syndrome

Bezold–Jarisch syndrome is basically a severe and ingravescent syndrome with a strong vagal component, characterized by bradycardia and hypotension to the point of apnoea. It responds poorly to atropine and better to ephedrine and ethylephrine (Effortil-R), to mention those drugs that are always present and ready on the trolley for regional anesthesia. It obviously also responds to the major catecholamines such as adrenaline and isoproterenol, which, however, are generally hardly ever readily at hand when needed; adrenaline usually has to be fetched from the refrigerator and isoproterenol from the hospital pharmacy.

The first to describe the syndrome was Albert von Bezold in 1867, who, in the Physiology Laboratory of the University of Würzburg, studied the effects of a glucoside alkaloid extracted from a fairly common plant in Europe belonging to the Liliaceae family, namely *Veratrum album*.

This alkaloid activates all the vagal receptors at the cardiopulmonary level. These early studies were later taken up again and developed in greater depth by Adolf Jarisch Junior in 1940.

The syndrome may occur in two apparently very different types of anesthetic block, that is to say subarachnoid anesthesia and interscalene blocks. There are those, like Kinsella and Tuckey, who deny that this is a vasovagal syndrome. In any event, its occurrence is made more severe by the presence of conditions of hypovolemia and, for the same reason, is favored by the seated position which gives rise to hypovolemic stasis in the lower limbs. It may also occur as a result of intravascular injection of local anesthetic.

But how do we explain its occurrence in two so very different anesthetic blocks as the subarachnoid block and the proximal block of the brachial plexus? One of the mechanisms whereby the syndrome may occur consists in the involvement of the cardiac sympathetic system. This is known to derive from the three cervical ganglia—upper, middle and lower (or stellate)—which give rise to the three cardiac nerves

—superior, middle and inferior. The thoracic sympathetic system, starting from the metameres of the lateral horns of T3, T4 and T5, also makes a substantial contribution. We are, however, well aware of the anatomical variability and of how approximate the neurovegetative innervation can be: it is by no means impossible that the competent paravertebral ganglia may be T2, T3 and T4, or T4, T5 and T6. This is what Winnie would call a prefixed or postfixed cardiac sympathetic plexus.

So, a hyperbaric anesthetic introduced at the level of L2–L3, if the patient is lying in the supine position, rises towards the upper metameres following the clivus of the lumbar lordosis and stops at the level of the dorsal kyphosis, T6. If, for anatomical or clinical reasons (even a slight Trendelenburg position), the anesthetic rises beyond that limit, it may easily enter the area of competence of the cardiac sympathetic system, possibly postfixed.

On the other hand, a considerable volume of anesthetic, injected at the interscalene level, may find a cleavage plane at the level of the deep cervical fascia, descending along which, under the effect of gravity, it may reach the first thoracic segments of the paravertebral sympathetic chain, above all in a patient in the seated position. It is no accident that the syndrome may set in even as much as an hour after performing the block—the time it takes to make its way towards the thoracic portion of the cardiac sympathetic system—and this may come on top of other contributory factors such as hypovolemic stasis in the lower limbs (due to sympathetic lumbar block in spinal anesthesia or in the 'beach-chair' position, often used in operations on the shoulder) (Fig. 8.1).

The therapy, as mentioned above, consists in the administration of vagolytic and sympathicomimetic drugs, simultaneously accelerating the fluid infusion rate, this latter being an

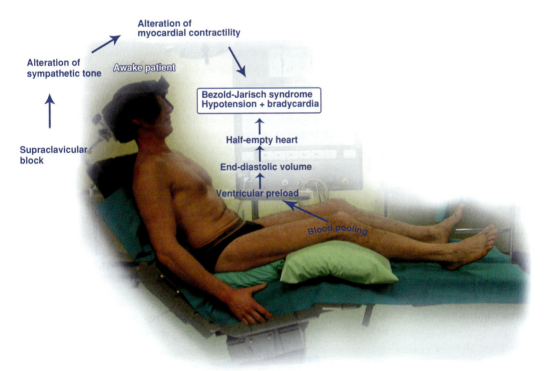

Fig. 8.1 Etiopathogenetic mechanism of Bezold–Jarisch syndrome. The patient is reclining in the 'beach-chair' position. Therapy: pharmacological treatment + Trendelenburg position, if necessary

inadequate measure when used alone, but one which is implemented in the sense of 'every little helps', also because the increased fluid flow rate in the venous system of the arm acts as a vehicle for the rapid delivery of the drugs to the heart. If necessary, the patient should be transferred in the Trendelenburg position; obviously, not in the case of spinal anesthesia, where only the legs may be raised.

As far as the drugs are concerned, we make abundant use of atropine above the classically recommended dose of 0.01 mg/kg; in certain situations, a 1 mg bolus is perfectly justified. If this administration fails to work within one minute, and in severe cases immediately afterwards, we resort to the use of ephedrine, the sympatheticomimetic agent of choice and first-line drug in these situations. Ephedrine acts in two ways: it increases the release of noradrenaline, the depletion of which in the presynaptic deposits explains the tachyphylaxis of the drug; it also acts as a monoamine oxidase inhibitor (MAOI) which does not cross the blood–brain barrier and therefore has no unwanted central effects. This second mechanism explains the relatively long duration of the effects achieved. The best way of using the drug is in low repeat doses at brief time intervals until the desired effect is obtained and without running the risk of exaggerating. Other drugs can be used if ephedrine fails to yield an adequate response and to prolong the results obtained. On the basis of our experience, these may be dopamine, metaraminol and adrenaline. If cardiac arrest occurs, we refer the reader to the classic treatises of resuscitation.

8.9 Claude Bernard-Horner Syndrome (Miosis–Ptosis–Enophthalmos)

Claude Bernard-Horner... who was he? But was he just one person... with two French Christian forenames and a German surname.... or were they two people, or perhaps even three?

Our textbooks never explain this.

Claude Bernard (1813–1878) was French, a disciple of Magendie, at whose death he took over the post of Professor of Experimental Medicine in Paris. He described the syndrome in 1862.

Johann Friedrich Horner (1831–1886) was a Swiss ophthalmologist and Professor at Zurich University. He described the syndrome in 1869.

Rather than a complication, this sequela is regarded as a side effect, which normally regresses within 24 h. It is attributable to a block of the cervical sympathetic system. For this reason, the afferences to the ciliary ganglion are severed, which explains the miosis. Obviously, in the case of multiple traumas, with the simultaneous presence of head injuries, the block is to be avoided because, after an anesthetic block performed for surgery of the humerus and/or shoulder, the patient would present with a certain anisocoria persisting for several hours, which would seriously confound the neurosurgeon. As regards the drooping eyelid, it is not a real ptosis; the third cranial nerve, the common oculomotor nerve, is intact and, more specifically, the palpebral ramus of its upper terminal branch is intact. Palpebral 'ptosis', in contrast, is due to sympathetic block of the superior tarsal nerve, which innervates the smooth muscle fibres of the tarsus (a fibroelastic lamina endowed with Müller's tarsal muscles), thus giving rise not so much to ptosis as to a relaxation of the eyelid and therefore a narrowing of the palpebral rim.

And what about the enophthalmos? The same explanation goes for this problem, too. Tenon's capsule, which is attached to the circumference of the eye socket and envelops the eyeball in a manner resembling a truncated cone, is endowed with smooth muscle fibres innervated by the sympathetic nervous system, which gives them a more or less constant tone. In the eventuality of hyperthyroidism, in fact, characterized by sympathetic hypertonia, exophthalmos may occur; the formation of primary retrobulbar fat, which is often regarded as being the cause of exophthalmos, is only secondary to the space created by the protrusion of the eyeball (*natura abhorret vacuum*—'Nature abhors a vacuum'). In the case of a sympathetic block, the opposite to what happens in hyperthyroidism occurs, namely enophthalmos.

There is no treatment for Claude Bernard-Horner syndrome; one can only warn the patient that the syndrome will probably occur and that, as in Murphy's law, even if one were able to take all and heaven knows what imaginable precautions, it would happen all the same. Obviously, the patient must also be reassured that the syndrome will disappear by the following morning (amyelinic fibres remain anesthetized longer than myelinic fibres). The statistical incidence of the syndrome varies according to the different authors and block techniques. According to Al-Khafaji & Elias, it ranges from 18 to 98 %.

As far as the middle interscalene block is concerned, in a study of ours in 692 patients, the incidence of Claude Bernard-Horner syndrome was 93.5 %.

8.10 Recurrent Nerve Block (Some Good May Come of it)

The right recurrent laryngeal nerve stems from the vagus nerve at the base of the neck in front of the subclavian artery and, after looping around it from front to back, travels medially following the right margin of the oesophagus. After emitting the middle cardiac branches, the tracheal, pharyngeal and oesophageal branches, it terminates in a portion called the inferior laryngeal nerve. The latter splits into an anterior and a posterior branch: the anterior branch innervates the cricoarytenoid, oblique thyroarytenoid, aryepiglottic, thyroepiglottic and vocal muscles; the posterior branch travels to the posterior cricoarytenoid and the transverse arytenoid muscles, anastomosing finally with the internal branch of the superior laryngeal nerve to form Galen's loop. The left recurrent laryngeal nerve stems from the vagus nerve at the level of the aortic arch and after looping around it, as the right recurrent nerve does with the subclavian artery, it ascends along the anterior surface of the oesophagus, behaving and terminating in the same way as its right-side counterpart.

The spread of the anesthesia to the inferior laryngeal nerve is relatively infrequent and, in any case, unpredictable. The various authors report differing statistical data. According to Ward, recurrent nerve block is present in 3 % of cases. According to Urmey, the dysphonia is due not so much to the recurrent nerve block as to the concomitant block of the sympathetic system: by giving rise to secondary vasodilation of the pharyngeal and laryngeal vessels, this may cause oedema of the vocal cords (true and false) on the same side as the block with impairment of the vocal mechanisms.

In our study of 692 patients, using the middle interscalene block, we registered the phenomenon in 0.9 % of cases. Intuitively, it seems more likely to occur with the techniques that involve a closer approach to the cervical spine and in proportion to the volume of anesthetic used. A recurrent nerve block is generally resolved by the day after the intervention, again depending on the anesthetic used. Rather than being a complication, it is an embarrassing side effect. It is embarrassing for the patient who finds it hard to communicate with relatives who come to see him or her and for the anesthetist who has to reassure them that the phenomenon is only transitory. I remember the case of a loquacious lady whose husband forestalled any attempt at reassurance on my part by asking me: 'She's going to stay that way, isn't she?'

8.11 Bronchospasm

In epidural or subarachnoid anesthesia, the rare cases of bronchospasm are explicable in terms of an extension of the anesthetic block to the thoracic metameres, which nullifies the sympathetic innervation of the bronchial system by boosting vagal activity. It is, however, more difficult to find this mechanism responsible in the case of a proximal block of the brachial plexus, postulating an extension of the block in a caudal direction along the thoracic paravertebral sympathetic chain. If this were the case, as Shah and Hirschman have pointed out, the phenomenon would be unilateral. In any event, this eventuality, albeit rare, makes it even more inadvisable to subject patients who have a positive history for episodes of an asthmatic type to a supraclavicular block of the brachial plexus.

Bibliography

Aiazzi Mancini M, Donatelli L (1969) Trattato di farmacologia. Vallardi Editore, Milano

Alemanno F, Egarter-Vigl E (2010) Lesioni Nervose. In: Pippa P, Busoni P (eds) Anestesia Locoregionale. Verduci Editore, Roma

Al-Khafaji JM, Ellias MA (1986) Incidence of Horner's syndrome with interscalene brachial plexus block and its importance in the management of head injury. Anesthesiology 64:127–131

Baciarello M, Danelli G, Fanelli G (2009) Real-time ultrasound visualization of intravascular injection of local anesthetic during a peripheral nerve block. Reg Anesth Pain Med 34:278–279

Barutell C, Vidal F, Raich M, Montero A (1980) A neurological complication following brachial plexus block. Anesthesia 35:365–367

Benumof JL (2000) Permanent loss of cervical spinal cord function associated with interscalene block performed under general anesthesia. Anesthesiology 93:1541–1544

Bernard C (1862) Des phénomènes oculo-pupillaires produits par la section du nerf sympathique cervical: ils sont indépendants des Phénomènes vasculaires calorifiques de la tête. Comptes rendus de l'Accamédie des sciences, Paris 55:381–388

Borgeat A, Blumenthal S (2007) Unintended destination of local anesthetics. In: Neal JM, Rathmell JP (eds) Complications in regional anesthesia & pain medicine. Saunders Elsevier, Philadelphia, p 196

Charbonneau H, Marcou TA, Mazoit JX, Zetlaoui PJ, Benhamou D (2009) Early use of lipid emulsion to treat incipient mepivacaine intoxication. Reg Anesth Pain Med 34:277–278

Finucane BT (1999) Complications of regional anesthesia. Churchill Livingstone, New York, Edinburgh, Philadelphia, San Francisco

Ganong WF (1971) Fisiologia medica. Piccin Editore, Padova

Gasparetto A, Torelli L (1964) Il 4-idrossibutirrato di sodio come "farmaco base" in anestesie cliniche plurimedicamentose. Acta Anaesthesiologica It 15(I):27–51

Gnaho A, Erieuz S, Gentili M (2009) Cardiac arrest during an ultrasound-guided sciatic nerve block combined with nerve stimulation. Reg Anesth Pain Med 34:278

Horner JF. Über eine Form von Ptosis. Klinische Monatsblätter für Augenheilkunde, Stuttgart 7:193–198

Kinsella SM, Tuckey JP (2001) Perioperative bradycardia and asystole: Relationship to vasovagal syncope and the Bezold-Jarisch reflex. Br J Anaesth 86:859–868

Knoblanche GE (1979) Incidence and aetiology of phrenic nerve blockade associated with supraclavicular brachial plexus block. Anaesth Intens Care 7:346–349

Liguori GA (2007) Hemodynamic complications. In: Neal JM, Rathmell JP (eds) Complications in regional anesthesia & pain medicine. Saunders Elsevier, Philadelphia

Litz RJ, Popp M, Stehr SN, Koch T (2006) Successful resuscitation of a patient with ropivacaina-induced asystole after axillary plexus block using lipid infusion. Anesthesia 61:800–801

Meneghelli V, Nussdorfer GG (1977) Il sistema nervoso dell'uomo. Edizioni CLEUP, Padova

Moore DC (1969) Anestesia regionale. Piccin Editore, Padova

Neal JM, Moore IM, Kopacz DJ, Liu SS, Kramer DJ, Plorde JJ (1998) Quantitative analysis of respiratory, motor and sensory function after supraclavicular block. Anesth Analg 86:1239–1244

Neal JM, Rathmell JP (2007) Complications in regional anesthesia & pain medicine. Saunders Elsevier, Philadelphia

Neal JM (2007) Neuraxis mechanical injury. In: Neal JM, Rathmell JP (eds) Complications in regional anesthesia & pain medicine. Saunders Elsevier, Philadelphia

Paqueron X (2006) Guida pratica di anestesia locoregionale. Fogliazza Editore, Milano

Rice ASC, Mc Mahon SB (1992) Peripheral nerve injury caused by injection needles used in regional anaesthesia: influence of bevel configuration studied in a rat model. Br J Anaesth 69:433

Rosenblatt MA, Abel M, Fischer GW, Itzkovich CJ, Eisenkraft JB (2006) Successful use of a 20% lipid emulsion to resuscitate a patient after a presumed ropivacaina-related cardiac arrest. Anesthesiology 105:217–218

Santayana G (1903) The life of reason: reason in common science. Scribner, New York

Selander D, Dhunér KG, Lundborg G (1977) Peripheral nerve injury due to injection needles used for regional anaesthesia. Acta Anaesthsiol Scand 21:182

Shah MB, Hirschman DA (1985) Sympathetic blockade cannot explain bronchospasm following interscalene brachial plexus block. Anesthesiology 62:847–848

Sites BD, Brull R, Chan VW, Spence BC, Gallagher J, Beach ML, Sites VR, Abbas S, Hartman GS (2010) Artifacts and pitfall errors associated with ultrasound-guided regional anesthesia: Part II: A pictorial approach to understanding and avoidance. Reg Anesth Pain Med 35(2 Suppl):S81–S92

Sites BD, Brull R, Chan VW, Spence BC, Gallagher J, Beach ML, Sites VR, Abbas S, Hartman GS (2007) Artifacts and pitfall errors associated with U.S. guided regional anesthesia. Part II: a pictorial approach to understanding and avoidance. Reg Anesth Pain Med 32(5):419–433

Sonsino DH, Fischler M (2009) Immediate intravenous lipid infusion in the successful resuscitation of ropivacaine-induced cardiac arrest after infraclavicular brachial plexus block. Reg Anesth Pain Med 34:276–277

Stiller B (1907) Die asthenische Konstitutionskrankheit. Enke, Stuttgart

Thompson GE, Rorie DK (1983) Functional anatomy of the brachial plexus sheaths. Anesthesiology 59:117–122

Urmey W (2000) Tecniche di Anestesia Loco-Regionale e di Terapia Antalgica. Promo Leader Service Editore, Firenze, Settembre

Urmey WF (2007) Pulmonary Complications. In: Neal JM, Rathmel IP (eds) Complcations in regional anesthesia & pain medicine. Saunders Elsevier, Philadelphia

Ward ME (1974) Interscalene approach to brachial plexus. Anesthesia 29:147–157

Weinberg GL, VadeBoncouer T, Ramaraju GA, Garcia-Amaro MF, Cwik MJ (1998) Pretreatment or resuscitation with a lipid infusion shifts the dose-response to bupivacaine-induced asystole in rats. Anesthesiology 88:1071–1075

Winnie AP, Nader AM (2001) Santayana's prophecy fulfilled. Reg Anesthesia Pain Med 26(6):558–564

Zetlaoui PJ, Labbe JP, Benhamou D (2008) Ultrasound guidance for axillary plexus block does not prevent intravascular injection. Anesthesiology 108:761

Infraclavicular Brachial Plexus Block

9

M. Bosco and A. Clemente

9.1 Introduction

The ideal brachial plexus block should rapidly produce complete anesthesia of the upper arm, forearm and hand, permit stable positioning of a catheter and be almost entirely free of side effects and complications. It should be possible to perform the block without having to place the arm in any particular position and be effective even with just a single puncture. The infraclavicular brachial plexus block is a good candidate.

In this chapter, we will be adopting a scheme illustrated in a previous review by Tran et al. distinguishing between the term 'approach', meaning the access route to the brachial plexus (interscalene, supraclavicular, infraclavicular, axillary, midhumeral), and the term 'technique', referring to the mode whereby the plexus is located (paraesthesia, neurostimulation, ultrasonography), or the endpoint, that is to say the target predetermined before injecting the local anesthetic (type of contraction elicited, one or more injections, etc.).

The various aspects that make up the vast subject matter of infraclavicular blocks will be analysed paying particular attention to what has been described and demonstrated in the literature in keeping with the dictates of evidence-based medicine. Anesthetists have always shown a certain amount of interest in this approach to the brachial plexus, asking themselves numerous questions for which they have come up with answers in the course of recent decades on the basis of a whole series of targeted, increasingly accurate scientific studies.

In this chapter, we have attempted to collect these answers and summarize them from the vast body of literature on the subject, as shown by the very substantial suggested reading listed below. We are confident that both the reader approaching the practice of regional anesthesia for the first time and the more experienced anesthetist may find interesting insights here capable of improving their clinical practice to the benefit of the patient and for their own personal and professional satisfaction.

9.2 Anatomy of the Infraclavicular Region

'Regional anesthesia is simply an exercise in applied anatomy' claims Winnie, one of the founding fathers of this discipline, in order to stress the importance of a profound knowledge of anatomy for performing safe and effective peripheral anesthesia.

M. Bosco (✉)
Department of Anesthesiology and Critical Care Medicine, Catholic University of the Sacred Heart, Largo A. Gemelli 1, 00168, Rome, Italy
e-mail: mbosco@rm.unicatt.it

A. Clemente
Anesthesiology, Intensive Care and Pain Therapy Service, IRCCS—Immacolata Dermopathic Institute (IDI), Via dei Monti di Creta 104, 00167, Rome, Italy
e-mail: antonio.clemente@idi.it

The infraclavicular region is clearly delimited superiorly by the bony edge of the clavicle, and inferiorly by the border of the pectoralis major muscle; the deltopectoral groove marks the outer limit, whereas a vertical line from the bony edge proximal to the internal border of the pectoralis major muscle closes off the area medially. From externally to internally, we recognize a surface layer of loose cutaneous and subcutaneous tissue below which we find the aponeurosis of the fascia of the pectoralis major muscle, which, via the deltopectoral groove, extends towards the deltoid muscle. The subsequent plane is identified as the pectoralis major muscle beneath which runs the clavipectoral fascia containing the middle axillary artery and the subclavian muscle and extends to the pectoralis minor muscle. Its deepest part goes on to constitute the anterior wall of the axillary fossa; in the latter, in its more medial part, runs the neurovascular bundle with the axillary vein followed by the artery and the three cords of the brachial plexus that gradually wind around the artery as it travels distally.

Various authors have described different procedures for reaching the brachial plexus by an infraclavicular route, proposing landmarks and indicating connection lines identifying the most suitable point of insertion of the needle. For a deeper understanding of the course of the nerve fibres, it is useful to describe the teaching instrument consisting in the existence of a hypothetical 'anesthetic line' that connects the various points identified by the different approaches to the brachial plexus, ranging from the interscalene to the axillary approach. With the patient in the supine position, with the head turned towards the side contralateral to the side to be anesthetized and the arm abducted 45° in relation to the thorax, a line is traced joining the points on the skin identifying: (A) the apex of the scalene triangle at the level of C5, (B) the mid-point of the clavicle, (C) the deltopectoral groove between the coracoid process and the thorax, and (D) the axillary artery pulse in the armpit (Figs. 9.1 and 9.2).

The visualization of the plexus as a linear structure crossing the fixed anatomical landmarks makes it possible to develop variant versions of the standard techniques, according to clinical needs, for example, by modifying the inclination of the needle in order to obtain a more suitable spread of the local anesthetic or to facilitate the insertion of a perineural catheter.

To the two-dimensional view of the anesthetic line, we can add the third dimension of the depth of the plexus by introducing the concept of

Fig. 9.1 Anesthetic line on the patient (P. Pippa, P. Busoni)

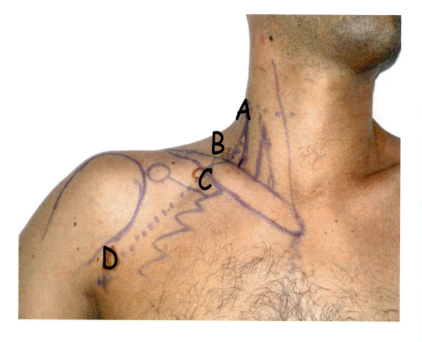

Fig. 9.2 Anesthetic line on a cadaver

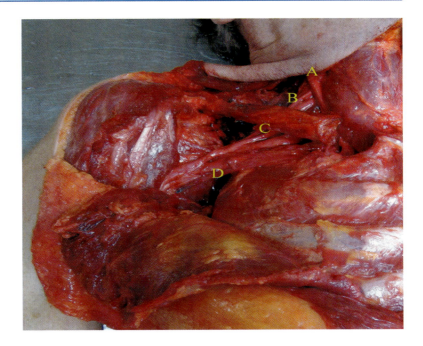

'depth gauging', that is to say the possibility of estimating the depth of the brachial plexus on the basis of surface landmarks, particularly the clavicle. The latter has a sigmoidal shape with the lateral terminal part wider and flatter and an almost cylindrical medial part connected by a curvilinear central section, which covers a segment of the neurovascular bundle, the first rib and the thoracic wall. The application of simple geometric principles to the constant relationship between clavicle and brachial plexus in the vicinity of the coracoid process enables its depth to be gauged with a margin of error of 1 cm. It has been seen, in fact, that as the brachial plexus has an oblique trend, the divergence between its course and that of the clavicle varies on the sagittal plane, proving more constant, however, at 1 cm medially to the coracoid process. In other words, at this point, the plexus finds itself more consistently directly below the clavicle, and therefore, if we imagine a rectangle extending with its longer side from the clavicle to the point of insertion, the shorter side will correspond to the depth of the brachial plexus (Figs. 9.3 and 9.4).

As regards the location of the lung, the more laterally one proceeds, the greater will be the distance between the skin surface and the rib cage, as well as that between the brachial plexus and the parietal pleura.

Knowledge of the anatomical relationships of the structures making up the infraclavicular region helps to identify the most appropriate entry point of the needle for performing a thoroughly safe block. It should not be forgotten, however, that not only the depth but also other variables must be carefully evaluated in the execution of the block, such as the direction of the needle and its inclination in relation to the chest wall.

9.3 Bazy's Technique

The first description of an infraclavicular plexus block dates back to the second decade of the twentieth century just a few years after the advent of Hirschel's and Kulenkampff's techniques. The aim at the time was to overcome the limitations of their techniques such as the incomplete nature of the block in the case of

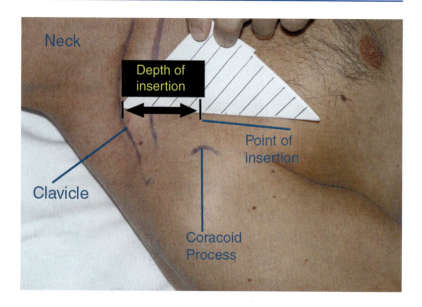

Fig. 9.3 For explanation see text

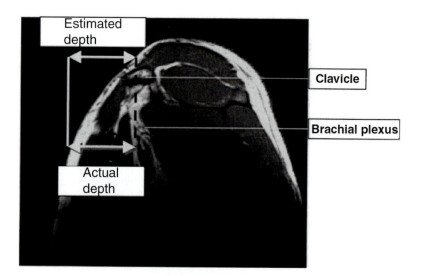

Fig. 9.4 For explanation see text

Hirschel's technique and the frequent reports of complications, particularly pulmonary lesions, with the Kulenkampff's technique.

The French physician Bazy proposed a technique for approaching the brachial plexus at a higher level by inserting the needle below the clavicle in a position immediately medial to the coracoid process. After placing the patient in the supine position with the shoulders resting upon a pillow, the arm was moderately abducted (about 45°) to bring the plexus into a more superficial position and to render the coracoid process more prominent. The anesthetist's position is alongside the patient on the side to be operated on, between the torso and the arm, from where he identifies the so-called anesthetic line, that is, the line from the apex of the coracoid process to Chassaignac's tubercle. The needle, measuring at least 9 mm in length, is directed according to this line in such a way that it barely skirts the posterior edge of the clavicle. Immediately after the needle passes beyond the upper edge, 10 ml of local anesthetic is injected. Without moving the needle, the arm is then flexed and adducted in order to approach closer to the plexus, and a further 10 ml of drug is then injected.

Slight modifications were subsequently made to this procedure, but none of them succeeded in undermining the popularity of the Kulenkampff's technique, which continued to be the technique of choice, relegating the infraclavicular approach to no more than the role of an alternative.

9.4 Raj Technique

A more widespread use of the infraclavicular brachial plexus block came about after the technique was included in Labat's celebrated 1930 textbook entitled *Regional Anesthesia*. It was, however, in 1973 that Raj proposed a new approach for the purposes of overcoming a number of limitations accompanying the most widespread type of block via the axillary route, namely the need to have the patient's arm abducted by even as much as more than 90°; the difficulty encountered in anesthetizing the musculocutaneous or the axillary nerve; and the need to administer additional infiltrations to anesthetize the intercostobrachial nerve, if a tourniquet is used. In the method described by Raj, the patient remains supine with the arm preferably but not necessarily abducted 90°. The needle entry point is determined at a distance of 2.5 cm below the lower edge of the clavicle and particularly on the paramedian line that crosses the point where one succeeds in palpating the pulse of the subclavian artery before it travels deeper beneath the clavicle, or on the line passing through the mid-point of the clavicle. The needle is then directed at a 45° angle to the skin, laterally towards the brachial artery, tracing the so-called Raj line. The success of the block is reported in 95 % of more than 200 patients with no increase in complications such as vascular puncture compared to other approaches.

A more recent study by Wilson et al. conducted with magnetic resonance in volunteers has revealed, however, a substantial degree of anatomical imprecision with this approach, showing an average 26 mm deviation of the 'Raj line' from the target with the consequent need to redirect the needle, increasing the patient's discomfort as well as the risk of complications. Moreover, on evaluating the two landmarks, it was noted that the mid-point of the clavicle is situated approximately 17 mm (9–23 mm) laterally to the subclavian artery pulse, at the edge of the clavicle. The landmarks therefore are not interchangeable in the clinical setting.

This technique has not enjoyed the hoped-for popularity, and few data are available from the clinical studies in which it has been used. There have therefore been many other authors who have proposed different descriptions of new approaches, modifying the needle entry site and reporting various different success and complication rates.

9.5 Coracoid Approach

Again in 1998, Wilson stated that the infraclavicular approach, though effective, was little used owing to the lack of experience of anesthetists who preferred the more familiar axillary block. Verifying this with the study of the anatomy of the infracoracoid region by means of magnetic resonance, he introduced a very simple and safe technique for performing an infraclavicular block. Taking the tip of the coracoid process as a landmark and shifting 2 cm caudally and 2 cm medially, the needle is then introduced in a posterior direction. The needle will thus come into contact with the cords of the brachial plexus, where they surround the second part of the axillary artery at a depth of 4.24 ± 1.49 cm (2.25–7.75 cm) in men and 4.01 ± 1.29 (2.25–6.5 cm) in women (Fig. 9.5).

The validity of this approach has been confirmed in a descriptive study conducted in 150 consecutive patients who were administered 40 ml of 1.5 % mepivacaine plus adrenaline 5

Fig. 9.5 Coracoid approach

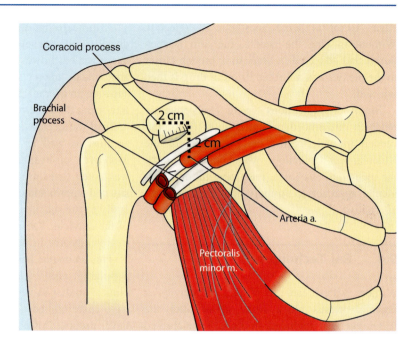

mcg/ml. Wilson et al. stressed the comfortable position of the patient's arm for performing the block, the importance of an easily palpable bony landmark even in obese subjects and the high success rate evaluated as analgesia in the areas of the five terminal nerves of the plexus, particularly when a distal contraction (e.g. movement of the hand or fingers) is sought as an endpoint using the nerve stimulator.

9.5.1 Modified Coracoid Approaches

The renewed interest in infraclavicular blocks has prompted the search for new technical solutions. Minville et al. using clearly identifiable bony landmarks and electrical nerve stimulation, have experimented with a new procedure in 300 patients. They indicated the entry point as lying at a distance of 1 cm below the clavicle and 1 cm medially to the coracoid process. The needle was then directed towards the apex of the axillary fossa at an angle of 45°. Generally speaking, the first contraction elicited was that of the musculocutaneous nerve, when 10 ml of 1.5 % lidocaine was injected with 1:400,000 adrenaline. The needle was then withdrawn 1–2 cm and redirected medially and posteriorly in search of a distal contraction (hand or wrist) with a current intensity ranging from 0.3 to 0.5 mA where another 30 ml of the same solution was administered (Figs. 9.6 and 9.7).

The simplicity of this proposed technique was emphasized by a French study, which demonstrated the remarkable rapidity of the learning curve. In fact, on comparing the characteristics of the block performed by anesthetists with at least two years of experience with those of the block performed by postgraduate students to whom the infraclavicular block had only been explained theoretically, it was seen that there were no differences in success rates, but only in execution times, which, moreover, were not clinically significant.

A modified Raj approach was proposed by Borgeat et al. With the patient in the supine position and the arm in a natural position alongside the body, two landmarks were defined: one lateral, the ventral portion of the acromial process of the scapula; and the other medial, the jugulum. On tracing a line through these two points, one then identifies the pulse of the subclavian artery in the armpit. The patient's head is turned slightly towards the side opposite the one to be operated

9 Infraclavicular Brachial Plexus Block

Fig. 9.6 Minville's coracoid approach (landmarks)

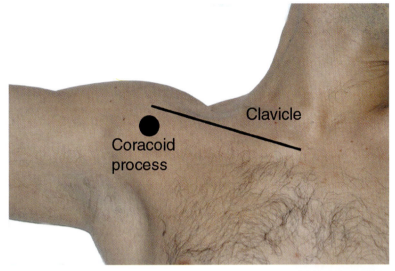

Fig. 9.7 Minville's coracoid approach (anatomical projection)

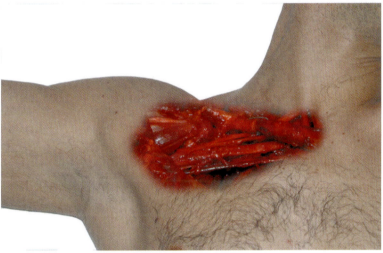

on, while the arm is abducted 90° and raised approximately 30°; the outline of the clavicle is then palpated and marked along its entire length. The entry point lies at a distance of 1 cm caudad to the lower edge of the clavicle at its mid-point. The needle (a 50-mm needle is sufficient) is directed laterally at an angle of 45–60° to the skin towards the point where the axillary artery emerges in the armpit, as close as possible to the lateral border of the pectoralis major muscle (Fig. 9.8).

The injection, after eliciting a distal contraction, yielded an optimal 97 % successes rate without causing pneumothorax and with only 2 % of vascular punctures in 150 patients. The best results were obtained with the distal contraction of the median nerve (flexion of the fingers) because this indicated that the needle tip was approximately in the central region of the plexus, from which the local anesthetic could spread more easily to the ulnar and radial nerves.

The limitations of this technique are the 90° abduction of the arm which may prove painful in traumatized patients and the pain caused by the needle when crossing the pectoralis major

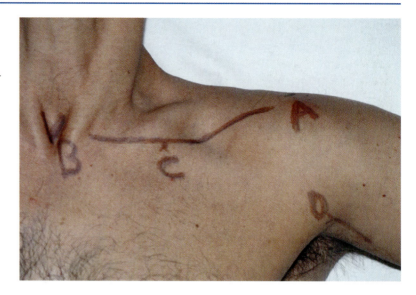

Fig. 9.8 Landmarks for Raj's modified approach. *A* ventral part of the acromial process of the scapula; *B* jugulum; *C* mid-point between *A* and *B*; *D* point of emergence of the axillary artery

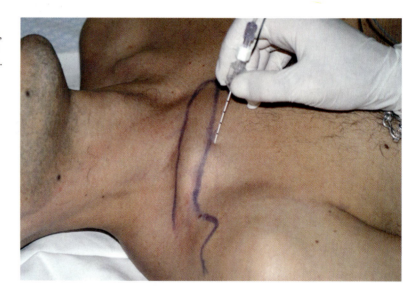

Fig. 9.9 The needle is inserted at the Kilka point, the mid-point between the jugulum and the acromion. The needle orientation is vertical (anteroposterior)

muscle. Mild sedation is particularly indicated with this technique.

9.6 Vertical Approach

The vertical infraclavicular block described by Kilka et al. is performed with the patient in the supine position, with the limb to be anesthetized adducted and the hand on the abdomen. Two landmarks are identified: the jugulum and the ventral part of the acromion. The entry point of the needle (Kilka point) is at the mid-point of the line joining the two landmarks, immediately below the clavicle. The needle is inserted in an anteroposterior direction, perpendicularly to the horizontal plane (Fig. 9.9).

It is estimated that the plexus lies at a depth of 3–4 cm, whereas the pleura lies at a depth of not less than 6 cm. If no contraction is identified at the Kilka point, the needle can be reinserted, again in an anteroposterior direction immediately caudad to the clavicle at a distance of 0.5–1 cm first more laterally and then more medially. If the mid-point of the jugulum–acromion line is lower than the edge of the clavicle, the needle entry point is defined as the crossover point of the lower edge of the clavicle and the sagittal plane passing through the mid-point. Important for the purposes of reducing the risk of pneumothorax is to maintain the perpendicular direction of the needle, avoiding medial deviations. What is more, an excessively medial direction will more easily lead to an accidental vascular puncture.

A radiological study of this approach, conducted by Klaastad et al. using magnetic resonance, in 20 healthy volunteers has confirmed the validity of the indications and precautions suggested. In particular, the authors emphasize the need to pay attention to the risk of pneumothorax, inasmuch as it is impossible to define the safety limits in terms of depth (within a 4–6 cm range, both the plexus and the pleura are to be found), nor can they be predicted on the basis of the patient's anthropometric characteristics, the only definite fact being a greater risk in female subjects. Furthermore, it may be that, in the needle paths suggested, one may encounter vessels, nerves and the first rib that may act as warning signs or barriers before reaching the lung.

9.7 Lateral Approach

For the purposes of substantially reducing the risk of pneumothorax, a technique has been proposed that involves the insertion of the needle in a more lateral site, in order to bring it closer to the cords and further away from the pleura. The lateral approach was studied preliminarily by Klaastad et al. in healthy volunteers in a non-invasive manner with magnetic resonance. The safety profile of the block was confirmed, observing that to make contact with the pleura, it is necessary to double the recommended 45° entry angle of the needle in relation to the skin plane, with both 45° and 90° abduction of the arm, although the authors advise the use of 90° abduction so as to have greater precision of the needle path in reaching the cords as well as a greater distance from the pleura. In that position, a further improvement is offered by a 65° rather than a 90° inclination, or by starting with 40° and gradually increasing the angle to 80°.

The same authors have also attempted to further perfect the lateral infraclavicular block by studying the best inclination of the needle and the risk of coming into contact with the pleura and vessels, leaving the patient's arm alongside the body. The patient is placed in the supine position with the shoulders relaxed, the arm to be operated on adducted, the hand on the abdomen and the head turned slightly towards the contralateral side. The anesthetist takes up position to the rear of the patient's shoulders and, running a finger laterally below the lower edge of the clavicle, identifies the first bony prominence corresponding to the medial surface of the coracoid process. This landmark is easily detectable even in obese patients or in patients with tonic musculature and identifies a sagittal plane in which the needle movements will take place. The needle is inserted tangentially to the antero-inferior edge of the clavicle and directed posteriorly at an angle of 0–30° to the coronal plane. On analysing the images obtained with magnetic resonance, the authors suggest directing the needle initially at an angle of 15° posteriorly and not inserting it to a depth of more than 6.5 cm (Fig. 9.10).

The depth of the plexus and vessels is significantly reduced with age, while the cephalic vein is located more anteriorly in obese patients. However, though the nerve cords often protect the axillary vessels from the needle, the physiological variability advises against performing the block in patients with frank coagulopathy.

The validity of the anatomical assumptions on which the rationale for the lateral infraclavicular block is based has been confirmed also in clinical practice. Ninety-one per cent success, defined as complete anesthesia or analgesia of the area from the elbow downwards, within

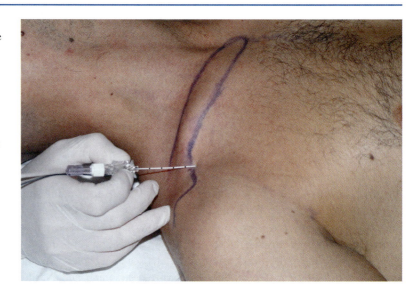

Fig. 9.10 Right infraclavicular region: The coracoid process and the clavicle are clearly observable. The needle is directed at an angle of approximately 15° posterior to the coronal plane. The plexus is estimated to lie at a depth of 4–6.5 cm

20 min of executing the block and a vascular puncture rate of 2 % is among the main advantages observed. The use of the approach in patients has confirmed the depth at which the plexus is detected, but requires an insertion angle greater than 10–12° indicated by the radiological study (as much as 23° on average). The cephalocaudal direction of the needle reduces the risk of accidental haematoma because, while the vascular structures present an anterocaudal course in relation to the plexus, the needle approaches the plexus from the posterior part, as indicated by Koscielniak-Nielsen et al. The results of a study by Gurkan et al. along the same lines in a much larger population of patients, in whom the most effective angle was 25° and the depth at which the plexus was detected 51 mm, showed a success rate of 89.7 %, but also a 6.6 % accidental vascular puncture rate. In both studies, better results were obtained by injecting the local anesthetic at the level of the posterior cord (contraction due to radial nerve stimulus with extension of the wrist and fingers). It should be stressed that the advantages that the lateral infraclavicular block affords can also be exploited in the paediatric population in which it has proved effective and safe both in case reports by Sedeck and Goujard and in studies in larger populations conducted by Gurkan et al.

9.8 Infraclavicular Block Using Neurostimulation

9.8.1 Which Current Threshold?

The use of the electrical nerve stimulator to identify cords of the brachial plexus makes the execution of the infraclavicular block safer when compared to eliciting paraesthesias, but what is the appropriate current threshold for the injection of local anesthetic?

In an editorial by Joseph Neal published in 2001 in the second edition of *Regional Anesthesia and Pain Medicine*, the author wondered how 'near' sufficiently near was and came to the conclusion that a current of 0.5 mA constituted a safe threshold for avoiding neuronal damage while at the same time ensuring that the needle was close enough to the plexus to enable the block to be successful. Attempts to reduce it failed to lead to better success rates. Even so, for the infraclavicular block, this indication has been called into question in an attempt to lower the threshold to 0.3 mA with the idea of increasing the success rate of the technique by approaching closer to the cords, without, however, inducing neurological damage. In fact, in a group of 188 patients submitted to coracoid infraclavicular block, Wilson reported that the patient group in which the stimulation current was reduced to 0.1–0.3 mA presented a higher success rate than in patients stimulated with current values ranging from 0.3 to 0.5 mA (84.7 % vs. 67.1 %, $p < 0.05$), findings later confirmed by Gu et al. In an observational study conducted by Keschner et al. the authors stress that the 0.3 mA threshold induced no neurological damage in 288 patients, with a success rate of 94 %. In a telephone interview 24 h postoperatively, a number of patients complained of mild disturbances but all of these had resolved by the time of the first postoperative visit, carried out at most 7 days later. Thus, the execution of an infraclavicular block with a low current threshold (0.2–0.3 mA) is a safe and efficacious method.

9.8.2 Which Type of Contraction?

The infraclavicular block, if it is to be successful, needs to anesthetize all three of the cords that make up the plexus at that level. It is important to recognize which type of contraction identifies the cord that innervates the relevant area of the surgical operation, but this association is not as simple a task as it might seem. Our understanding of the anatomy of the bronchial plexus is incomplete. In the infraclavicular space, the brachial plexus is remodelled and the various terminal branches depart from the three cords at different, non-constant levels varying from person to person. What is more, in the course of this transition the nerve fibres rotate around the axillary artery, taking up different positions as they move distally.

To simplify the understanding of the association between muscle contraction and stimulation of a given cord, the analysis made in a technical report by Borene et al. proves very effective and elegant, concluding with the observation that the direction of movement of the fifth finger in a limb in the anatomical position, and indicates which cord is being stimulated. In detail, the lateral cord is the result of the merging of the anterior divisions of the upper and middle trunks. From this, the following nerves depart: the musculocutaneous nerve (biceps muscle, coracobrachialis muscle, flexor muscles of the arm and the medial portion of the brachialis muscle), the lateral portion of the median nerve (pronator teres muscle, flexor carpi radialis muscle, flexor pollicis longus muscle, flexor digitorum profundus muscle, from the lateral half to the second finger, the first two lumbricals and the abductor pollicis brevis muscle) and the lateral pectoral nerve. Its stimulation causes flexion of the elbow, pronation of the forearm, contraction of the lumbricals and of the muscles of the thenar eminence with consequent movement of the fifth finger laterally. The medial cord proceeds from the anterior division of the lower trunk and forms the medial pectoral nerve, the medial brachialis nerve, the anterior brachial cutaneous nerve, the medial part of the median nerve and the ulnar nerve (flexor carpi ulnaris, palmar brevis, flexor digitorum profundus, from the medial part to the fourth and fifth fingers, the palmar and dorsal interosseous muscles, the third and fourth lumbrical and the hypothenar eminence). The primary contraction of this cord is precisely that of the ulnar nerve which, by stimulating all these flexor muscles of the hand with an ulnar deviation of the wrist, induces the fifth finger to move medially. Lastly, the posterior cord stems from the merging of the posterior divisions of all three trunks, giving rise to the subscapular nerves (teres major muscle and subscapularis muscle), the thoracodorsal nerve (latissimus dorsi muscle), the axillary nerve (deltoid and teres minor muscles) and the radial nerve (triceps brachii muscle, lateral portion of the brachialis muscle, the group of extensor supinator muscles). Its stimulation will induce contraction of the extensor muscles of the forearm, hand and fingers with stimulation also of the deltoid muscle. The fifth finger will then appear to move posteriorly in relation to its anatomical position.

Borgeat, in his previously analysed description of the variant of the Raj technique, had underlined that searching for a 'distal' contraction, defined as the movement of the wrist or fingers, when compared to a 'proximal' contraction (contraction of the biceps, triceps, flexor carpi muscles), yielded a distinctly better success rate (97 vs. 44 %). An attempt was therefore made to analyse any difference in the choice of cord to be stimulated in order to obtain an efficacious block with distal contraction. Comparison between proximal stimulation of the musculocutaneous nerve and a distal contraction due to stimulation of the median nerve, revealed a reduced onset time and greater efficacy in the latter group. Yet, despite the fact that the majority of the patients did not request any supplement for surgery, either in the group with 'distal' contraction or in that with 'proximal' contraction, the percentages of paralysis and complete anesthesia of the upper limb after 20 min were low (paralysis 40 vs. 24 %, anesthesia 19 vs. 8 %, respectively). More promising results were obtained with stimulation of the posterior cord, even with minimal current thresholds (0.3 mA), presenting an earlier onset and a reduced failure rate when compared to stimulation of the medial or lateral cords according to Lecamwasam et al. Similarly, Bloc et al. reported that eliciting a distal contraction due to stimulation of the radial nerve achieved a greater success rate of the block defined as complete anesthesia of the limb, compared with distal contractions due to stimulation of the median or ulnar nerves (90 vs. 74 and 68 %, respectively). A radial-type contraction was confirmed as being the most effective also in those cases in which a double stimulation technique was opted for. In fact, using the first to block the musculocutaneous nerve, the choice of the second proved to have an effect on the efficacy of the block and, in particular, a second, radial-type contraction was associated with a 96 % success rate when compared to 89 % with median nerve stimulation and 90 % with ulnar nerve stimulation, as reported by Minville et al.

9.8.3 How Many Stimulations?

Being able to perform a block with a single injection would certainly be simpler and faster to execute, would cause less tissue trauma and risk of vascular puncture and would prove less painful for the patient. Furthermore, when performing a continuous block, the standard technique typically envisages a single injection. Despite the good success rates of blocks performed with a single injection, in an attempt to improve the efficacy even more, the effects of a larger number of stimulations were evaluated. In particular, Rodriguez et al. studied the differences between single, double and triple stimulation using the same total dose of local anesthetic. The injection of 40 ml of 1.5 % mepivacaine in a single administration proved less efficacious in terms of both sensory and motor blockade compared to two injections of 20 ml each. In addition, Rodriguez et al. comparing a single injection of 42 ml with two injections of 21 ml or three injections of 14 ml each, found that the groups receiving double or triple stimulation achieved better results, though presenting statistically significant differences between them. In both these studies, however, no particular type of contraction was sought nor did the authors specify which contractions were effectively found. The same objection can be levied against another study, conducted by Gaertner et al. comparing a single aspecific injection of 30 ml of a mixture of 0.5 % bupivacaine and 2 % lidocaine with triple stimulation, revealing a substantial increase in the success rate from 40 to 72.5 % with the triple stimulation ($p < 0.0001$).

Whereas, in the case of single stimulation, it is particularly the posterior cord that is sought and therefore the contractions typical of the radial nerve; comparing this with a double stimulation of the other main nerves excluding the radial nerve, interesting results are reported. In the single radial stimulation group, Rodrigiez et al. observed that significantly higher rates of complete anesthesia of the upper limb below the elbow were obtained compared with the double injection.

9.9 Infraclavicular Block and Ultrasound

The advent of ultrasound in the context of regional anesthesia has enormously stimulated the search for its possible applications in peripheral nerve blocks. The infraclavicular block was one of the first to be revisited in the light of the promising innovation of direct visualization of the anatomical structures, which previously could only be located by guesswork on the basis of surface landmarks and by electrical nerve stimulation. Moreover, we know that these landmarks may sometimes be hard to identify in certain types of patients, for example, in obese subjects, just as there may be anatomical variations that increase the difficulty of identifying nerves, thus increasing the risk of puncturing blood vessels. As regards the infraclavicular block in particular, we have seen that eliciting a peripheral contraction is necessary for the success of the block and the search for this contraction may mean that the block takes longer to perform.

If the visualization of anatomical structures helps to avoid complications such as vascular puncture and pneumothorax, can we safely use a more proximal approach in such a way as to anesthetize the three cords before they distance their course from that of the subclavian artery?

Ootaki et al. were among the first to apply ultrasonography in conjunction with infraclavicular blocks using a 7 MHz linear probe to visualize the vascular structures below the midpoint of the clavicle. Taking as their landmark the image of the subclavian artery, they surrounded the latter with local anesthetic by injecting 30 ml of 1.5 % lidocaine to the right and left of the artery, assuming that the cords, at that level, would be very close to the vessel. Ninety-five per cent of the patients underwent the operation without additional supplementation 30 min after execution of the block, and no complications occurred in any of them.

Instead of the 'perivascular' injection, a further proposal was to perform a 'perineural' injection, possibly at a more distal level where the three cords could be better identified and distinguished from the subclavian artery. A 3.5 MHz transthoracic ultrasonographic probe was used at the coracoid level to visualize the vessels and the three cords of the brachial plexus below the pectoralis minor muscle (Fig. 9.11).

Again under ultrasound guidance, an 18-gauge Tuohy needle was then inserted and directed in such a way as to inject approximately 10 ml of 2 % lidocaine around each of the three cords of the plexus. Sandhu and Capan reported that the onset time with this method was considerably reduced, complete anesthesia being

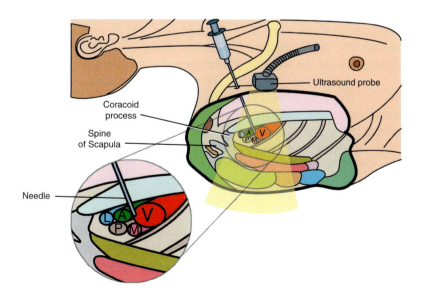

Fig. 9.11 Ultrasound-guided infraclavicular block

obtained after 6.7 ± 3.2 min in approximately 91 % of patients.

In the study by Ootaki et al. the arm to be operated on was positioned resting comfortably alongside the patient's body, whereas in the study by Sandhu and Capan, the arm was abducted 90°. When using ultrasonography, the problem of the position of the arm to be operated on is of practically no account, since the anatomical structures are in any case identified, and the anesthetist seeks to maintain his view of the needle as it advances in real time. For the sake of completeness, we should add that a study has effectively been conducted by Wang et al. to assess the influence of four different arm positions on the topographical anatomy of the infraclavicular region ultrasonographically, showing that 90° abduction with external rotation of the shoulder causes the brachial plexus to approach much closer to the skin (1.67 cm) and further away from the pleura (1.15 cm).

9.9.1 How Many Injections and on Which Cords?

Even with ultrasonography, we can still aim at performing a single administration of local anesthetic or at directing the needle in such a way as to inject the drug in two or three different positions. As in the case of electrical nerve stimulation, any movement of the needle, despite being under ultrasound guidance, may increase the possibility of damaging the surrounding tissues and reducing patient comfort.

In a randomized controlled study of 88 patients, Tran et al. studied the results of double versus single injection without observing any differences in terms of onset times, block execution times, success rates or incidence of adverse events. Even a triple injection failed to prove in any way superior to a single injection, particularly when performed directly on the posterior cord of the plexus, according to Desgagnes et al. On the contrary, in a study by Fredrickson et al. the injection of 30 ml of 2 % lidocaine posteriorly to the subclavian artery compared to three injections of 10 ml each aimed separately at the three cords of the plexus was associated not only with a faster execution time but also with a greater efficacy rate at 20 min on all the nerves involved.

Even with the use of electrical nerve stimulation alone, it has been demonstrated that contraction of the distal muscles innervated by the radial nerve is predictive of higher success rates compared to contractions due to stimulation of the median or ulnar nerve. Ultrasonography has revealed that the injection of local anesthetic, when the contractions due to radial nerve stimulation are induced with a current intensity of approximately 0.3 mA, corresponds to a spread of the anesthetic posteriorly to the artery (or on the posterior cord of the plexus) with a shift of the artery upwards and medially (Bloc et al.). This produces a block with a higher success rate compared to a contraction induced by the median nerve which, however, gives rise to a more superficial spread of local anesthetic. A study conducted in 218 patients was specifically designed to evaluate ultrasonographically and with the aid of the electrical nerve stimulator the difference in success rates of blocks aimed selectively at one cord of the brachial plexus in particular. Injection in the central area on the posterior cord produced an effective block in 96 % of cases compared to the 85 % of more peripheral locations: In particular, the success rates for the single cords were 99 % for the posterior cord, 92 % for the lateral cord and only 84 % for the medial cord, as reported by Bowens et al.

With these premises, Tran et al. proposed the so-called double bubble technique for the infraclavicular block. Under ultrasound guidance with a sterile coated 5–10-MHz linear probe, the infracoracoid region is visualized according to a coronal section with the patient in the supine position and with the arm comfortably resting alongside the body. A 100 mm needle is introduced in a downward direction according to the long axis of the probe ('in-plane' technique) and is directed below the subclavian/axillary artery. The injection of local anesthetic will produce a roundish hypoechoic image exactly below the circular, non-

9 Infraclavicular Brachial Plexus Block

Fig. 9.12 Ultrasound 'double bubble' sign after injection of local anesthetic (LA) posteriorly to the axillary artery (A). Note the roundish, non-compressible axillary artery image unlike the axillary vein (V)

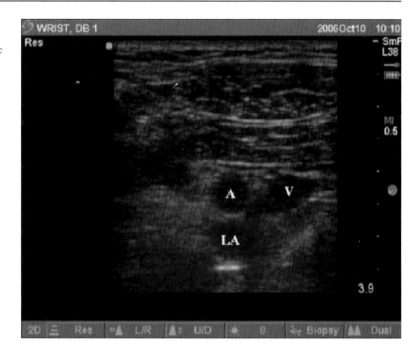

compressible cross section of the artery which will then be enveloped by the spread of the anesthetic (Fig. 9.12). This 'double bubble' ultrasound sign has proved to be indicative of the success of the infraclavicular block.

When directing the needle towards the posterior cord, one often encounters a resistance corresponding anatomically to a fascia investing the axillary artery which must be overcome in order to obtain an adequate spread of local anesthetic with an effective block, as indicated by Morimoto et al. This fascia might also explain the cases of failure of the block with neurostimulation alone despite a good elicited contraction. In addition, Dolan points out that it may be present not only in the posteromedial quadrant but also in the superior quadrant.

9.9.2 Other Proposed Techniques

We can summarize the main ultrasound-guided techniques suggested for performing infraclavicular blocks as belonging to three categories: lateral, medial and posterior.

The lateral approach is performed with the patient in the supine position with the arm adducted close to the side and using the coracoid process as a surface landmark. The probe is positioned below this, and the vascular and nerve structures are identified. The needle is introduced 2–4 cm above the probe at an angle of 45° to the skin in a caudal direction. With the medial approach, on the other hand, the patient's arm is abducted by up to 110°, the shoulder is rotated externally, and the elbow flexed 90°. The probe is placed at the apex of the deltopectoral groove and, in this case too, the needle entry point is 2–4 cm above the probe at an angle of 45° to the skin and in a caudal direction. Both approaches afford excellent anesthesia, but with the medial approach, the plexus is closer to the surface and easier to visualize, which makes for shorter block execution times. The lateral approach, however, certainly presents the advantage of reducing the risk of pneumothorax, but increases that of vascular puncture. Nevertheless, according to Bigeleisen and Wilson, it remains the approach to be preferred in those cases in which the patient is unable to abduct the arm.

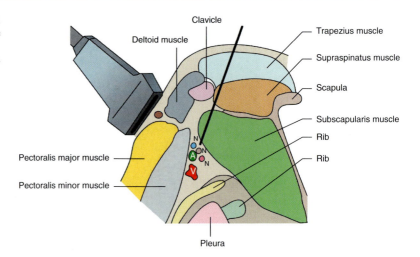

Fig. 9.13 Coronal section showing the position of the probe and the needle inserted as far as the cords of the brachial plexus

In both the preceding approaches, the needle is introduced at an angle of about 45°, which gives rise to a loss of definition in visualizing the body and tip of the needle as it gradually penetrates more deeply. To avoid this problem, a posterior approach has been proposed. The probe is positioned longitudinally below the edge of the clavicle and medially to the coracoid process. The needle insertion point is over the trapezius muscle, posteriorly enough to permit the passage between the clavicle and the scapula, maintaining a close alignment with the long axis of the probe (Fig. 9.13).

9.10 Ultrasound Versus Neurostimulation

Various authors have wondered whether or not the advent of ultrasonography in the execution of peripheral blocks can replace the consolidated use of electrical nerve stimulation. Undoubtedly, the choice of one or the other of these techniques cannot be made without considering the economic aspects. Not all care centres can afford to purchase an ultrasound appliance despite the fact that the cost of such equipment has decreased considerably in recent years. An attempt has been made by Sandhu et al. to quantitate the cost of the two techniques, showing that the use of ultrasonography, in at least 5,000 blocks, may in the final analysis prove advantageous, in that it reduces the costs of operating room times (calculated in terms of rates per minute).

In a study by Tabaoda et al. in which the use of ultrasonography with injection below the posterior cord was compared with the neurostimulation technique with a coracoid approach (2 cm caudad and 2 cm medially), it was found that there was a saving of block execution times of a few minutes (3 ± 1 min compared to 6 ± 2 min; $p < 0.0001$). Comparison with the lateral approach also demonstrated that ultrasound is not only a valid alternative to nerve stimulation with excellent clinical results, as claimed by Sauter et al. but is also associated, in a report by Gurkan et al. with a better quality of the block itself. In a study by Brull et al. the use of double stimulation furnished no advantages in terms of success rates when compared with ultrasound and, indeed, caused an increase in evoked paraesthesias (45 vs. 6 %, respectively; $p < 0.001$) with lengthier technical execution times (median 10–5 vs. 5 min; $p < 0.001$).

We will attempt now to view the question from a different perspective and, instead of trying necessarily to eliminate one or the other of these two techniques, ask ourselves whether or not the combined use of neurostimulation and ultrasound may yield advantages in terms of enhancing the efficacy of the block and reducing side effects. Various studies, such as those conducted by Dingemans et al., Gurkan et al., and Tekin et al. have addressed this issue with very similar results. In fact, they have proved incapable of finding statistically significant differences between the study groups, and the success rates obtained are comparable. The main limitation of these studies is that, in the ultrasound group, the target has always been the posterior cord, whereas, in the neurostimulation group, none of the authors have sought any particular specific contractions, but have made do with a generic distal contraction, thus probably underestimating the possible success. The last word on the ultrasound–neurostimulation combination therefore has still to be pronounced, but common sense may guide the clinician with regard to the most appropriate use of the technologies available.

9.11 Comparison of Approaches

9.11.1 Infraclavicular Versus General Anesthesia

Before analysing the studies comparing the infraclavicular block with the other approaches to the brachial plexus, let us consider for a moment a study conducted by Hadzic et al. in patients undergoing day-case surgery below the elbow, randomized to receiving regional anesthesia with an infraclavicular block or general anesthesia with a laryngeal mask. The use of a short-acting local anesthetic such as chloroprocaine followed by sedation with propofol proved to be distinctly more advantageous than general anesthesia with desflurane and infiltration of the surgical wound with 0.25 % bupivacaine. In fact, as many as 79 % of patients receiving regional anesthesia were able to avoid having to pass via the recovery room compared to only 25 % in the general anesthesia group ($p < 0.001$). Of those who had to spend time in the recovery room, the patients undergoing infraclavicular blocks presented less postoperative pain and none required additional painkillers, whereas 48 % of the general anesthesia group needed additional analgesic agents. Lastly, the latter group also required lengthier periods for recovering the ability to walk and, consequently, longer discharge times compared to patients undergoing peripheral blocks (145 ± 79 vs. 82 ± 41 min and 218 ± 93 min and 121 ± 37 min, respectively; both parameters with $p < 0.001$).

9.11.2 Infraclavicular Versus Interscalene Block

There are no studies comparing these two approaches to the brachial plexus. Their clinical indications are, in fact, also different in that the infraclavicular block is preferably performed for distal operations on the upper limb (below the elbow), whereas the interscalene block is performed for more proximal operations such as those involving the shoulder and upper arm.

9.11.3 Infraclavicular Versus Supraclavicular Block

Theoretically, the supraclavicular block presents the anatomical advantage of being performed in an area where the brachial plexus is more superficial and its branches are more closely grouped together, thus permitting rapid, complete anesthesia of the upper limb with a single injection of local anesthetic. In clinical practice, however, randomized controlled studies have failed to confirm any significant advantages compared to the infraclavicular block.

With the use of electrical nerve stimulation alone, comparison between the two approaches in a study conducted by Yang et al. in 100 patients showed no substantial differences in execution and onset times, or in the quality of the block and patient satisfaction, but revealed a reduction in side effects such as Claude Bernard-Horner syndrome in the infraclavicular group. According to Rodriguez et al. the spread of local anesthetic in the infraclavicular block remains confined below the clavicle, thus reducing also the incidence of hoarseness and paralysis of the phrenic nerve. Arcaud et al. additionally used nerve stimulation to confirm the position of the needle inserted under ultrasound guidance in a randomized controlled study in 80 patients, but they, too, found similar success rates and execution times.

Although the lesser depth of the brachial plexus at the supraclavicular level should make for optimal ultrasound visibility, this does not necessarily mean better clinical results. In fact, the visualization of the needle and the spread of local anesthetic after a single administration in patients randomized to receiving a supraclavicular, infraclavicular or axillary block showed the same success rates, incidence of pain during the procedure, and incidence of vascular puncture in all three study groups (Tran et al.). In favour of the infraclavicular approach, on the other hand, are the results obtained by Fredrickson et al. who randomly assigned 60 patients to receiving a supraclavicular block with a single administration of local anesthetic in the 'corner pocket' according to the technique described by Soares et al. or an infraclavicular block with injections on each of the three cords of the brachial plexus. Although a similar sensory block was obtained at 30 min in both groups, better surgical anesthesia was achieved with the infraclavicular approach with more complete cover of the ulnar territory. No better results were obtained by Koscielniak-Nielsen et al. with the supraclavicular block even when attempting to administer two injections for each approach so as to visualize a spread of local anesthetic completely enveloping the cords of the plexus in both groups. In this study, too, the authors observed both a more rapid onset and a more efficient block were produced via the infraclavicular route owing to the superior analgesia in the ulnar and median nerve territories, the greater efficacy of the motor block and the lower incidence of side effects.

9.11.4 Infraclavicular Versus Axillary Block

Since the block via the axillary route is one of the most widely used approaches to the brachial plexus, there are numerous studies comparing it to the infraclavicular block and, although various different techniques and landmarks have been used for the latter, the results always tend to be in favour of the infraclavicular approach despite the different definitions used to define the success of the block. In three randomized controlled studies by Kapral et al., Fleischmann et al., and Rettig et al. comparing the two approaches with single nerve stimulation and a single administration of local anesthetic, the infraclavicular approach presented onset times similar to those of the axillary approach, but a better success rate (97–100 % vs. 80–85 %) probably due to better analgesia of the radial, axillary and musculocutaneous nerves. The success rates prove comparable if we are talking about an axillary block with three or four stimulations. The increased number of needle passes, however, compared with the infraclavicular single-administration approach, entails a lengthier execution time, greater patient discomfort and a higher incidence of adverse events (paraesthesias and vascular punctures) according to Deleuze et al., and Koscielniak-Nielsen et al.

The use of ultrasound has further improved the performance of the infraclavicular block. One randomized controlled study by Tran et al. in fact, has shown that the infraclavicular block is associated with more rapid execution times and less pain related to the procedure when compared with an axillary block with triple injections. In line with these results are those obtained by Tedore et al. in 232 patients randomized to receiving a US-guided infraclavicular block or an axillary block with the transarterial technique. The greater pain and paraesthesias associated with the latter technique have prompted patients to opt for the infraclavicular approach for further future anesthesia.

If we compare both approaches used in conjunction with ultrasound guidance, the results prove more homogeneous with similar success rates, as reported by Tran et al. and with nonsignificant pain values perceived by the patient in the course of the procedure, according to Fredrickson et al. so much so as to suggest that the choice can be made only on the basis of the anesthetist's experience and the patient's preferences.

9.11.5 Infraclavicular Versus Midhumeral Block

In the literature, we find only two randomized controlled studies, both conducted by Minville et al. comparing the midhumeral block with the infraclavicular block with double stimulation. Both approaches had similar success rates (90–95 %). It should be noted that the infraclavicular approach was associated with a shorter technical execution time but with a slower onset time of the block, thus equalling the midhumeral block in terms of total anesthesia time. The midhumeral approach, however, presented more intense pain in the course of skin puncture and electrical nerve stimulation (VAS 35 ± 27 mm vs. 19 ± 18 mm; $p < 0.011$).

9.12 Local Anesthetics and Infraclavicular Block

9.12.1 Which and at What Concentrations?

All local anesthetics can obviously be used in the execution of an infraclavicular block. The choice may be dictated by patient-related factors, the type of surgery planned and the patient admission regimen (hospital, day surgery, outpatient surgery).

In a study by Tran et al., lidocaine, even when used alone, has proved efficacious at the concentration of 1.5 % in single administration in the US-guided block. The idea of exploiting the rapid onset of lidocaine anesthesia and the longer-lasting duration of the more recently employed local anesthetics underlies the choice of the constituent elements of the so-called mixtures. In an observational study in 360 patients, the most suitable combination of lidocaine plus bupivacaine was evaluated, similar efficacy being found for the 2 % lidocaine plus 0.5 % bupivacaine and the 1.5 % lidocaine plus 0.375 % bupivacaine combinations, both of which with epinephrine 1:200,000. By contrast, the anesthesia induced by 1 % lidocaine plus 0.25 % bupivacaine proved inadequate in a study by Salazar and Espinosa. Valid results were also obtained by Jiang et al. with 2 % lidocaine plus 0.75 % ropivacaine in the coracoid approach in 160 patients. The use of mixtures, however, remains a matter of controversy, in that the calculation of the toxic dose of local anesthetic that can be used in any given patient is less predictable. There can be no doubt that drugs such as ropivacaine and levobupivacaine can be used successfully alone, respecting the different onset times. An Italian study conducted by Piangatelli et al. compared the effects of 30 ml of 0.75 % ropivacaine with those of 0.5 % levobupivacaine, revealing a greater onset time for the motor block in the group treated with ropivacaine, but a significantly longer sensory block in the levobupivacaine group without any increase in side effects.

9.12.2 What Volume?

Traditionally, studies with electrostimulation and a single injection have used volumes of 30 ml and sometimes pushing the volume as far as 40 ml. The advent of ultrasonography has prompted anesthetists to use increasingly low volumes, relying on the visualization of the spread of local anesthetic as a reliable indicator of success of the block. Reducing the amount of local anesthetic is not merely a matter of personal preference but may have practical repercussions in terms of reducing the costs of a single block and fewer side effects due to systemic absorption. For the US-guided infraclavicular block with a single injection, Tran et al. showed the minimum effective volume for 90 % of patients (MEV 90) to be 35 ml (95 % CI, 30–37.5 ml). Alternatively, the use of ultrasonography enables the local anesthetic to be injected in a targeted manner around each of the cords constituting the brachial plexus at this level. On the basis only of the observation of an adequate spread of local anesthetic around the cords, without referring to predetermined volumes, some authors found, in 14 patients, that the total volume for an adequate anesthesia was 16.1 ± 1.9 ml, whereas in 4 patients, the additional drug requirement meant that a total volume of 19.5 ± 7.1 ml was needed. Similar results were found in a larger sample of 160 patients in whom Jiang et al. studied the effects of predetermined volumes (5, 6, 7 or 8 ml) of local anesthetic (2 % lidocaine plus 0.75 % ropivacaine) for each of the cords of the brachial plexus. The group receiving 6 ml volumes and therefore a total of 18 ml induced a good analgesic effect without any side effects and without adversely affecting onset times.

9.13 Complications

9.13.1 Pneumothorax

The occurrence of pneumothorax is the adverse event that more than any other has limited the popularity of the infraclavicular block performed with electrical nerve stimulation alone. In a study by Neuburger, an incidence ranging from 0.2 to 0.7 % was determined despite correct technique and precise identification of the landmarks. A number of expedients suggested by Sanchez et al. regarding the maximum needle insertion depth or the inclination of the needle in relation to the plane of the skin may prove helpful, as may the use of techniques that identify more distal landmarks, but the most efficacious improvement is unquestionably the use of ultrasound guidance. The identification of the pleural dome and, above all, the visualization of the needle path with the 'in-plane' insertion technique are indispensable prerequisites in order to operate safely. The use of ultrasound, in fact, in itself unfortunately does not guarantee complete avoidance of this much feared complication, as pointed out by Koscielniak-Nielsen et al.

9.13.2 Claude Bernard–Horner Syndrome

When performing the infraclavicular block, a Claude Bernard-Horner syndrome may occur due to paralysis of the sympathetic ganglia of the cervical chain caused by high concentrations and volumes of local anesthetic penetrating beyond the natural barrier of the clavicle and reaching the cervical vertebrae. In studies conducted in large numbers of patients, this complication may not even be mentioned or may be present with an incidence of as much as 7 % for more proximal approaches. According to Salengros et al., we may reasonably estimate the incidence as approximately 5 % in blocks with a single injection of 40 ml of local anesthetic. One case of Claude Bernard-Horner syndrome was even reported by Hosten et al. for a block performed via a lateral approach. This rare side effect does not necessarily give rise in itself to major clinical consequences, but induces anxiety and discomfort, thus causing reduced patient acceptance of the anesthesia technique. We should bear in mind the fact that the cranial spread of local anesthetic, in addition to a Claude Bernard-Horner syndrome, may lead to alterations of respiratory function, the first of which is a warning sign that suggests the need for more thorough monitoring of the patient's condition.

9.13.3 Ventilatory Dysfunction

The spread of local anesthetic towards the cervical roots may lead to a reduced functionality of the diaphragm as is always observed in interscalene blocks and in the majority of supraclavicular blocks. Rodriguez et al. found no evidence of changes in forced expiratory volume compared to basal levels in patients after infraclavicular block with a single administration of 40 ml of 1.5 % mepivacaine. The same conclusions were reached by Dukkenkopf et al. in a study conducted in 20 patients with a modified Raj technique with 40–50 ml of 0.5 % ropivacaine. Rettig et al., however, conducted an ultrasonographic study of the diaphragmatic excursions after a block with 0.75 % ropivacaine for a volume of 5 ml/kg, revealing changes in hemidiaphragmatic movement (reduced or paradoxical) in 26 % of patients with a reduction in total forced expiratory volume and in forced expiratory volume in 1 s (FEV_1), despite the fact that no clinically significant signs of ventilatory dysfunction were noticed. All in all, we cannot entirely rule out effects on ventilatory dynamics as a result of the execution of an infraclavicular block. Certainly, as suggested by Blumenthal et al., the incidence of such complications can be greatly reduced by preferring techniques with continuous infusion when compared to the injection of a single bolus of local anesthetic.

9.13.4 Other Complications

The introduction of a needle in the proximity of nerve structures may accidentally damage these structures, causing neurological lesions due to mechanical trauma or to intraneural injection of local anesthetic. Although the use of ultrasound guidance could reduce the incidence of such complications, there are no randomized controlled trials with a number of recruited patients sufficient to detect statistically significant differences in the incidence of complications related to the various block techniques. One study by Fredrickson and Kilfoyle in more than 1,000 peripheral blocks for orthopaedic surgery revealed an 8.2 % rate of new neurological symptoms (6.3–10.4 %) by postoperative day 10, 3.7 % (2.7–5.0) after one month and a 0.6 % rate (0.27–1.3 %) 6 months postoperatively. These percentages are not very different from those observed with more traditional techniques, but this may also mean that the origin of the damage is not so much due to the anesthesia technique as to the type of surgery performed. It has been seen, however, that eliciting paraesthesias during the execution of the block is a risk factor independent of the development of neurological damage. Brachial plexopathy at the infraclavicular level has been noted both postblock and after axillary arteriography. In an investigation by Tsao and Wilbourn, histological analysis of 13 patients with this complication showed an axonal loss particularly affecting the median nerve, along with severe electrophysiological damage. In these cases, the term used is 'medial brachial fascial compartment (MBFC) syndrome', characterized by a neurological deficit and by pain resulting from a haematoma within a compartment of the upper arm.

The development of a haematoma of the axillary artery is a rare complication but is one that may prove dangerous in patients with mycotic aneurisms at the level of the upper limbs. According to Gleeton et al., an echo-Doppler study prior to execution of the block may help to identify this and possibly also other anatomical abnormalities present.

Rodriguez et al. have reported a case of dislocation of the shoulder after an infraclavicular coracoid block. This event may be the result of a number of concomitant causes, ranging from an undiagnosed glenohumeral instability to paralysis of the shoulder muscles and positioning of the arm under the torso. The authors suggest that particular attention should be paid to the position of the arm when annulling the motor function of the shoulder muscles with a peripheral block.

9.14 Continuous Infraclavicular Block

A perineural catheter positioned via the infraclavicular route theoretically presents a number of advantages: The more compact anatomy of the brachial plexus at this level facilitates the success of the block with a single injection; the technique does not require any particular positions of the arm which may remain adducted close to the torso; there is less possibility of catheter dislodgment as a result of the patient's daily movements; it facilitates the monitoring of the medication with a reduction in the risk of infection. Unfortunately, perineural continuous blocks with traditional non-stimulating catheters have yielded success rates as low as only 40 %, as reported by Salinas. Two technical innovations introduced recently are greatly improving the success rates of the technique, namely the use of stimulating catheters and the assistance provided by real-time ultrasound guidance of the catheter movements.

An interesting semiquantitative systematic review has been published by Morin et al. in an attempt to summarize the data furnished by randomized controlled studies comparing the use of traditional non-stimulating catheters with that of stimulating catheters. Although the analysis included different types of block and drugs used, the stimulating catheters were found to afford superior analgesia and, in particular, a reduction, ranging from 8 to 56 %, in the need for painkillers on demand in the postoperative period.

Mariano et al. have shown that the possibility of visually following the insertion of the catheter has also yielded decisive advantages compared to the classic technique using non-stimulating catheter. It not only permits shorter execution times but also leads to an increase in success rates, reducing side effects such as accidental vascular puncture. The same conclusions were reached in a study by Dhir and Ganapathy in 66 patients in whom the concomitant use of ultrasonography and electrical nerve stimulation proved superior both to the traditional insertion of a non-stimulating catheter and to the insertion of a stimulating catheter without ultrasound and neurostimulation assistance. In fact, it revealed a higher success rate of the block with a lower probability of dislodgment without any differences in block execution times. Slater et al., using ultrasound guidance, wondered whether the anesthesia administered directly through the needle, before inserting the catheter, was superior to that obtained by administering the local anesthetic after placing the catheter. The latter procedure involved 4 min longer technical execution times without any adverse effect on patient comfort. Despite the fact that the through-the-needle anesthesia technique enabled the tip to be directed in such a way as to facilitate a satisfactory spread of local anesthetic, surprisingly the percentage of complete blocks in this group was lower. One possible explanation is that, in the through-the-catheter technique, the catheter, with its multiple orifices, succeeds in inducing a more complete distribution of the anesthetic around the cords of the brachial plexus.

A further aid to the correct positioning of the tip of the catheter may be provided by the use of an ultrasonographic contrast medium which, when injected in small amounts, creates new ultrasound signals thus permitting a more precise identification of the disposition of the structures examined. The most suitable medium for this purpose is a 5 % glucose solution, which presents electroneutrality characteristics, thus preserving the use of electrical nerve stimulation also after its injection. Dhir et al. achieved 100 % success rates by simultaneously combining the use of ultrasound with contrast medium enhancement (5 % glucose solution) and a stimulating catheter.

9.14.1 Continuous Infusion at Home

According to Klein, continuous perineural infusion is associated with a more complete postoperative analgesia with a reduced consumption of opioids, a reduction in side effects, better rehabilitation and a greater sense of well-being on the part of the patient. These considerations, together with the increase in indications for outpatient surgery, have led anesthesiologists to assess the hypothesis of administering continuous infusion outside the hospital setting. The most controversial issues involved have to do with discharging a patient with an anesthetized limb prone to involuntary damage, the degree of trust to be accorded the patient with regard to the pharmacological management of his or her postoperative pain, and the possible risk of local anesthetic toxicity. Ilfeld et al. have studied the effects of different dosage regimens in continuous infusion at home, using programmable pumps, equipped with a mechanism for the infusion of boluses at the patient's request. They found that, when compared to the continuous infusion of saline, a significant reduction in postoperative pain was achieved (VAS after one day: 2.5 ± 1.6 vs. 6.1 ± 2.3) as well as a reduction in narcotic use and related side effects, and as much as a tenfold reduction in sleep disturbance scores and therefore greater patient satisfaction.

9.14.2 Pharmacological Notes: Volumes, Concentrations, Doses

The correct calculation of the volume of local anesthetic to be used, that is, of an efficacious but safe dosage, and therefore of the final concentration is indispensable, particularly for continuous blocks in which both the monitoring of the patient and the volume of the reservoir of the portable infusion pumps are limited. For the purposes of identifying an adequate volume to be administered, Ilfeld et al., in 30 recruited patients, compared three different 0.2 % ropivacaine infusion regimens: a 'basal' group at an infusion rate of 12 ml/h with a patient-controlled bolus of 0.05 ml; a 'basal + bolus' group at a rate of 8 ml/h with a bolus of 4 ml; and a 'bolus' group at a rate of 0.03 ml/h with a bolus of 9.9 ml. The 'basal' group required more oral analgesics and had a shorter median infusion duration compared to the other two. The 'bolus' group had the longest median infusion duration but also presented a significant increase in intense breakthrough pain episodes. The 'basal + bolus' group was associated with the greatest overall degree of patient satisfaction, thus proving the recommended regimen for orthopaedic surgery from the elbow downwards. The same authors also attempted to reduce the volume to be delivered even further, testing a more concentrated solution of local anesthetic and leaving the total dosage unaltered, that is to say maintaining a total dosage of 16 mg/h, they compared an infusion of 0.2 % ropivacaine at 8 ml/h and a bolus of 4 ml with an infusion of 0.4 % ropivacaine at 4 ml/h and a bolus of 2 ml. The results showed that the patients treated with the first regimen presented good analgesia with a high percentage of completely numb sensation of the limb, and therefore less risk of accidental damage, that is, approximately three times less than in patients treated with a more concentrated anesthetic. The possible explanation for this is that at the infraclavicular level, the plexus is distributed in three cords separated by the axillary artery. The greater concentration of the anesthetic and its lower volume renders only part of the plexus insensitive, giving rise to an unpleasant and clinically dangerous sensation. The greater volume, albeit at a lesser concentration, on the other hand, reaches all the cords, but it is less likely that its dilution will give rise to total numbness. The same authors also attempted to improve the postoperative analgesia of this technique by adding clonidine 1 mcg/ml to the local anesthetic solution by continuous infusion. Although this drug showed an increase in the duration of the analgesia in blocks with a single administration, it failed to yield the same degree of efficacy in continuous blocks, showing no clinically significant difference compared to the use of the local anesthetic alone.

9.14.3 Catheter-Related Complications

In addition to the risks related to the infraclavicular block technique itself, which we have already discussed, those relating to the use of a perineural catheter include infections, neurological damage, catheter migration and local anesthesia toxicity. Various studies have evaluated the presence of infectious complications in continuous blocks in general, the consensus of opinion being that these are rare events the incidence of which increases with the duration of the infusion, as claimed by Neuburger et al.

In the literature, we also find a description by Tran et al. of a clinical case in which a stimulating catheter inserted via the infraclavicular route needed to be removed surgically. In fact, the authors, encountering difficulty in withdrawing it, cut the proximal part and when withdrawing the distal part, the catheter came away, whereas the metal stimulating guide was retained. To avoid such an occurrence, it is advisable not to tamper with perineural catheters by cutting them.

Bibliography

Arcand G, Williams SR, Chouinard P, Boudreault D, Harris P, Ruel M, Girard F (2005) Ultrasound-guided infraclavicular versus supraclavicular block. Anesth Analg 101(3):886–890

Bigeleisen P, Wilson M (2006) A comparison of two techniques for ultrasound guided infraclavicular block. Br J Anaesth 96(4):502–507

Bloc S, Garnier T, Komly B, Asfazadourian H, Leclerc P, Mercadal L, Morel B, Dhonneur G (2007) Spread of injectate associated with radial or median nerve-type motor response during infraclavicular brachial-plexus block: an ultrasound evaluation. Reg Anesth Pain Med 32(2):130–135

Bloc S, Garnier T, Komly B, Leclerc P, Mercadal L, Morel B, Dhonneur G (2006) Single-stimulation, low-volume infraclavicular plexus block: influence of the evoked distal motor response on success rate. Reg Anesth Pain Med 31(5):433–437

Blumenthal S, Nadig M, Borgeat A (2004) Combined infraclavicular plexus block with suprascapular nerve block for humeral head surgery in a patient with respiratory failure: is an alternative approach really the best option for the lungs? Anesthesiology 100(1):190 (author reply 190–191)

Borene SC, Edwards JN, Boezaart AP (2004) At the cords, the pinkie towards: Interpreting infraclavicular motor responses to neurostimulation. Reg Anesth Pain Med 29(2):125–129

Borgeat A, Ekatodramis G, Dumont C (2001) An evaluation of the infraclavicular block via a modified approach of the Raj technique. Anesth Analg 93(2):436–441

Bowens C Jr, Gupta RK, O'Byrne WT, Schildcrout JS, Shi Y, Hawkins JJ, Michaels DR, Berry JM (2010) Selective local anesthetic placement using ultrasound guidance and neurostimulation for infraclavicular brachial plexus block. Anesth Analg 110(5):1480–1485

Brull R, Lupu M, Perlas A, Chan VW, McCartney CJ (2009) Compared with dual nerve stimulation, ultrasound guidance shortens the time for infraclavicular block performance. Can J Anaesth 56(11):812–818

Cornish PB, Nowitz M (2005) A magnetic resonance imaging analysis of the infraclavicular region: can brachial plexus depth be estimated before needle insertion? Anesth Analg 100(4):1184–1188

De Tran QH, Bertini P, Zaouter C, Munoz L, Finlayson RJ (2010) A prospective, randomized comparison between single- and double-injection ultrasound-guided infraclavicular brachial plexus block. Reg Anesth Pain Med 35(1):16–21

De Tran QH, Clemente A, Doan J, Finlayson RJ (2007) Brachial plexus blocks: a review of approaches and techniques. Can J Anaesth 54(8):662–674

Deleuze A, Gentili ME, Marret E, Lamonerie L, Bonnet F (2003) A comparison of a single-stimulation lateral infraclavicular plexus block with a triple-stimulation axillary block. Reg Anesth Pain Med 28(2):89–94

Desgagnes MC, Levesque S, Dion N, Nadeau MJ, Cote D, Brassard J, Nicole PC, Turgeon AF (2009) A comparison of a single or triple injection technique for ultrasound-guided infraclavicular block: a prospective randomized controlled study. Anesth Analg 109(2):668–672

Desroches J (2003) The infraclavicular brachial plexus block by the coracoid approach is clinically effective: an observational study of 150 patients. Can J Anaesth 50(3):253–257

Dhir S, Ganapathy S (2008) Comparative evaluation of ultrasound-guided continuous infraclavicular brachial plexus block with stimulating catheter and traditional technique: a prospective-randomized trial. Acta Anaesthesiol Scand 52(8):1158–1166

Dhir S, Ganapathy S (2008) Use of ultrasound guidance and contrast enhancement: a study of continuous infraclavicular brachial plexus approach. Acta Anaesthesiol Scand 52(3):338–342

Dingemans E, Williams SR, Arcand G, Chouinard P, Harris P, Ruel M, Girard F (2007) Neurostimulation in ultrasound-guided infraclavicular block: a prospective randomized trial. Anesth Analg 104(5):1275–1280

Dolan J (2009) Fascial planes inhibiting the spread of local anesthetic during ultrasound-guided infraclavicular brachial plexus block are not limited to the posterior aspect of the axillary artery. Reg Anesth Pain Med 34(6):612–613

Dullenkopf A, Blumenthal S, Theodorou P, Roos J, Perschak H, Borgeat A (2004) Diaphragmatic excursion and respiratory function after the modified Raj technique of the infraclavicular plexus block. Reg Anesth Pain Med 29(2):110–114

Fleischmann E, Marhofer P, Greher M, Waltl B, Sitzwohl C, Kapral S (2003) Brachial plexus anaesthesia in children: lateral infraclavicular vs. axillary approach. Paediatr Anaesth 13(2):103–108

Frederiksen BS, Koscielniak-Nielsen ZJ, Jacobsen RB, Rasmussen H, Hesselbjerg L (2010) Procedural pain of an ultrasound-guided brachial plexus block: a comparison of axillary and infraclavicular approaches. Acta Anaesthesiol Scand 54(4):408–413

Fredrickson MJ, Kilfoyle DH (2009) Neurological complication analysis of 1,000 ultrasound guided peripheral nerve blocks for elective orthopaedic surgery: a prospective study. Anaesthesia 64(8):836–844

Fredrickson MJ, Patel A, Young S, Chinchanwala S (2009) Speed of onset of 'corner pocket supraclavicular' and infraclavicular ultrasound guided brachial plexus block: a randomised observer-blinded comparison. Anaesthesia 64(7):738–744

Fredrickson MJ, Wolstencroft P, Kejriwal R, Yoon A, Boland MR, Chinchanwala S (2010) Single versus triple injection ultrasound-guided infraclavicular block: confirmation of the effectiveness of the single injection technique. Anesth Analg 111(5):1325–1327

Gaertner E, Estebe JP, Zamfir A, Cuby C, Macaire P (2002) Infraclavicular plexus block: multiple injection versus single injection. Reg Anesth Pain Med 27(6):590–594

Gleeton D, Levesque S, Trepanier CA, Gariepy JL, Brassard J, Dion N (2010) Symptomatic axillary hematoma after ultrasound-guided infraclavicular block in a patient with undiagnosed upper extremity mycotic aneurysms. Anesth Analg 111(4):1069–1071

Grossi P (2001) Brachial plexus block. The anesthetic line is a guide for new approaches. Minerva Anestesiol 67(9 Suppl 1):45–49

Gu HH, Che XH, Li PY, Liang WM (2007) Low minimal stimulating current improves infraclavicular brachial plexus block efficacy. Zhonghua Yi Xue Za Zhi 87(21):1470–1473

Gurkan Y, Acar S, Solak M, Toker K (2008) Comparison of nerve stimulation vs. ultrasound-guided lateral sagittal infraclavicular block. Acta Anaesthesiol Scand 52(6):851–855

Gurkan Y, Hosten T, Solak M, Toker K (2008) Lateral sagittal infraclavicular block: clinical experience in 380 patients. Acta Anaesthesiol Scand 52(2):262–266

Gurkan Y, Ozdamar D, Solak M, Toker K (2008) Lateral sagittal infraclavicular block is a clinically effective block in children. Eur J Anaesthesiol 25(11):949–951

Gurkan Y, Tekin M, Acar S, Solak M, Toker K (2010) Is nerve stimulation needed during an ultrasound-guided lateral sagittal infraclavicular block? Acta Anaesthesiol Scand 54(4):403–407

Hadzic A, Arliss J, Kerimoglu B, Karaca PE, Yufa M, Claudio RE, Vloka JD, Rosenquist R, Santos AC, Thys DM (2004) A comparison of infraclavicular nerve block versus general anesthesia for hand and wrist daycase surgeries. Anesthesiology 101(1):127–132

Hosten T, Gurkan Y, Solak M, Toker K (2008) A case of Horner's syndrome following lateral sagittal infraclavicular block. Agri 20(4):45–48

Ilfeld BM, Le LT, Ramjohn J, Loland VJ, Wadhwa AN, Gerancher JC, Renehan EM, Sessler DI, Shuster JJ, Theriaque DW et al (2009) The effects of local anesthetic concentration and dose on continuous infraclavicular nerve blocks: a multicenter, randomized, observer-masked, controlled study. Anesth Analg 108(1):345–350

Ilfeld BM, Morey TE, Enneking FK (2004) Infraclavicular perineural local anesthetic infusion: a comparison of three dosing regimens for postoperative analgesia. Anesthesiology 100(2):395–402

Ilfeld BM, Morey TE, Enneking FK (2002) Continuous infraclavicular brachial plexus block for postoperative pain control at home: a randomized, double-blinded, placebo-controlled study. Anesthesiology 96(6):1297–1304

Ilfeld BM, Morey TE, Enneking FK (2003) Continuous infraclavicular perineural infusion with clonidine and ropivacaine compared with ropivacaine alone: a randomized, double-blinded, controlled study. Anesth Analg 97(3):706–712

Jiang XB, Zhu SZ, Jiang Y, Chen QH, Xu XZ (2009) Optimal dose of local anesthetic mixture in ultrasound-guided infraclavicular brachial plexus block via coracoid approach: analysis of 160 cases. Zhonghua Yi Xue Za Zhi 89(7):449–452

Kapral S, Jandrasits O, Schabernig C, Likar R, Reddy B, Mayer N, Weinstabl C (1999) Lateral infraclavicular plexus block vs. axillary block for hand and forearm surgery. Acta Anaesthesiol Scand 43(10):1047–1052

Keschner MT, Michelsen H, Rosenberg AD, Wambold D, Albert DB, Altman R, Green S, Posner M (2006) Safety and efficacy of the infraclavicular nerve block performed at low current. Pain Pract 6(2):107–111

Kilka HG, Geiger P, Mehrkens HH (1995) Infraclavicular vertical brachial plexus blockade. A new method for anesthesia of the upper extremity. An anatomical and clinical study. Anaesthesist 44(5):339–344

Klaastad O, Lilleas FG, Rotnes JS, Breivik H, Fosse E (2000) A magnetic resonance imaging study of modifications to the infraclavicular brachial plexus block. Anesth Analg 91(4):929–933

Klaastad O, Lilleas FG, Rotnes JS, Breivik H, Fosse E (1999) Magnetic resonance imaging demonstrates lack of precision in needle placement by the infraclavicular brachial plexus block described by Raj et al. Anesth Analg 88(3):593–598

Klaastad O, Smedby O, Kjelstrup T, Smith HJ (2005) The vertical infraclavicular brachial plexus block: a simulation study using magnetic resonance imaging. Anesth Analg 101(1):273–278

Klaastad O, Smith HJ, Smedby O, Winther-Larssen EH, Brodal P, Breivik H, Fosse ET (2004) A novel infraclavicular brachial plexus block: the lateral and sagittal technique, developed by magnetic resonance imaging studies. Anesth Analg 98(1):252–256

Klein SM (2002) Beyond the hospital: continuous peripheral nerve blocks at home. Anesthesiology 96(6):1283–1285

Koscielniak-Nielsen ZJ, Frederiksen BS, Rasmussen H, Hesselbjerg L (2009) A comparison of ultrasound-guided supraclavicular and infraclavicular blocks for upper extremity surgery. Acta Anaesthesiol Scand 53(5):620–626

Koscielniak-Nielsen ZJ, Rasmussen H, Hesselbjerg L, Gurkan Y, Belhage B (2005) Clinical evaluation of the lateral sagittal infraclavicular block developed by MRI studies. Reg Anesth Pain Med 30(4):329–334

Koscielniak-Nielsen ZJ, Rasmussen H, Hesselbjerg L, Nielsen TP, Gurkan Y (2005) Infraclavicular block causes less discomfort than axillary block in ambulatory patients. Acta Anaesthesiol Scand 49(7):1030–1034

Koscielniak-Nielsen ZJ, Rasmussen H, Hesselbjerg L (2008) Pneumothorax after an ultrasound-guided lateral sagittal infraclavicular block. Acta Anaesthesiol Scand 52(8):1176–1177

Lecamwasam H, Mayfield J, Rosow L, Chang Y, Carter C, Rosow C (2006) Stimulation of the posterior cord predicts successful infraclavicular block. Anesth Analg 102(5):1564–1568

Mariano ER, Loland VJ, Bellars RH, Sandhu NS, Bishop ML, Abrams RA, Meunier MJ, Maldonado RC, Ferguson EJ, Ilfeld BM (2009) Ultrasound guidance versus electrical stimulation for infraclavicular brachial plexus perineural catheter insertion. J Ultrasound Med 28(9):1211–1218

Minville V, Amathieu R, Luc N, Gris C, Fourcade O, Samii K, Benhamou D (2005) Infraclavicular brachial plexus block versus humeral approach: comparison of anesthetic time and efficacy. Anesth Analg 101(4): 1198–1201

Minville V, Asehnoune K, Chassery C, N'Guyen L, Gris C, Fourcade O, Samii K, Benhamou D (2005) Resident versus staff anesthesiologist performance: coracoid approach to infraclavicular brachial plexus blocks using a double-stimulation technique. Reg Anesth Pain Med 30(3):233–237

Minville V, Fourcade O, Bourdet B, Doherty M, Chassery C, Pourrut JC, Gris C, Eychennes B, Colombani A, Samii K et al (2007) The optimal motor response for infraclavicular brachial plexus block. Anesth Analg 104(2):448–451

Minville V, Fourcade O, Idabouk L, Claassen J, Chassery C, Nguyen L, Pourrut JC, Benhamou D (2006) Infraclavicular brachial plexus block versus humeral block in trauma patients: a comparison of patient comfort. Anesth Analg 102(3):912–915

Minville V, N'Guyen L, Chassery C, Zetlaoui P, Pourrut JC, Gris C, Eychennes B, Benhamou D, Samii K (2005) A modified coracoid approach to infraclavicular brachial plexus blocks using a double-stimulation technique in 300 patients. Anesth Analg 100(1):263–265

Morimoto M, Popovic J, Kim JT, Kiamzon H, Rosenberg AD (2007) Case series: Septa can influence local anesthetic spread during infraclavicular brachial plexus blocks. Can J Anaesth 54(12):1006–1010

Morin AM, Kranke P, Wulf H, Stienstra R, Eberhart LH (2010) The effect of stimulating versus nonstimulating catheter techniques for continuous regional anesthesia: a semiquantitative systematic review. Reg Anesth Pain Med 35(2):194–199

Neal JM (2001) How close is close enough? Defining the "paresthesia chad". Reg Anesth Pain Med 26(2):97–99

Neuburger M, Buttner J, Blumenthal S, Breitbarth J, Borgeat A (2007) Inflammation and infection complications of 2,285 perineural catheters: a prospective study. Acta Anaesthesiol Scand 51(1):108–114

Neuburger M, Landes H, Kaiser H (2000) Pneumothorax in vertical infraclavicular block of the brachial plexus. Review of a rare complication. Anaesthesist 49(10):901–904

Ootaki C, Hayashi H, Amano M (2000) Ultrasound-guided infraclavicular brachial plexus block: an alternative technique to anatomical landmark-guided approaches. Reg Anesth Pain Med 25(6):600–604

Piangatelli C, De Angelis C, Pecora L, Recanatini F, Cerchiara P, Testasecca D (2006) Levobupivacaine and ropivacaine in the infraclavicular brachial plexus block. Minerva Anestesiol 72(4):217–221

Raj PP, Montgomery SJ, Nettles D, Jenkins MT (1973) Infraclavicular brachial plexus block–a new approach. Anesth Analg 52(6):897–904

Rettig HC, Gielen MJ, Boersma E, Klein J, Groen GJ (2005) Vertical infraclavicular block of the brachial plexus: effects on hemidiaphragmatic movement and ventilatory function. Reg Anesth Pain Med 30(6):529–535

Rettig HC, Gielen MJ, Boersma E, Klein J (2005) A comparison of the vertical infraclavicular and axillary approaches for brachial plexus anaesthesia. Acta Anaesthesiol Scand 49(10):1501–1508

Rodrguez J, Barcena M, Alvarez J (2003) Shoulder dislocation after infraclavicular coracoid block. Reg Anesth Pain Med 28(4):351–353

Rodriguez J, Barcena M, Alvarez J (2003) Restricted infraclavicular distribution of the local anesthetic solution after infraclavicular brachial plexus block. Reg Anesth Pain Med 28(1):33–36

Rodriguez J, Barcena M, Lagunilla J, Alvarez J (2004) Increased success rate with infraclavicular brachial plexus block using a dual-injection technique. J Clin Anesth 16(4):251–256

Rodriguez J, Barcena M, Rodriguez V, Aneiros F, Alvarez J (1998) Infraclavicular brachial plexus block effects on respiratory function and extent of the block. Reg Anesth Pain Med 23(6):564–568

Rodriguez J, Barcena M, Taboada-Muniz M, Lagunilla J, Alvarez J (2004) A comparison of single versus multiple injections on the extent of anesthesia with coracoid infraclavicular brachial plexus block. Anesth Analg 99(4):1225–1230

Rodriguez J, Taboada M, Oliveira J, Ulloa B, Barcena M, Alvarez J (2010) Single stimulation of the posterior cord is superior to dual nerve stimulation in a coracoid block. Acta Anaesthesiol Scand 54(2):241–245

Rodriguez J, Taboada-Muniz M, Barcena M, Alvarez J (2004) Median versus musculocutaneous nerve response with single-injection infraclavicular coracoid block. Reg Anesth Pain Med 29(6):534–538 (discussion 520–533)

Salazar CH, Espinosa W (1999) Infraclavicular brachial plexus block: variation in approach and results in 360 cases. Reg Anesth Pain Med 24(5):411–416

Salengros JC, Jacquot C, Hesbois A, Vandesteene A, Engelman E, Pandin P (2007) Delayed Horner's syndrome during a continuous infraclavicular brachial plexus block. J Clin Anesth 19(1):57–59

Salinas FV (2003) Location, location, location: Continuous peripheral nerve blocks and stimulating catheters. Reg Anesth Pain Med 28(2):79–82

Sanchez HB, Mariano ER, Abrams R, Meunier M (2008) Pneumothorax following infraclavicular brachial plexus block for hand surgery. Orthopedics 31(7):709

Sandhu NS, Bahniwal CS, Capan LM (2006) Feasibility of an infraclavicular block with a reduced volume of lidocaine with sonographic guidance. J Ultrasound Med 25(1):51–56

Sandhu NS, Capan LM (2002) Ultrasound-guided infraclavicular brachial plexus block. Br J Anaesth 89(2):254–259

Sandhu NS, Sidhu DS, Capan LM (2004) The cost comparison of infraclavicular brachial plexus block by nerve stimulator and ultrasound guidance. Anesth Analg 98(1):267–268

Sauter AR, Dodgson MS, Stubhaug A, Halstensen AM, Klaastad O (2008) Electrical nerve stimulation or ultrasound guidance for lateral sagittal infraclavicular blocks: a randomized, controlled, observer-blinded, comparative study. Anesth Analg 106(6):1910–1915

Sedeek KA, Goujard E (2007) The lateral sagittal infraclavicular block in children. Anesth Analg 105(1):295–297

Slater ME, Williams SR, Harris P, Brutus JP, Ruel M, Girard F, Boudreault D (2007) Preliminary evaluation of infraclavicular catheters inserted using ultrasound guidance: through-the-catheter anesthesia is not inferior to through-the-needle blocks. Reg Anesth Pain Med 32(4):296–302

Soares LG, Brull R, Lai J, Chan VW (2007) Eight ball, corner pocket: the optimal needle position for ultrasound-guided supraclavicular block. Reg Anesth Pain Med 32(1):94–95

Taboada M, Rodriguez J, Amor M, Sabate S, Alvarez J, Cortes J, Atanassoff PG (2009) Is ultrasound guidance superior to conventional nerve stimulation for coracoid infraclavicular brachial plexus block? Reg Anesth Pain Med 34(4):357–360

Tedore TR, YaDeau JT, Maalouf DB, Weiland AJ, Tong-Ngork S, Wukovits B, Paroli L, Urban MK, Zayas VM, Wu A et al (2009) Comparison of the transarterial axillary block and the ultrasound-guided infraclavicular block for upper extremity surgery: a prospective randomized trial. Reg Anesth Pain Med 34(4):361–365

de Tran QH, Charghi R, Finlayson RJ (2006) The "double bubble" sign for successful infraclavicular brachial plexus blockade. Anesth Analg 103(4):1048–1049

de Tran QH, Clemente A, Tran DQ, Finlayson RJ (2008) A comparison between ultrasound-guided infraclavicular block using the "double bubble" sign and neurostimulation-guided axillary block. Anesth Analg 107(3):1075–1078

de Tran QH, Dugani S, Dyachenko A, Correa JA, Finlayson RJ (2011) Minimum effective volume of lidocaine for ultrasound-guided infraclavicular block. Reg Anesth Pain Med 36(2):190–194

de Tran QH, Russo G, Munoz L, Zaouter C, Finlayson RJ (2009) A prospective, randomized comparison between ultrasound-guided supraclavicular, infraclavicular, and axillary brachial plexus blocks. Reg Anesth Pain Med 34(4):366–371

Tran QD, Gordon A, Asenjo JF, de la Cuadra-Fontaine JC (2005) Retained and cut stimulating infraclavicular catheter. Can J Anaesth 52(9):998–999

Tsao BE, Wilbourn AJ (2004) Infraclavicular brachial plexus injury following axillary regional block. Muscle Nerve 30(1):44–48

Wang FY, Wu SH, Lu IC, Hsu HT, Soo LY, Tang CS, Chu KS (2007) Ultrasonographic examination to search out the optimal upper arm position for coracoid approach to infraclavicular brachial plexus block–a volunteer study. Acta Anaesthesiol Taiwan 45(1):15–20

Wilson JL, Brown DL, Wong GY, Ehman RL, Cahill DR (1998) Infraclavicular brachial plexus block: parasagittal anatomy important to the coracoid technique. Anesth Analg 87(4):870–873

Yang CW, Kwon HU, Cho CK, Jung SM, Kang PS, Park ES, Heo YM, Shinn HK (2010) A comparison of infraclavicular and supraclavicular approaches to the brachial plexus using neurostimulation. Korean J Anesthesiol 58(3):260–266

Axillary Brachial Plexus Block

M. Bosco and A. Clemente

10.1 Historical Note

From the Heidelberg Surgical Clinic (Director: Prof. Dr. Wilms)

Anesthesia of the brachial plexus in upper limb surgery (Private Lecturer: Dr. Georg Hirschel)

In recent years local anesthesia has made very rapid progress, increasingly gaining ground in many areas and involving almost the whole of the body, whereas its application in major operations on the extremities has tended to lag behind. It is now customary to operate under local anesthesia on the fingers and toes, as well as on the hands and feet. The anesthetization of nerve trunks covering extensive territories at the level of the arms and legs is also practiced. Nevertheless, conduction anesthesia of all the extremities is still associated with substantial complications and is therefore rarely used. As regards surgery of the lower limbs in patients for whom narcotic treatment may be life-threatening, one may at a push resort to the use of spinal anesthesia. On the arms this is impossible.

There has been no lack of partly successful attempts, for example, in amputations of the arm under local anesthesia. Reclus injected his low-dose cocaine solution, starting from the skin and proceeding as far as the bone, finally obtaining anesthesia. Crile attempted to anesthetize the brachial plexus, for this purpose making a cut in the posterior border of the sternocleidomastoid muscle. At this point he went in search of the nerve trunks and injected a certain amount of cocaine into each trunk.

These, however, are isolated attempts under local anesthesia, which subsequently failed to yield any useful procedure. The preparations were too complex and caused the patient too much anxiety. The search for the individual nerves was in itself a major intervention.

Encouraged by my experience with the emptying of the armpit under local anesthesia in cases of cancer of the breast, I attempted to anesthetize the brachial plexus so as to be able to operate without anesthesia at the level of the arm and hand.

For the emptying of the armpit at that time an injection of 1 % novocaine was sufficient with the addition of a few drops of

M. Bosco (✉)
Department of Anesthesiology and Critical Care Medicine, Catholic University of the Sacred Heart, Rome, Italy
e-mail: mbosco@rm.unicatt.it

A. Clemente
Anesthesiology, Intensive Care and Pain Therapy Service, IRCCS—Immacolata Dermopathic Institute (IDI), Rome, Italy
e-mail: antonio.clemente@idi.it

tätigkeit durch den Extrakt der antagonistischen Hypophyse herabgesetzt und dadurch indirekt die Blutung eingeschränkt wird, und so Dauerwirkungen erzielbar sind, das sind heute noch offene Fragen. Begnügen wir uns für heute mit dem Ergebnis, dass wir in dem Pituitrin ein Mittel kennen gelernt haben, **dessen praktische Verwertbarkeit bei gynäkologischen Uterusblutungen jedenfalls weitere Nachprüfung verdient.** Der Satz von Hofbauer: „Für gynäkologische Zwecke scheint nach wenigen orientierenden bisherigen Versuchen das Mittel wenig wirksam zu sein" besteht augenscheinlich **nicht zu Recht**.

Aus der Heidelberger chirurgischen Klinik (Direktor: Prof. Dr. Wilms).

Die Anästhesierung des Plexus brachialis bei Operationen an der oberen Extremität.

Von Privatdozent Dr. Georg Hirschel.

Während die Lokalanästhesie in den letzten Jahren rapide Fortschritte machte und sich immer mehr Terrain eroberte, das fast den ganzen Körper betraf, war ihre Anwendung bei grösseren Eingriffen an den Extremitäten bisher zurückgeblieben. Wohl ist man jetzt gewöhnt, an Fingern und Zehen, auch an Händen und Füssen mit Lokalanästhesie zu operieren, auch Leitungsanästhesien einzelner grösserer Nervengebiete an Beinen und Armen auszuführen, allein eine Leitungsanästhesie der ganzen Extremität ist immer mit grossen Umständen verknüpft und wird deshalb selten zur Ausführung gebracht. Am Beine kann man sich in Fällen, wo eine Narkose für den Patienten gefahrbringend ist, mit der Spinalanästhesie behelfen, am Arme ist dies nicht möglich.

Es hat nicht an Versuchen gefehlt und solche sind teilweise auch gelungen, z. B. Amputationen am Oberarm in Lokalanästhesie zur Ausführung zu bringen. Reclus ging von der Haut bis auf den Knochen mit seiner Kokainlösung schrittweise vor und erreichte schliesslich eine Anästhesie. Crile versuchte den Plexus brachialis zu anästhesieren und machte zu diesem Zwecke einen Schnitt am hinteren Rande des Kopfnickers, dann suchte er die Nervenstämme auf und injizierte in jeden einzelnen derselben eine gewisse Menge Kokains.

Alle diese Versuche stehen vereinzelt da und ein brauchbares Verfahren hat sich aus ihnen nicht herausgebildet. Die Vorbereitungen waren zu umfangreich und für den Patienten zu beängstigend und das Aufsuchen der einzelnen Nerven bedeutete an und für sich schon einen grösseren Eingriff.

Angeregt durch meine Erfahrungen[1]), die ich bei der Anwendung der Lokalanästhesie bei der Ausräumung der Achselhöhle beim Mammakarzinom machte, versuchte ich nun, den Plexus brachialis zu anästhesieren, um am Arme und der Hand ohne Narkose operieren zu können.

Für die Ausräumung der Achselhöhle genügte damals das 1 proz. Novokain mit einigen wenigen Tropfen Adrenalin. Die Technik der Injektion habe ich genau beschrieben. Die Anästhesie reichte weit nach oben bis zur ersten Rippe, so dass alle sichtbaren Drüsen und Lymphstränge schmerzlos entfernt werden konnten. Die Berührung der grossen Nervenstämme löste keinerlei Schmerz aus. Allerdings war diese Anästhesie nur oberflächlich, die Extremität selbst hatte normale Empfindung.

Auf Grund dieser Erfahrungen nahm ich nun eine 2 proz. Lösung von Novokain und spritzte diese nach derselben Methode in den Plexus brachialis ein. Um eine zu rasche Resorption des Anästhetikums zu verhindern, machte ich vorher eine leichte Stauung durch eine Pelotte, die auf die Gefässstämme gelegt und durch zwei elastische Bänder um die Schulter und die Brust fixiert war (Fig. 1). Nach eingetretener

---

[1]) Hirschel: Die Anwendung der Lokalanästhesien bei grösseren Operationen an Brust und Thorax (Mammakarzinom, Thorakoplastik). Münch. med. Wochenschr. No. 10, 1911.

Anästhesie wurde die Stauung abgebrochen und zum Zwecke der Operation in Blutleere der Oberarm abgeschnürt.

Auf diese Art konnten in 3 Fällen bei völliger Anästhesie des ganzen Armes grössere Operationen ausgeführt werden.

Im ersten Falle handelte es sich um einen 28 jährigen Mann, bei dem eine Kugel in der Ellbogenbeuge direkt über dem Gelenke entfernt

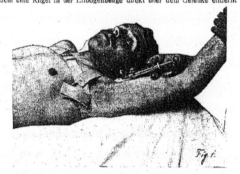

Fig. 1.

wurde. Eingespritzt wurden 25 ccm der 2 proz. Novokainlösung mit einigen Tropfen Adrenalin. Die völlige Anästhesie trat nach ½ Stunde ein und dauerte etwa 1½ Stunden.

Der zweite Fall betraf eine alte, schwache Frau von 70 Jahren mit

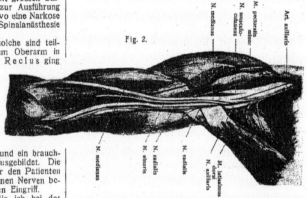

Fig. 2.

einer ausgedehnten Tuberkulose des rechten Ellbogengelenkes. Eingespritzt wurden 30 ccm der Lösung. Die Anästhesie trat nach 20 bis 25 Minuten ein. Ohne den geringsten Schmerz konnte die Amputation etwas über der Mitte des Oberarmes vorgenommen werden.

Beim dritten Falle handelte es sich um einen 58 jährigen Mann mit tuberkulöser Osteomyelitis der distalen Ulnaepiphyse. Gebraucht wurden auch 30 ccm der Lösung. Das Eintreten der Anästhesie dauerte in diesem Falle etwa 40 Minuten, doch war dieselbe dann auch vollständig.

Um die Aufregung der Patienten zu vermindern, wurde bei fast allen Lokalanästhesien vorher Morphium oder Pantopon injiziert; der alten Frau wurde zur Beruhigung die Maske zur Sauerstoffinhalation vorgehalten, besonders als der Knochen durchsägt wurde. Sie hatten während der Operation keinerlei Schmerz empfunden.

Was die Technik der Injektion betrifft, so ist zu dem oben Gesagten noch folgendes zu bemerken:

Der Arm wird, wie auch aus Fig. 1 ersichtlich ist, stark abduziert und dann die Pelotte angelegt, die einen mässigen Druck ausübt auf die gut palpablen Gefässe. Damit man zur Injektion genügend Spielraum hat, muss sie möglichst weit nach oben unter den Pektoralis geschoben werden. Dann fixiert man mit der einen Hand die Arterie und geht mit der Injektionsnadel möglichst weit oben unter dem Pectoralis major in der Richtung des Armes ein (Fig. 1). Beim Vordringen der Nadel muss sofort gespritzt werden, um die Gefässe zum Ausweichen zu bringen und ihre Verletzung zu vermeiden. Man umspült so mit einigen

adrenaline. The technique of this injection has been described by me in the greatest possible detail. The anesthesia extended upwards as far even as the first rib, with the result that all the visible lymph nodes and glands could be removed painlessly. The stimulation of the large nerve trunks was also painless. It was, however, only a superficial anesthesia, the limb itself continuing to present normal sensitivity.

On the basis of this experience, I took a 2 % novocaine solution and injected it by the same method into the brachial plexus. To prevent an excessively rapid absorption of the anesthetic I brought about a slight stasis by applying a compression belt on the vascular trunks fixed to the shoulder and chest with two elastic bands (Fig. 1). When the anesthesia had set in, I interrupted the stasis and applied a tourniquet on the arm in order to be able to operate in a state of ischemia.

In three cases, the complete anesthesia obtained with this procedure made it possible to perform major surgery on the entire arm.

The first of these was the case of a 28-year-old man who required surgery for the removal of a bullet that had lodged in the cubital tunnel of the elbow just above the joint. I injected 25 cc. of 2 % novocaine solution with the addition of a few drops of adrenaline. After half an hour and for a period lasting an hour and a half the anesthesia was total.

The second case was one of an elderly 70-year-old lady greatly debilitated by diffuse tuberculosis at the level of the right elbow. We injected 30 cc. of solution. The anesthesia set in after 20-25 min. The arm could be amputated painlessly just above the middle part of the humerus.

The third case was one of a 58-year-old man with tubercular osteomyelitis of the distal ulnar epiphysis. In this case, too, we used an injection of 30 cc. of solution, and the anesthesia set in after 40 min, but then proved total.

To reduce the patient's anxiety, prior to almost all the local anesthesias administered, we injected morphine or Pantopon. To put the elderly lady's mind at rest, we applied an oxygen mask, particularly when sawing the bone.

During the interventions the patients experienced no pain sensations.

As far as the injection technique is concerned, I would like to add the following observations:

As may be seen in Fig. 1, the arm is substantially abducted in order to apply the compression belt that exerts a moderate compression on the easily palpable vessels. To make room for the injection the needle must be pushed upwards as far as possible to a point below the pectoralis muscle. At this point the artery is fixed with one hand, pushing the needle upwards as far as possible to a point below the pectoralis major muscle and in the direction of the arm (Fig. 1). To keep the vessels at a safe distance and avoid injuring them the liquid must be injected right from the outset when advancing the needle. In this way the median and ulnar nerves are bathed with just a few injections of the solution. It is then necessary to deliver a further injection below the artery at approximately the level of the insertion of the latissimus dorsi muscle. Here the needle mainly comes into contact with the radial nerve. In this way the artery is bathed and with just a little careful attention one avoids damaging the artery and vein.

The anesthetist must take great care to make sure when pressing the needle upwards that it goes beyond the first rib, because otherwise it will not make contact with the axillary and musculocutaneous nerves. As can be seen in Fig. 2, (according to Spalteholz) departing, more or less at the same level from the head of the humerus, which is palpable, are the musculocutaneous nerve superiorly and the axillary nerve inferiorly. Figure 3 shows their ramification at the level of the skin of the arm. Both the nerves can be reached easily by the injection: in my three cases they were anesthetized.

With gentle massaging after the injection the anesthetic can be spread by increasing the pressure.

The needle did not damage the vessels either in the three cases described above, or in another three cases described previously. In any event, vascular lesions are always a possibility and it is essential that a complex local anesthesia should not be entrusted to non-experts. It may be that the consequences of an injury to an artery due to puncture with a thin needle may not be important. I am of the opinion that, even with the addition of adrenaline, the application of a tourniquet to the limb is fundamental for the success of the anesthesia. Probably, the novocaine would otherwise be reabsorbed instead of infiltrating the large nerve trunks. In the three cases described from 20 to 40 min elapsed before the onset of the anesthesia. It is likely that this time period may be reduced by improving the technique.

We used a 2 % solution, bearing in mind the thickness of the nerve trunks, and we consumed on average approximately 0.6 grams of novocaine. This high concentration was excellently tolerated by the patients none of whom ever manifested any kind of adverse reaction or disturbance. The amount of adrenaline added was relatively low, 1 drop of adrenaline 1:1,000 in 30 cc. of solution. As I observed previously, isolated cases of nausea and vomiting after local anesthesia are due mainly to the addition of adrenaline: larger amounts of novocaine were always well tolerated. In case of necessity, the concentration of the novocaine solution could probably be further increased, thus shortening the anesthesia onset time.

In all major surgeries performed under local anesthesia, I believe it is of the utmost importance to carefully monitor the psychological state of the individual patients. The anesthetist is making a grave mistake if he submits unsuitable, fearful or psychologically disturbed patients to local anesthesia. One cannot rule out the possible occurrence of severe states of shock that may have serious consequences. There must be a well defined indication, not only for the choice and execution of surgery, but also for the administration of local anesthesia.

In any case, it is good policy, as already mentioned above, to administer morphine or Pantopon or scopomorphine. Good sedation is obtained with such premedication. An oxygen mask can also be applied or a few drops of ether or chloroform can be administered. Assuming these precautions are taken, local anesthesia will make important progress in future.

10.2 Introduction

One of the purposes of this monographic study was to commemorate, at a distance of about a century, the first brachial plexus blocks, namely Kulenkampff's supraclavicular block and Hirschel's axillary block. What better way to do this than to reproduce the original articles accurately translated from the German into English? (for the translation of the Kulenkampff article, see Chap. 6).

On glancing at the texts, one has the impression, on the one hand, that the authors are experimenting with new paths that had never previously been explored, introducing the needle more or less blindfold, identifying the drug and the right concentration for the anesthesia, and basing these attempts on their knowledge of anatomy; on the other hand, one is impressed by the topicality of certain concepts, such as the cranial administration of the anesthetic, the downstream compression and massaging to facilitate its spread and the combination of the peripheral anesthetic technique with the need to sedate the patient.

The Hirschel text reproduced here in translation does not show its 100-year age and, above all, does not appear to be the document that marked the start of a long story. The axillary block is something of a paradox, because everything seems to have already been known right from the outset, yet enormous progress has been made over the years, particularly in the last two decades, with regard to identifying more precise techniques safer and more effective drugs and adjuvants, and devices facilitating the execution of the blocks.

Since the advent of ultrasound techniques, we have been able to easily recognize the anatomical elements, the needle position in relation to the nerve structures and the spread of the anesthetic, and finally, it is now possible to appreciate the many details acquired over the years in the 'blind' techniques to improve the efficacy rates and discover the reasons for a number of previously inexplicable failures.

In this chapter, we will attempt to present a succinct yet complete account of the axillary block—from Hirschel's initial efforts to the present-day ultrasound-guided techniques—which we hope will be of use both to experts for establishing the links and possible synergies between old and new techniques, and to novices for familiarizing themselves with techniques they will never perform, but which have contributed to the success of one of the most commonly executed anesthetic blocks.

10.3 Indications

The indications for the axillary block constitute surgical operations involving the skin, muscles, bones and nerves from the hand to the elbow.

In addition, it is indicated for the treatment of postoperative pain, in cases presenting chronic pain in complex regional pain syndromes, in cases of deafferentation pain, neuropathy and pain due to accidental intra-arterial injection of drugs with arterial spasm.

10.4 Contraindications

There are very few local contraindications to the axillary block. These include the impossibility of abducting the arm for traumatic reasons or due to chronic diseases; the presence of lymphadenopathies or infections of the axillary region; and previous surgery responsible for altering the anatomy (e.g. lymphadenectomy).

The relative systemic contraindications refer above all to anticoagulant treatment, haemorrhagic diseases, nervous system diseases and peripheral nerve injuries.

As in all types of regional anesthesia, refusal of the procedure, in the absence of contraindications to general anesthesia, constitutes an absolute contraindication to execution of the block.

10.5 Comparison of Approaches to the Brachial Plexus

There are various different methods that the anesthetist can choose to achieve anesthesia and analgesia of the upper limb inducing a sensory and motor block of the regions from the distal part of the humerus downwards. In the present age of evidence-based medicine, one cannot disregard what the scientific publications state in order to be able to provide qualified performance for the good of the patient and for ensuring greater safeguards, also of a legal nature, on the part of the anesthetist. We will therefore examine what the literature has produced in recent years with regard to the evolution of brachial plexus block by the axillary route, highlighting the technical suggestions best supported by scientific evidence. In this and in the following section, we intend to avail ourselves of a schematization already used in a recent review (Tran et al.) involving the use of the term 'approach' when referring to the site at which access is gained to the brachial plexus, that is to say the supraclavicular, infraclavicular, axillary and midhumeral approaches. The term 'technique' will be used to refer to the modalities whereby the nerve branches are identified (eliciting paraesthesias, loss of resistance, fascial click, transarterial puncture, neurostimulation, ultrasound) and to the endpoints selected before injecting the local anesthetic (type of twitches elicited, single or multiple twitches, etc.).

10.5.1 Axillary Versus Supraclavicular Approach

Only two randomized controlled studies have compared the axillary and supraclavicular blocks. The first of these, conducted by Fleck et al. recruited 40 patients randomized to receiving a transarterial axillary block or a supraclavicular block with neurostimulation, finding no significant difference in the percentage of patients requiring supplementary anesthesia (80 vs. 65 %, respectively). Kapral et al. on the other hand, using a US-guided supraclavicular approach, obtained a more satisfactory block of the musculocutaneous nerve compared to the axillary block (100 vs. 75 %, respectively). We can conclude that, on the basis of the limited evidence available, the supraclavicular block is capable of achieving results comparable to those obtained with the axillary approach.

10.5.2 Axillary Versus Infraclavicular Approach

The axillary and the infraclavicular approaches share very similar indications, and for this reason, in the literature, there is no lack of studies attempting to demonstrate the superiority of one technique over the other. Although the infraclavicular approach uses different landmarks and there may be different success rates of this type of block, the results are fairly constant and would appear to favour this approach.

It has been demonstrated that the infraclavicular approach with a single stimulation produces satisfactory surgical anesthesia in a higher percentage of patients compared to the axillary approach with a single stimulation (97–100 vs. 80–85 %; $p = 0.05$) as a result of a better block of the territories of competence of the axillary and musculocutaneous nerves. Moreover, according to Chin et al. the infraclavicular approach affords better tolerance of tourniquet-induced pain.

When compared to the axillary approach with three or four stimulations, the infraclavicular approach with a single administration showed comparable success rates (85–92 %) in two studies conducted by Koscielniak-Nielsen et al. in a total of 180 patients. The infraclavicular approach, however, according to Deleuze, et al. required fewer needle insertions and thus presented shorter execution times and proved more comfortable for the patients, reducing both the pain associated with the procedure and the incidence of side effects such as paraesthesias and vascular puncture.

The advent of ultrasound guidance has renewed interest in the infraclavicular block, increasing its safety margins. Transarterial axillary block has been compared with the ultrasound-guided infraclavicular block in 232 patients, with similar results in terms of execution times or adequacy of anesthesia, but the infraclavicular block presented a lower incidence of paraesthesias and less pain at the site of the block at two and ten days. This explains the greater number of patients reported by Tedore et al. that expressed a desire to opt for the infraclavicular block as a future anesthesia approach. In line with these results are those reported by Tran et al. who evaluated the ultrasound-guided infraclavicular block versus the axillary block with triple stimulation. The two approaches presented similar success rates (91 vs. 89 %, respectively), but the infraclavicular approach yielded shorter execution times (3.90 ± 2.27 vs. 8.03 ± 3.92 min; $p < 0.001$) and lower VAS values (2.70 ± 2.02 vs. 4.17 ± 2.57; $p < 0.01$). Lastly, the same authors compared the infraclavicular and axillary approaches, both US-guided, no appreciable differences being found in terms of anesthesia-related times (23–25 min), success rates (95–97 %) and incidence of side effects such as paraesthesias and vascular puncture. The axillary approach, however, required a greater number of needle insertions and needle movements during execution of the block.

10.5.3 Axillary Versus Midhumeral Approach

In a study by Bonaziz et al. the midhumeral injection of local anesthetic into the terminal branches of the brachial plexus has yielded a higher success rate compared to the axillary approach with dual stimulation (88 vs. 54 %; $p < 0.01$). These results, however, were not confirmed in the study conducted by Fuzier et al. who found a similar degree of efficacy, although the musculocutaneous nerve was better anesthetized in the midhumeral group. The axillary block with dual stimulation, moreover, presented shorter execution and onset of anesthesia times, thus proving better tolerated by the patients.

Comparison between the midhumeral and a triple injection axillary block was conducted by March et al. in 96 patients. The triple injection axillary approach yielded a higher success rate (94 vs. 79 %; $p < 0.05$), reduced performance times (8 ± 4 vs. 11 ± 4 min; $p < 0.01$) and onset times (16 ± 6 vs. 21 ± 9 min), but caused a higher incidence of vascular puncture (22 vs. 8 %; $p < 0.05$).

Two studies, on the other hand, have compared the midhumeral approach and the axillary approach with quadruple stimulation, finding no difference in success rates. The axillary approach, however, was associated, in one study by Koscielniak-Nielsen et al. with shorter times to achieve adequate anesthesia for surgery (26 ± 8 vs. 30 ± 6 min; $p = 0.04$), while in the other study by Sia et al. it was associated with less pain related to the procedure (VAS = 16 ± 9 vs. 22 ± 12 mm; $p < 0.005$).

10.6 Axillary Brachial Plexus Block Techniques

The localization of the terminal branches of the brachial plexus at the axillary level can be achieved with indirect methods such as the stimulation of paraesthesias or appropriate twitches, or with direct-view methods such as ultrasound guidance. These techniques are not mutually exclusive and can be integrated in order to improve the results. We will therefore examine the eliciting of paraesthesias, the loss of resistance, fascial clicks, transarterial puncture and ultrasound guidance.

10.6.1 Eliciting Paraesthesias

Contact of the needle with the peripheral nerve branches produces a sensation of sudden, intense tingling, tickling, burning or formication in the area they innervate, which is termed paraesthesia. Before the advent of the electrical nerve stimulator in regional anesthesia practice, eliciting paraesthesias was the most valid empirical method for establishing how near the needle tip was to the brachial plexus.

The success rate reported in the literature for this technique is variable according to the different parameters with which the success of a block is defined and the various factors related to the technique in question that are capable of influencing its success. For example, when the use of this technique correlates positively with the number of paraesthesias elicited, it has been seen, in a report by Baranowski and Pither, that the eliciting of one, two or three paraesthesias is associated with success rates of 60, 82 and 100 %, respectively. These results, however, need to be considered with caution, inasmuch as the patients were not randomly assigned to the groups examined. What is more, the success rate may be related to the inclination imparted to the needle during the injection. An insertion perpendicular to the axillary artery compared to one tangential to the artery presented a higher success rate and better quality block. Rucci et al. moreover, have demonstrated that a slower local anesthetic injection speed (30 s) also yields better results than a faster injection rate (10 s).

On the other hand, three randomized controlled studies conducted by Youssef and Degrand, Turkan et al., and Goldberg et al. have assessed attempts to elicit paraesthesias with the transarterial puncture technique.

We refer the reader to the specific section addressing this technique, briefly recalling here that no significant differences were found compared to the eliciting of just a single paraesthesia.

The advent of electrical nerve stimulation has supplanted the search for paraesthesias in clinical practice, yet not many randomized controlled studies have analysed the differences. We will mention three such studies, in two of which the techniques investigated showed no statistically significant differences in success rates. In the third, most recent of these studies, conducted by Sia et al. 96 patients were recruited and randomized to receiving two types of blocks, one with the eliciting of three paraesthesias plus local infiltration of the coracobrachialis muscle and the other with quadruple neurostimulation.

The latter technique yielded a higher success rate (91 vs. 76 %; $p < 0.05$) with a reduction in anesthesia onset times (25 ± 8 vs. 35 ± 9 min; $p < 0.001$) due to a simultaneous reduction in block execution and onset times.

10.6.2 Loss of Resistance

Alternative methods to the eliciting of paraesthesias were sought as early as the 1980s in order to reduce the incidence of nerve injuries and accidental vascular punctures in the search for the brachial plexus. On the strength of the 'loss of resistance' technique used to detect the epidural space, the sensation of 'loss of resistance' was also proposed at the axillary level as an endpoint for the injection of local anesthetic, which the anesthetist perceives when the needle penetrates the fascia investing the neurovascular bundle in that region.

This 'cannulation' of the neurovascular bundle was compared by Hill and Campbell with the widespread practice of eliciting paraesthesias at that time in a randomized controlled study in 60 patients. The loss of resistance technique not only presented a higher success rate (73 vs. 43 %; $p < 0.05$) but also a more complete block in the axillary, musculocutaneous and radial nerve regions along with a significant reduction in vascular punctures (7 vs. 33 %; $p < 0.01$).

10.6.3 Fascial Click

In the path taken by the needle in its descent from the skin to the deeper layers in search of the brachial plexus, the anesthetist is capable of perceiving several clicks due to the needle passing through the tissues. Recognizing the click that marks the entry of the needle into the neurovascular space of the axillary region will determine the success or failure of the technique.

In a study conducted in 100 patients, Baranowski and Pither observed a higher failure rate when positioning a catheter using the fascial click technique, compared to the eliciting of paraesthesias or the use of electrical nerve stimulation, due to incomplete block of the territories of the median and ulnar nerves. In line with these results are the results of a study conducted by Tuominen et al. who report a higher failure rate as compared with electrical nerve stimulation (13 vs. 0 %) and a lower incidence of complete blocks (60 vs. 73 %), although these differences are not statistically significant.

To improve the results, an attempt was made to combine the determination of the fascial click with other techniques. Rodriguez et al. for instance, combined the fascial click with the injection of saline, demonstrating that when cold (8–11 °C), saline proves capable of eliciting paraesthesias in a more consistent manner compared to room temperature saline, giving rise to increased success rates. The same group subsequently compared the fascial click plus the injection of cold saline versus the use of the electrical nerve stimulator (just a single distal twitch), finding a positive response and a success rate of around 95 % in both groups. By contrast, in a report by Fuzier et al. the combination with electrical nerve stimulation proved reliable and efficacious in the context of catheterization via the axillary route in emergency upper limb surgery in as many as 120 patients.

10.6.4 Transarterial Puncture

Transarterial puncture consists in perforating the axillary artery and injecting all the volume of local anesthetic (usually about 40 ml) posteriorly to it. Alternatively, you can also subdivide the dose and deposit half of it posteriorly and half anteriorly to the artery. The success rates range from 70 to 82 %, In particular, according to Hockey et al. the single injection posteriorly to the artery presents a slower onset of anesthesia and less involvement of the territories of the median nerve. The same study, however, failed to show any difference between a single injection anteriorly to the artery and the two injections, half in front and half to the rear of the artery. Particular attention must be paid to avoiding an intravascular injection, especially with this technique which, by increasing the pressure within the neurovascular compartment, may shift the walls of the vessels, moving them closer to the needle tip which itself remains immobile.

This technique, as reported by Pere et al. has proved to be equivalent to a single injection together with the use of the electrical nerve stimulator. A randomized controlled study conducted by Jones in 57 patients has even found that transarterial puncture is superior to double neurostimulation with a success rate of 66 vs. 47 % ($p < 0.05$). On the other hand, in two studies conducted by Koscielniak-Nielsen et al. in a total of 200 patients, a quadruple stimulation produced better results (success rates of 88–94 vs. 62–64 %; $p < 0.001$) with a reduction in time to anesthesia (23–30 vs. 37–38 min; $p < 0.001$) despite the longer performance times (10–11 vs. 7–8 min; $p < 0.001$), probably on account of a shorter latency and reduced demand for supplementation.

In a study by Goldberg et al. quadruple stimulation also proved superior to transarterial puncture and eliciting paraesthesias, with higher success rates (87 vs. 54 %; $p < 0.001$) and despite a longer execution period (11 vs. 7 min; $p < 0.05$), total anesthesia time was lower (32 vs. 39 min; $p < 0.05$).

10.6.5 Neurostimulation

Although neurostimulation may appear to be a recent innovation, as early as 1912 a nickel needle was used connected to an electrical nerve stimulator that evoked given muscle contractions when the needle tip was close to a nerve. The clinical use of the technique, however, became widespread only when it was possible to apply more advanced technologies that have permitted the development of portable stimulators and of needles made of more suitable materials, insulated electrically except for the tip. Since the 1990s, there has been a plethora of publications attempting to refine the electrical nerve stimulator technique, particularly for the axillary block, determining how many and which contractions should preferably be evoked in order to obtain an effective block.

With the single stimulation technique, the muscle twitch that, when elicited, yields the best results is the one related to the territories of the radial nerve. Rodriguez et al. in fact, have found that, as compared to stimulation of the median nerve, a radial twitch indicates similar anesthetic cover of the territories of the median nerve but significantly superior efficacy with regard to the territories of the ulnar and radial nerves. The use of a single injection for the axillary block is based on the concept of a single neurovascular compartment delimited also by a connective or fibrous sheath. Pressure exerted downstream of the injection site is thought to allow the local anesthetic to spread more proximally. This hypothesis has been analysed in a study by Koscielniak-Nielsen et al. in 98 patients which, as a result of radiographic monitoring of the spread of the injectate, showed no differences between the group in which pressure was exerted and the control group, similar success rates being registered in both groups.

A recent review article by Chin and Handoll, published in the *Cochrane Database of Systematic Reviews,* has analysed all the studies comparing groups with different numbers of stimulations. There are 11 clinical trials comparing double stimulation with single stimulation, showing that the former significantly reduces the anesthesia failure rate. In particular, it is stressed that in a study by Rodriguez et al. of 60 patients, it has been demonstrated that the combination of radial and musculocutaneous nerve contractions is associated with a better quality of anesthesia compared to that associated with twitches of the ulnar and musculocutaneous nerves. In the paediatric population, however, Carre et al. report less uniform results. Although double stimulation yielded earlier onset times, this technique failed to produce a more complete block. The hypothesis adduced to explain this difference versus adults may be that the local anesthetic may have a better circumferential spread due to the anatomy of the neurovascular bundle in that age bracket.

The differences between the technique eliciting multiple contractions (more than two) and that using only a single stimulation were analysed in 7 trials. The first of these showed that the multiple stimulation technique not only reduced the anesthesia failure rate but also the percentage of incomplete motor blocks. Another 11 compared multiple stimulations with double stimulation, showing that eliciting multiple contractions, in this case too, reduces the anesthesia failure rate and the percentage of incomplete motor blocks and significantly reduces the pain caused by the tourniquet.

Sia et al. in 81 patients, evaluated a triple injection technique (with stimulation of the radial, median and musculocutaneous nerves) versus a technique involving four stimulations, reporting similar success rates for the blocks (90 vs. 92 %). Moreover, the study showed comparable results also for the latency (17 vs. 19 min) and the anesthesia onset times (approximately 25 min) despite the fact that the triple stimulation technique involved shorter performance times (5 ± 2 vs. 8 ± 3 min; $p < 0.01$). The quadruple stimulation technique presents the drawback that it induces significantly greater pain values related to the procedure (VAS = 13 ± 2 vs. 8 ± 2 mm; $p < 0.01$). The same authors in two later randomized controlled trials attempted to better define which contraction pattern in triple stimulation was more effective, demonstrating that the radial–median–musculocutaneous combination achieved a higher success rate than the ulnar–median–musculocutaneous combination (91 vs. 73 %; $p < 0.05$), despite taking longer to perform (7.8 ± 1.8 vs. 6.5 ± 1.7 min; $p < 0.01$). Furthermore, they showed that, in the case of radial stimulation, eliciting a distal contraction (such as the supination of the hand or the extension of the fingers) permits a better sensory block and a reduction in onset times compared to injection involving a proximal contraction, despite the fact that its localization takes longer (8.4 ± 1.9 vs. 7 ± 1.7 min; $p < 0.01$).

10.6.6 Ultrasound Guidance

The advent of the use of ultrasound in medicine opened up new horizons also in the regional anesthesia sector. After the various different techniques that permitted the anesthetist by guesswork to indirectly locate the presence of a nerve, inserting the needle on the basis of external landmarks, with ultrasound guidance it now proves possible to view the anatomical structures, the direction of the needle and the spread of local anesthetic directly. The anesthetist is called upon to apply his or her knowledge of anatomy to the two-dimensional ultrasound image in which the different grey scales or the compactness or otherwise of colour identifies very precise structures, which it is of fundamental importance to be familiar with and to be able to recognize.

The brachial plexus when approached via the axillary route is observed by placing the probe transversely in relation to the arm abducted 90°. In this way, a scan parallel to the sagittal plane, or slightly oblique, is obtained. The marker present on the transducer is placed superiorly in relation to the operator or cranially in relation to the patient (Fig. 10.1).

The typical image obtained with a linear transducer has as its first landmark the axillary artery, which is usually accompanied by from one to four veins with a very variable disposition. The vessels and nerves are to be found in a loose, connective tissue space, rich in septa, with

10 Axillary Brachial Plexus Block

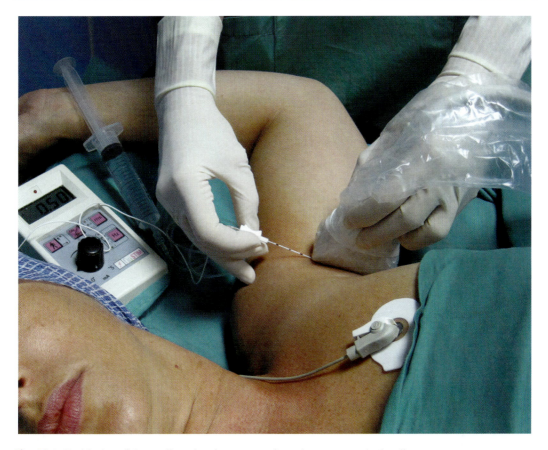

Fig. 10.1 Positioning of the needle and probe transversely to the neurovascular bundle

a hyperechoic appearance and a triangular shape. When the patient is positioned for scanning, these structures lie within a distance of 1–2 cm from the skin, even in grossly obese patients (Sheppard et al.) (Fig. 10.2).

At this level, the brachial plexus has branched out into its terminal branches, and the median, ulnar and radial nerves appear as well-defined bunches of hyperechogenic, vesicular structures. With high-resolution ultrasonographs, it is even possible to recognize the endoneurial structures that separate the individual fascicles. The radial nerve rests upon the underside of the neurovascular bundle enclosed by the two aponeuroses of the coracobrachialis and triceps brachii muscles. The humerus, which closes the field of vision in depth, has the appearance of a hyperechogenic arch with an acoustic void to its rear. Numerous studies have evaluated the position of the nerves around the brachial artery in order to understand what their normal distribution is. By way of reference, we may mention the study conducted by Chan et al. who have produced a schematic diagram of the ultrasound image, visualizing it as the face of a watch. The median nerve is situated in 58 % of cases between 7 and 8 o'clock (sectors 7 and 8), the ulnar nerve in 87 % of cases in sectors 1 and 2, and the radial nerve in 70 % of cases in sectors 3 and 4 (Fig. 10.3).

The radial nerve presents the most complex sonoanatomy both because it is distributed in a very variable manner and, above all, because its visibility is often reduced by the posterior acoustic reinforcement artefact due to the brachial artery (Fig. 10.4).

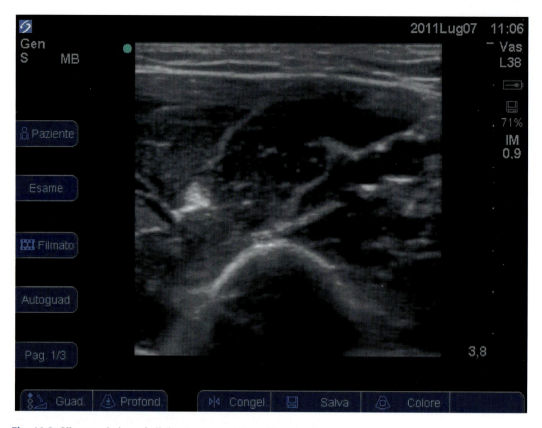

Fig. 10.2 Ultrasound view of all the structures at the axillary level

Moreover, the nerve is embedded in the connective tissue of the axillary fossa, unlike the other nerve trunks, which are surrounded mainly by muscle tissue.

Not infrequently, the injection of local anesthetic improves the local visibility posteriorly to the artery, reducing the reinforcement phenomenon, and improves the visualization of the branches of the radial nerve which were previously undetectable. The relative positions of the nerves are very variable not only individually but also in relation to the pressure exerted by the transducer on the arm.

The musculocutaneous nerve is not normally directly related to the brachial artery and is not found within the neurovascular compartment but is included within the belly of the coracobrachialis muscle and may sometimes lie between the aponeurosis of this same muscle and that of the biceps brachii muscle. The cross-section of the nerve at this level is characteristically streamlined, surrounded by muscular tissue, with the classic ultrasound appearance of honeycomb nerves (Fig. 10.5).

Ultrasound-guided axillary block was compared with the transarterial puncture technique in two studies: Soeding et al. found it produces a better sensorimotor block, a shorter onset time and a reduced incidence of paraesthesias compared to the blind injection of a half dose posteriorly and a half dose anteriorly to the artery. Also when applied in conjunction with the transarterial technique, ultrasound guidance made it possible to reduce the block performance time and the failure rate, as reported by Sites et al.

The issue as to whether the use of ultrasound is preferable to that of electrical nerve stimulation is still a matter of heated debate today. Despite the optimistic claims of those who anticipate a complete reduction in side effects, performance times, etc., no evidence has been

Fig. 10.3 Percentage detection of the different terminal branches in the ultrasound image (from Chan et al. modified)

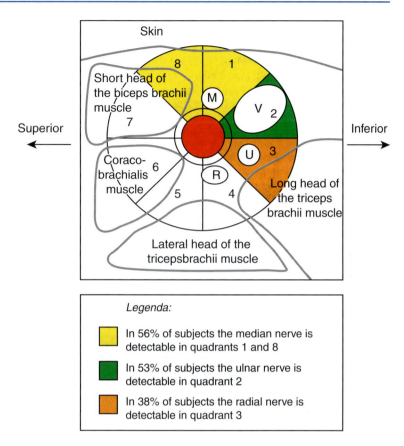

found to date of such clear-cut advantages in terms of success rates. As regards the learning curve of this new technique, according to Morros et al. it has been estimated that, for anesthetists with experience of the traditional axillary block, at least 15 US-guided blocks are needed to obtain clinically comparable results.

There are studies such as that by Schwemmer et al. in which ultrasound guidance and neurostimulation were compared in the operative management in axillary plexus blocks, revealing in the ultrasound group a higher success rate (98.2 vs. 83.1 %), enabling the surgical intervention to be started 15 min earlier (5 vs. 20 min; $p < 0.001$), with a lower duration of anesthesia (85 vs. 120 min; $p < 0.001$) and a reduced need for postoperative assistance (5.4 vs. 32.4 %; $p < 0.001$).

In a more recent axillary block study conducted by Blox et al. 120 patients were subdivided into three groups (neurostimulation, ultrasound guidance with an 'in-plane' approach and ultrasound guidance with an 'out-of-plane' approach). The authors' aim was to assess patient comfort in subjects undergoing axillary brachial plexus block with the three techniques and describing their experience of the anesthesia in terms of 'comfortable' or 'very comfortable'. 25 and 55 % of patients in the 'out-of-plane' ultrasound group reported feeling comfortable and very comfortable, respectively, as compared to 20 and 32 % in the 'in-plane' ultrasound group, and 8 and 25 % in the neurostimulation group.

On the other hand, neurostimulation and ultrasound guidance do not necessarily oblige the anesthetist to make a mutually exclusive choice between them. The axillary plexus block technique may avail itself of the concomitant use of both procedures for greater patient safety and a higher success rate.

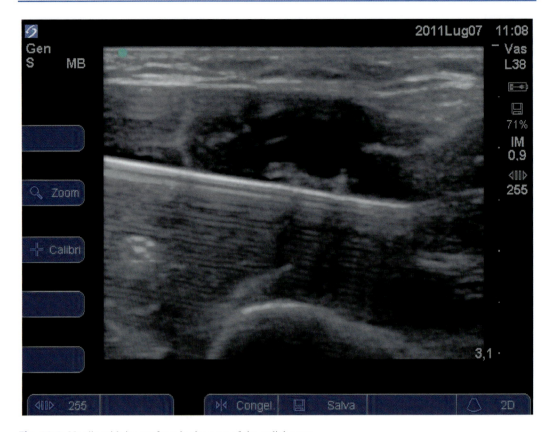

Fig. 10.4 Needle with its artefacts in the area of the radial nerve

10.7 Continuous Blocks

The continuous axillary block has been described by various authors, and it has been performed, according to the respective periods, using the devices available at the time, ranging from the early intravenous Teflon cannulas attached with plasters, to the latest dedicated kits.

The indications for this type of block are all included in the indications for the continuous infraclavicular block, which must be regarded as being first choice.

In actual fact though, the precarious stability of the catheter and the ease of infection of the exit point in the armpit have meant that these blocks have been practically abandoned in clinical practice.

A few anesthetists still use the procedure, adopting a tunnelling technique that allows the catheter to emerge in a position outside the axillary fossa.

This detail makes it possible to limit the percentage of infections, although it is difficult to maintain the catheter in place for more than 72 h.

10.8 Personal Notes Regarding Technique

I feel I should add a number of considerations in the light of my 25 years of clinical experience with this block.

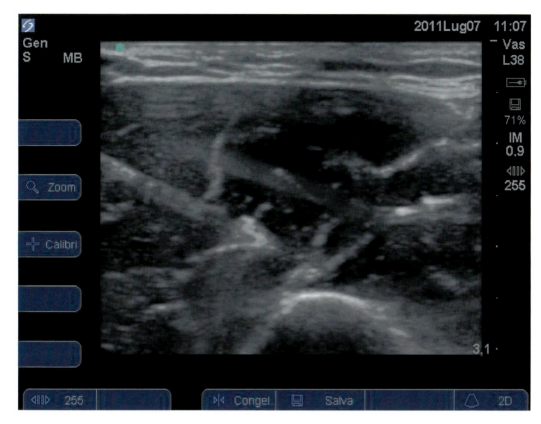

Fig. 10.5 The musculocutaneous nerve reached by the needle, well away from the neurovascular bundle

10.9 ENS

Perform the puncture as proximally as possible without involving the axillary fossa.

Insert the 50-mm needle tangentially to the artery and attempt first to find and stimulate the nerve branch that innervates the area on which surgery is to be performed and subsequently the contiguous branch.

Always search for and block the musculocutaneous nerve.

Search for the stimulation up to 0.2 mA. Do not administer the anesthetic if the stimulation persists below this threshold.

Apply downstream compression during the administration of the anesthetic.

Use local anesthetics at intermediate concentrations (e.g. mepivacaine 1.5 %, ropivacaine 0.75 %), up to a volume of 35–40 ml.

Immediately after the end of the administration, adduct the arm, maintain the compression downstream of the needle entry point for a few minutes and massage gently.

10.9.1 Ultrasound

Position the 35-mm high-frequency probe transversely to the neurovascular bundle below the point where it is crossed anteriorly by the pectoralis major muscle, as is visible in the anatomical illustration in Fig. 10.6.

Use an 80-mm needle and insert the needle 'in plane' 2 cm above or below the edge of the probe, according to the nerve branches that have to be reached first (Figs. 10.7, 10.8 and 10.10).

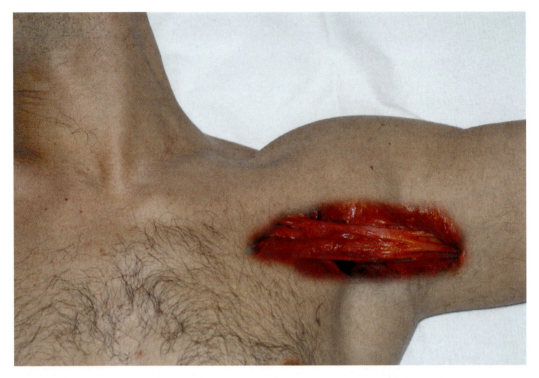

Fig. 10.6 Illustration of the anatomy of the neurovascular bundle at the axillary level with the removal of the pectoralis muscles

The 80-mm needle enables the anesthetist to maintain a position more parallel to the ultrasound beam, thus obtaining greater visibility and the ability to manoeuvre with a wider angle.

With a single superior access, block first the musculocutaneous nerve, then the median nerve, after which, using the décollement caused by the local anesthetic, the radial and ulnar zones are reached (Fig. 10.9).

The yellow arrows represent the three positions that the needle occupies during the performance of the block. Using the same needle entry site each time, the needle is retracted and repositioned without exiting from the skin. The red colour represents the spread of the anesthetic around the radial nerve and the musculocutaneous nerve.

The two vertical light blue lines indicate the projection on the skin of the musculocutaneous nerve and the needle entry point. The distance between these two lines must be such as to allow the needle to reach the musculocutaneous nerve at an adequate angle for it to be visualized by the ultrasonograph (45°).

With the inferior access, the radial nerve is blocked first below the artery within the fascia, then the ulnar zone, avoiding the axillary vein, after which one reaches the median nerve, passing above the artery and moving it using a few cc. of local anesthetic. Proceeding in the same direction, the musculocutaneous nerve can be reached (Fig. 10.10).

The utmost attention needs to be paid to the spread of the anesthetic, which must always be present and must be detectable ahead of the needle tip.

Using the ultrasound technique, the volume of local anesthetic can be reduced by 50 %.

Adduction of the arm, compression downstream of the puncture and light massaging constitute useful means of facilitating the spread of the local anesthetic and reducing the block onset time.

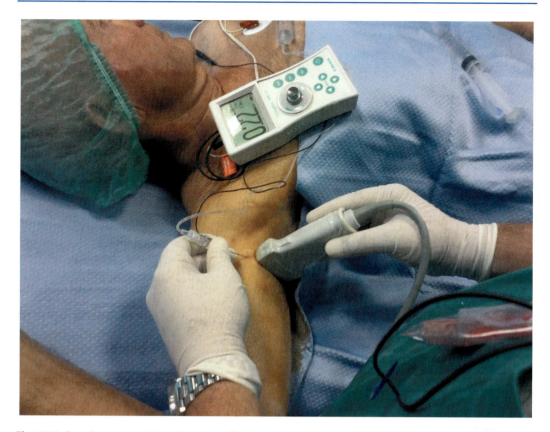

Fig. 10.7 Superior access with an 80-mm needle

10.10 Complications

The success of the axillary block is due not only to the simplicity of performance but also to the limited incidence and severity of complications.

10.10.1 Vascular Puncture

Accidental venous or arterial puncture is a common event with the use of ENS, but is much less frequent (approximately 5-fold less) with the use of ultrasound.

If the subject's coagulative condition is normal, moderate compression resolves the problem; in the presence of coagulative impairment, the formation of a haematoma is possible.

10.10.2 Acute Toxicity

In the eventuality of a vascular puncture, there may be an intravascular injection of local anesthetic, with the immediate onset of symptoms of acute toxicity, ranging from a metallic taste in the mouth to involuntary movements of the limbs, even to the point of a convulsive crisis.

The prevention of such events is based on aspiration every 5 cc. of anesthetic, slow administration and maintaining constant verbal contact with the patient.

For the purposes of rapidly detecting the symptoms related to acute toxicity, it is advisable to avoid the use of sedative drugs before performing the block or confining their use to sedation under vigilant monitoring, in case of excessive agitation.

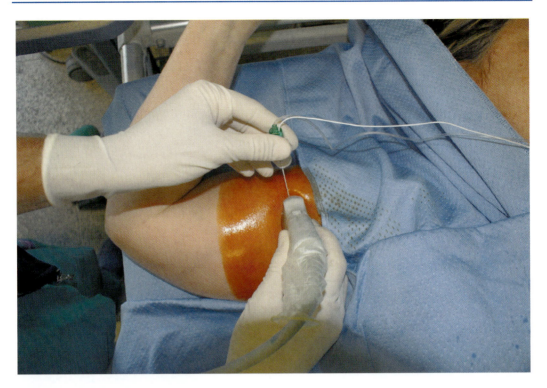

Fig. 10.8 Another example in an obese patient

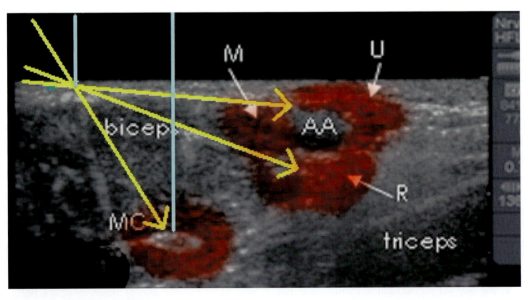

Fig. 10.9 Representation of the brachial plexus block execution technique with ultrasound guidance; we have proposed this technique in order to be able to distribute the local anesthetic both at the perivascular level and on the musculocutaneous nerve from the same needle entry site on the skin. M = median nerve; U = ulnar nerve; R = radial nerve; MC = musculocutaneous nerve; AA = axillary artery

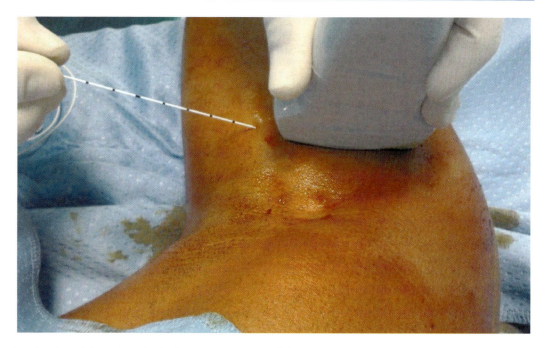

Fig. 10.10 Inferior entry point for better access to the radial nerve

10.10.3 Nerve Injuries

Nerve injuries as a result of axillary block are to be regarded as extremely rare events.

ENS has permitted a substantial reduction in nerve injuries compared to the techniques used previously, such as the eliciting of paraesthesias or the transarterial technique. Ultrasonography, if correctly employed, enables the anesthetist to visualize the nerve structures and the needle tip, thus making it possible to avoid direct contact with the nerve and the intraneural administration of local anesthetic.

From this point of view, the studies by Hadzic et al. have demonstrated that only administrations at high pressure in the nerve fascicles are capable of destroying the nerve cells and causing permanent injury.

Attention, however, must be paid to the presumed nerve injuries attributed to the anesthetic block, which are more likely to be the result of iatrogenic lesions or incorrect postures.

The use of short-bevel needles and ENS, which permits the monitoring of the stimulation intensity, in conjunction with ultrasound visualization, makes it possible to reduce nerve damage to a minimum.

Bibliography

Baranowski AP, Pither CE (1990) A comparison of three methods of axillary brachial plexus anaesthesia. Anaesthesia 45(5):362–365

Bloc S, Mercadal L, Garnier T, Komly B, Leclerc P, Morel B, Ecoffey C, Dhonneur G (2010) Comfort of the patient during axillary blocks placement: a randomized comparison of the neurostimulation and the ultrasound guidance techniques. Eur J Anaesthesiol 27(7):628–633

Bouaziz H, Narchi P, Mercier FJ, Labaille T, Zerrouk N, Girod J, Benhamou D (1997) Comparison between conventional axillary block and a new approach at the midhumeral level. Anesth Analg 84(5):1058–1062

Carre P, Joly A, Cluzel Field B, Wodey E, Lucas MM, Ecoffey C (2000) Axillary block in children: single or multiple injection? Paediatr Anaesth 10(1):35–39

Chan VW, Perlas A, McCartney CJ, Brull R, Xu D, Abbas S (2007) Ultrasound guidance improves success rate of axillary brachial plexus block. Can J Anaesth 54(3):176–182

Chin KJ, Handoll HH (2011) Single, double or multiple-injection techniques for axillary brachial plexus block for hand, wrist or forearm surgery in adults. Cochrane Database Syst Rev 7:CD003842

Chin KJ, Singh M, Velayutham V, Chee V (2010) Infraclavicular brachial plexus block for regional anaesthesia of the lower arm. Cochrane Database Syst Rev 2:CD005487

De Tran QH, Clemente A, Doan J, Finlayson RJ (2007) Brachial plexus blocks: a review of approaches and techniques. Can J Anaesth 54(8):662–674

Deleuze A, Gentili ME, Marret E, Lamonerie L, Bonnet F (2003) A comparison of a single-stimulation lateral infraclavicular plexus block with a triple-stimulation axillary block. Reg Anesth Pain Med 28(2):89–94

Fleck JW, Moorthy SS, Daniel J, Dierdorf SF (1994) Brachial plexus block. A comparison of the supraclavicular lateral paravascular and axillary approaches. Reg Anesth 19(1):14–17

Fuzier R, Fourcade O, Fuzier V, Arnold S, Torrie J, Olivier M (2006) The feasibility and efficacy of short axillary catheters for emergency upper limb surgery: a descriptive series of 120 cases. Anesth Analg 102(2):610–614

Goldberg ME, Gregg C, Larijani GE, Norris MC, Marr AT, Seltzer JL (1987) A comparison of three methods of axillary approach to brachial plexus blockade for upper extremity surgery. Anesthesiology 66(6):814–816

Hickey R, Hoffman J, Tingle LJ, Rogers JN, Ramamurthy S (1993) Comparison of the clinical efficacy of three perivascular techniques for axillary brachial plexus block. Reg Anesth 18(6):335–338

Hill DA, Campbell WI (1992) Two approaches to the axillary brachial plexus. Loss of resistance to saline or paraesthesia? Anaesthesia 47(3):207–209

Jones TS (1997) Comparison of axillary block techniques: is there a difference in success rates? AANA J 65(3):257–259

Kapral S, Krafft P, Eibenberger K, Fitzgerald R, Gosch M, Weinstabl C (1994) Ultrasound-guided supraclavicular approach for regional anesthesia of the brachial plexus. Anesth Analg 78(3):507–513

Koschielniak-Nielsen ZJ, Christensen LQ, Pedersen HL, Brusho J (1995) Effect of digital pressure on the neurovascular sheath during perivascular axillary block. Br J Anaesth 75(6):702–706

Koscielniak-Nielsen ZJ, Hesselbjerg L, Fejlberg V (1998) Comparison of transarterial and multiple nerve stimulation techniques for an initial axillary block by 45 mL of mepivacaine 1 % with adrenaline. Acta Anaesthesiol Scand 42(5):570–575

Koscielniak-Nielsen ZJ, Nielsen PR, Nielsen SL, Gardi T, Hermann C (1999) Comparison of transarterial and multiple nerve stimulation techniques for axillary block using a high dose of mepivacaine with adrenaline. Acta Anaesthesiol Scand 43(4):398–404

Koscielniak-Nielsen ZJ, Rasmussen H, Hesselbjerg L, Nielsen TP, Gurkan Y (2005) Infraclavicular block causes less discomfort than axillary block in ambulatory patients. Acta Anaesthesiol Scand 49(7):1030–1034

Koscielniak-Nielsen ZJ, Rasmussen H, Nielsen PT (2004) Patients' perception of pain during axillary and humeral blocks using multiple nerve stimulations. Reg Anesth Pain Med 29(4):328–332

March X, Pardina B, Torres-Bahi S, Navarro M, del Mar Garcia M, Villalonga A (2003) A comparison of a triple-injection axillary brachial plexus block with the humeral approach. Reg Anesth Pain Med 28(6):504–508

Morros C, Perez-Cuenca MD, Sala-Blanch X, Cedo F (2011) Ultrasound-guided axillary brachial plexus block: learning curve and results. Rev Esp Anestesiol Reanim 58(2):74–79

Pere P, Pitkanen M, Tuominen M, Edgren J, Rosenberg PH (1993) Clinical and radiological comparison of perivascular and transarterial techniques of axillary brachial plexus block. Br J Anaesth 70(3):276–279

Rodriguez J, Barcena M, Alvarez J (1996) Axillary brachial plexus anesthesia: electrical versus cold saline stimulation. Anesth Analg 83(4):752–754

Rodriguez J, Carceller J, Barcena M, Pedraza I, Calvo B, Alvarez J (1995) Cold saline is more effective than room temperature saline in inducing paresthesia during axillary block. Anesth Analg 81(2):329–331

Rodriguez J, Taboada M, Del Rio S, Barcena M, Alvarez J (2005) A comparison of four stimulation patterns in axillary block. Reg Anesth Pain Med 30(4):324–328

Rodriguez J, Taboada M, Valino C, Barcena M, Alvarez J (2006) A comparison of stimulation patterns in axillary block: part 2. Reg Anesth Pain Med 31(3):202–205

Rucci FS, Boccaccini A, Doni L, Pippa P (1995) The orthogonal two-needle technique: a new axillary approach to the brachial plexus. Eur J Anaesthesiol 12(4):333–339

Rucci FS, Pippa P, Boccaccini A, Barbagli R (1995) Effect of injection speed on anesthetic spread during axillary block using the orthogonal two-needle technique. Eur J Anaesthesiol 12(5):505–511

Schwemmer U, Schleppers A, Markus C, Kredel M, Kirschner S, Roewer N (2006) Operative management in axillary brachial plexus blocks: comparison of ultrasound and nerve stimulation. Anaesthetist 55(4):451–456

Sheppard DG, Iyer RB, Fenstermacher MJ (1998) Brachial plexus: demonstration at US. Radiology 208(2):402–406

Sia S, Bartoli M, Lepri A, Marchini O, Ponsecchi P (2000) Multiple-injection axillary brachial plexus block: a comparison of two methods of nerve localization-nerve stimulation versus paresthesia. Anesth Analg 91(3):647–651

Sia S, Bartoli M (2001) Selective ulnar nerve localization is not essential for axillary brachial plexus block using a multiple nerve stimulation technique. Reg Anesth Pain Med 26(1):12–16

Sia S, Lepri A, Campolo MC, Fiaschi R (2002) Four-injection brachial plexus block using peripheral nerve stimulator: a comparison between axillary and humeral approaches. Anesth Analg 95(4):1075–1079

Sia S, Lepri A, Magherini M, Doni L, Di Marco P, Gritti G (2005) A comparison of proximal and distal radial nerve motor responses in axillary block using triple stimulation. Reg Anesth Pain Med 30(5):458–463

Sia S (2006) A comparison of injection at the ulnar and the radial nerve in axillary block using triple stimulation. Reg Anesth Pain Med 31(6):514–518

Sites BD, Beach ML, Spence BC, Wiley CW, Shiffrin J, Hartman GS, Gallagher JD (2006) Ultrasound guidance improves the success rate of a perivascular axillary plexus block. Acta Anaesthesiol Scand 50(6):678–684

Soeding PE, Sha S, Royse CE, Marks P, Hoy G, Royse AG (2005) A randomized trial of ultrasound-guided brachial plexus anaesthesia in upper limb surgery. Anaesth Intensive Care 33(6):719–725

Tedore TR, YaDeau JT, Maalouf DB, Weiland AJ, Tong-Ngork S, Wukovits B, Paroli L, Urban MK, Zayas VM, Wu A et al (2009) Comparison of the transarterial axillary block and the ultrasound-guided infraclavicular block for upper extremity surgery: a prospective randomized trial. Reg Anesth Pain Med 34(4):361–365

de Tran QH, Clemente A, Tran DQ, Finlayson RJ (2008) A comparison between ultrasound-guided infraclavicular block using the "double bubble" sign and neurostimulation-guided axillary block. Anesth Analg 107(3):1075–1078

de Tran QH, Munoz L, Zaouter C, Russo G, Finlayson RJ (2009) A prospective, randomized comparison between single- and double-injection, ultrasound-guided supraclavicular brachial plexus block. Reg Anesth Pain Med 34(5):420–424

Tuominen MK, Pitkanen MT, Numminen MK, Rosenberg PH (1987) Quality of axillary brachial plexus block. Comparison of success rate using perivascular and nerve stimulator techniques. Anaesthesia 42(1):20–22

Turkan H, Baykal B, Ozisik T (2002) Axillary brachial plexus blockade: an evaluation of three techniques. Mil Med 167(9):723–725

Youssef MS, Desgrand DA (1988) Comparison of two methods of axillary brachial plexus anaesthesia. Br J Anaesth 60(7):841–844

Truncular Blocks

A. Barbati

11.1 Anatomical Considerations

Distally to the axilla, the terminal nerves of the brachial plexus take different courses according to their areas of competence.

The median nerve, along the entire length of the humeral canal (delimited anteriorly by the belly of the short head of the biceps brachii muscle and posteriorly by the medial head of the triceps brachii muscle), runs in a neurovascular compartment where it follows the brachial vessels positioned anteriorly in relation to the latter. At the level of the distal 3rd of the arm, it crosses the brachial artery and presents itself in the elbow region, medially to the medial margin of the biceps tendon and to the artery itself. It then proceeds down the forearm, posteriorly to the flexor digitorum superficialis muscle and the flexor longus pollicis muscle as far as the wrist and at this point passes into the carpal canal below the palmar aponeurosis, between the tendon of the flexor longus pollicis muscle (lateral) and the tendons of the flexor digitorum muscles (medial).

The ulnar nerve follows the vessels in a posterior position along the humeral canal (in the same compartment as the median nerve). At the level of the distal 3rd, it runs posteriorly in the olecranon canal, delimited medially by the medial epicondyle of the humerus and laterally by the olecranon. It then proceeds in the anteromedial part of the forearm and travels as far as the wrist medially to the ulnar artery in a neurovascular compartment delimited posteriorly by the flexor digitorum profundus muscle, anteriorly by the flexor digitorum superficialis muscle (laterally) and by the flexor carpi ulnaris muscle (medially).

The radial nerve already takes a posterior course in the axillary region, and at the level of the proximal 3rd–middle 3rd of the arm, following the torsion furrow of the humerus, it runs posteriorly, remaining between the brachial muscle and the lateral head of the triceps brachii muscle. It rotates around the humerus and, at the level of the middle–distal 3rd, reappears anteriorly, following the lateral head of the biceps brachii muscle in a posterior position, and, before reaching the lateral epicondyle of the humerus, gives rise to the deep and superficial branches that run along the forearm as far as the wrist and hand.

The musculocutaneous nerve, which has perforated the corobrachialis muscle in the axillary region, runs between the long head of the biceps brachii muscle (anterior) and the brachialis muscle (posterior). The motor fibres terminate with the innervation of the biceps brachii muscle, while the sensory branch, which runs superficially and laterally in relation to the lateral head of the biceps brachii muscle, enters the anterolateral region of the forearm in order to innervate the skin.

The medial cutaneous nerve of the forearm runs alongside the median nerve in the same neurovascular compartment, whereas the medial

A. Barbati (✉)
Pain Therapy Service, Padre Pio Hospital,
Mondragone, CE, Italy
e-mail: aldobarbati@hotmail.com

cutaneous nerve of the arm runs in the subcutaneous tissue of the same region. The medial cutaneous nerve of the arm innervates the skin of the medial region of the arm, and the medial cutaneous nerve of the forearm innervates that of the medial region of the forearm. NB Both of these nerves are exclusively sensory.

The innervation of the fingers is supplied by the terminal branches of the radial, median and ulnar nerves. They are usually four in number and run along the edges of the fingers, in the palmar and volar regions.

11.2 Truncular Block Techniques

11.2.1 Midhumeral Block (ENS)

Figures (11.1, 11.2).

Limb Position

Extended, abducted ca. 50° (as necessary for inserting the needle).

Landmarks

- Brachial gutter (delimited anteriorly by the belly of the short head of the biceps brachii muscle and posteriorly by the medial head of the triceps brachii muscle).
- Proximal 3rd–middle 3rd of the arm.
- Pulsation of the brachial artery.

Needle

50 mm, electrically insulated.

Local Anesthetic

20 ml for blocking all the components (3–6 ml per component).

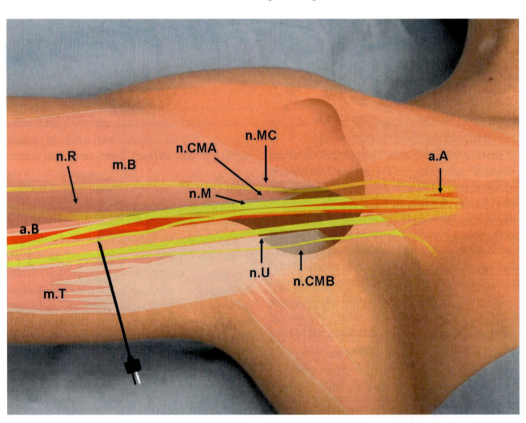

Fig. 11.1 Midhumeral block (proximal region of the arm): *n.M* = median nerve; *n.U* = ulnar nerve; *n.R* = radial nerve; *n. CMA* = medial cutaneous nerve of the forearm; *n. CMB* = medial cutaneous nerve of the arm; *n. MC* = musculocutaneous nerve; *a.B* = brachial artery; *a.A* = axillary artery; *m.B* = biceps brachii muscle; *m.T* = triceps brachii muscle

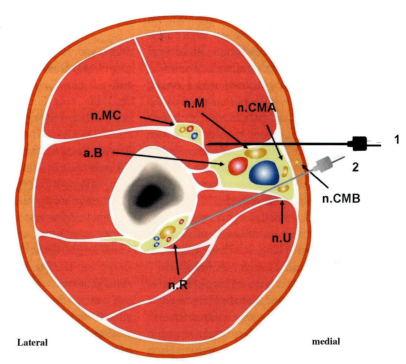

Fig. 11.2 Midhumeral block (cross section, *upper/middle* third of the arm) *n.M* = median nerve; *n.U* = ulnar nerve; *n.R* = radial nerve; *n, CMA* = medial cutaneous nerve of the forearm; *n. CMB* = medial cutaneous nerve of the arm; *n. MC* = musculocutaneous nerve; *a.B* = brachial artery

Technique

The anesthetist takes up position alongside the limb. With the non-dominant hand, he locates the pulsation off the brachial artery. He then inserts the needle perpendicularly to the skin and directs it downwards, anteriorly to the humerus, searching for the twitch due to stimulation of the musculocutaneous nerve (flexion of the forearm).

The needle is withdrawn as far as the subcutaneous tissues and is then redirected in depth, posterior to the humerus in order to elicit the twitches due to stimulation of the radial nerve (extension of the wrist, extension of the fingers, abduction of the thumb).

After blocking the deep branches, the needle is withdrawn again to the subcutaneous tissues and redirected, this time remaining very superficial, anteriorly to the pulsation of the brachial artery. On obtaining stimulation of the median nerve (flexion of the wrist, flexion of the fingers, opposition of the thumb), the needle is repositioned at the same depth posteriorly to the pulsation in order to elicit the twitches of the ulnar nerve (ulnar deviation of the wrist, flexion of the 4th and 5th fingers, adduction of the thumb). The local anesthetic injected is sufficient also to block the medial cutaneous nerve of the forearm. Before definitively extracting the needle, 2–3 ml of local anesthetic is injected into the subcutaneous tissue, for the medial cutaneous nerve of the arm.

Complications

Only the generic ones associated with the injection of local anesthetic.

11.2.2 Midhumeral Block (US)

Figures (11.3, 11.4, 11.5, 11.6, and 11.7).

Limb Position

Extended, abducted at least 50° (as necessary for positioning the probe).

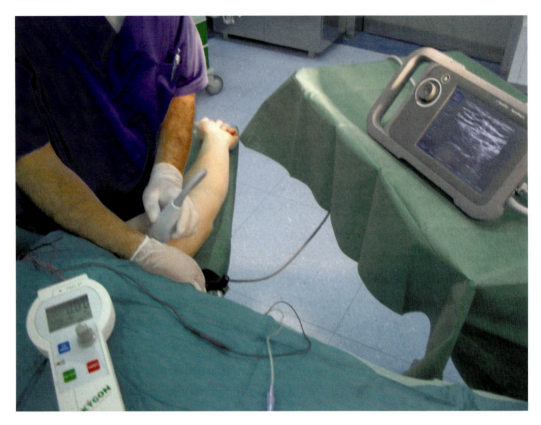

Fig. 11.3 Block with ultrasound guidance and ENS; NanoMaxx Ultrasound System and 10.5 MHz probe (SonoSite Inc., Bothell, USA); ENS Plexygon electrical nerve stimulator (Vygon Italia)

Probe
Linear, superficial view.

Approach
- Short axis:
- 'In plane' (Figs. 11.4, 11.5 or 'out of plane' (preferable on account of the shorter needle path).

Landmarks
- Brachial gutter (delimited anteriorly by the belly of the short head of the biceps brachii muscle and posteriorly by the medial head of the triceps brachii muscle).
- Proximal 3rd–middle 3rd of the arm.
- Brachial artery.

Needle
50 mm, electrically insulated or neutral.

Local Anesthetic
20 ml for blocking all the components (3–6 ml per component).

Technique
The anesthetist positions himself alongside the limb. With the non-dominant hand, he pilots the ultrasound probe and searches for the brachial vessels; he identifies the muscle bellies, visualizes the nerve trunks and chooses the most appropriate approach.

If the ENS technique is also used, the muscle twitches elicited will confirm the exact positioning of the needle.

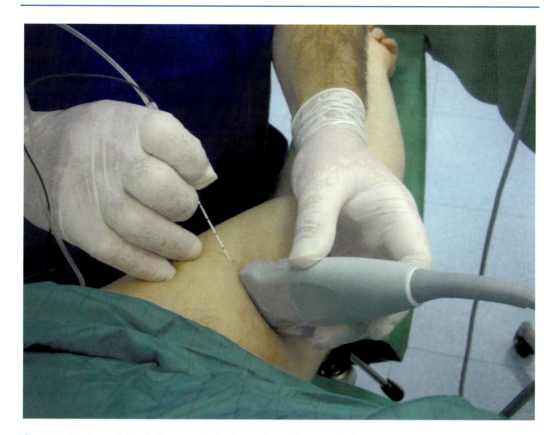

Fig. 11.4 Midhumeral block: linear probe in short axis position, needle direction 'in plane'; anterior approach

The local anesthetic injected is sufficient to block also the medial cutaneous nerve of the forearm.

The medial cutaneous nerve of the arm is blocked by injecting 2–3 ml of local anesthetic into the subcutaneous tissue at a point corresponding to the pulsation of the artery.

Complications

Only the generic ones associated with the injection of local anesthetic.

11.3 Elbow Region Blocks (ENS)

In this region, the nerves must be blocked singly because their courses are distant from one another (Fig. 11.8).

11.3.1 Median Nerve Block

Limb Position

Extended, supine.

Landmarks
- Medial and lateral epicondyles of the humerus.
- Biceps brachii muscle (medial border).
- Brachial artery pulsation (Fig. 11.8).

Needle

25–50 mm (depending upon the size of the limb), electrically insulated.

Local Anesthetic

3–5 ml.

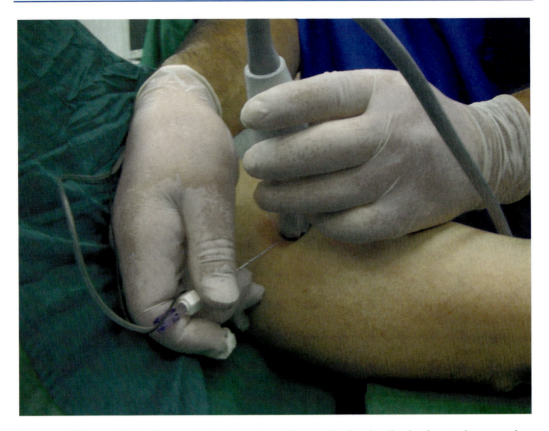

Fig. 11.5 Midhumeral block: linear probe in short axis position, needle direction 'in plane'; posterior approach

Technique
The anesthetist places himself alongside the limb. With the non-dominant hand, he locates the bony and vascular landmarks and identifies the medial border of the biceps brachii muscle. At a point corresponding to the pulsation of the brachial artery along the medial border of the muscle, he inserts the needle perpendicularly to the skin and directs it downwards advancing slowly, because the position of the nerve is not very deep. On obtaining the contraction of the flexor muscles of the hand, he injects the local anesthetic.

Complications
Only the generic ones associated with the injection of local anesthetic.

11.3.2 Radial Nerve Block

Limb Position
Extended, supine.

Landmarks
- Medial and lateral epicondyles of the humerus.
- Biceps brachii muscle (lateral border).

Needle
20–50 mm (depending upon the size of the limb), electrically insulated.

Local Anesthetic
3–5 ml.

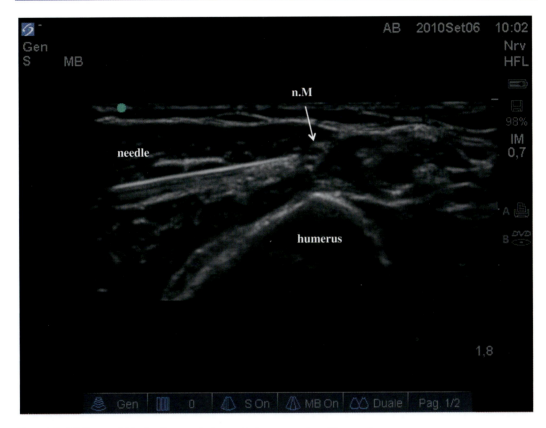

Fig. 11.6 Midhumeral block: ultrasound view, anterior approach; *n.M* = median nerve

Technique
The anesthetist places himself alongside the limb. With the non-dominant hand, he locates the bony landmarks and identifies the lateral border of the biceps brachii muscle. At a point corresponding to the border of the muscle, he inserts the needle perpendicularly to the skin and directs it downwards advancing slowly, because the position of the nerve is not very deep. On obtaining the contraction of the extensor muscles of the hand, he injects 3–5 ml of local anesthetic.

Complications
Only the generic ones associated with the injection of local anesthetic.

11.3.3 Ulnar Nerve Block
Figure (11.9).

Limb Position
Limb anteriorly extended and forearm flexed (hand on the contralateral shoulder).

Landmarks
Medial epicondyle of the humerus and olecranon (Fig. 11.9).

Needle
25 mm, electrically insulated.

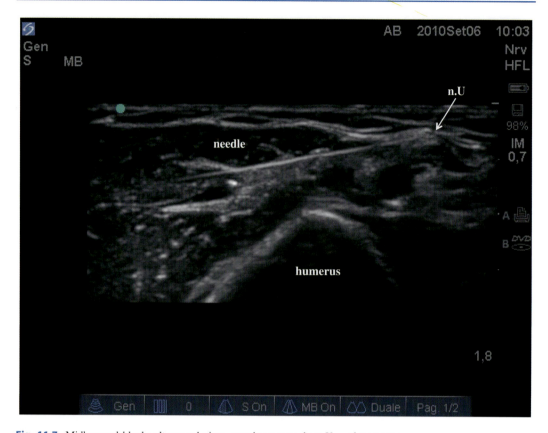

Fig. 11.7 Midhumeral block: ultrasound view, anterior approach; *n.U* = ulnar nerve

Local Anesthetic
2 ml.

Technique
The anesthetist places himself alongside the patient. With the non-dominant hand, he locates the bony landmarks and identifies the olecranon canal. He inserts the needle and penetrates into the canal in a proximal–distal direction. On obtaining the desired twitches, 2 ml of local anesthetic is injected.

Complications
Only the generic ones associated with the injection of local anesthetic.

Attention
Take care with the volumes injected in order not to compress the nerve on the non-extendable bony bed.

11.4 Elbow Region Blocks (US)

11.4.1 Median Nerve Block (US)

Figure (11.10).

Limb Position
Extended, supine.

Probe
Linear, superficial view.

Approach
- Short axis.
- 'In plane' or 'out of plane' (Fig. 11.10).

11 Truncular Blocks

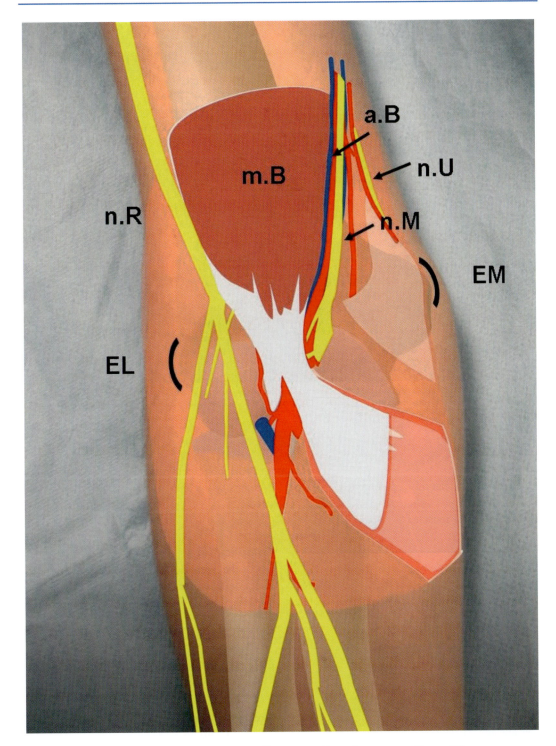

Fig. 11.8 Elbow block (anterior region): *n.M* = median nerve; *n.U.* = ulnar nerve; *r.N.* = radial

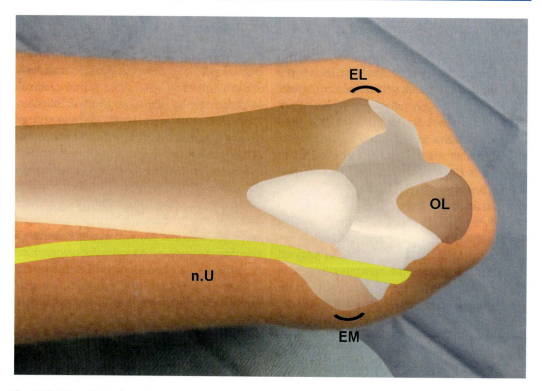

Fig. 11.9 Elbow block (posterior region): *n.U* = ulnar nerve; *OL* = olecranon; *EL* = lateral epiphysis; *EM* = medial epiphysis

Landmarks
- Medial and lateral epicondyles of the humerus.
- Biceps brachii muscle.
- Brachial artery.

Needle
50 mm, electrically insulated or neutral.

Local Anesthetic
3–5 ml.

Technique
The anesthetist takes up position alongside the patient. With the non-dominant hand, he pilots the ultrasound probe and identifies the muscle belly, the brachial artery and the nerve trunk. If the ENS technique is also used, the muscle twitches will confirm the exact position of the needle.

Complications
Only the generic ones associated with the injection of local anesthetic.

11.4.2 Radial Nerve Block (US)

Figure (11.11).

Limb Position
Extended, supine.

Probe
Linear, superficial view.

11 Truncular Blocks

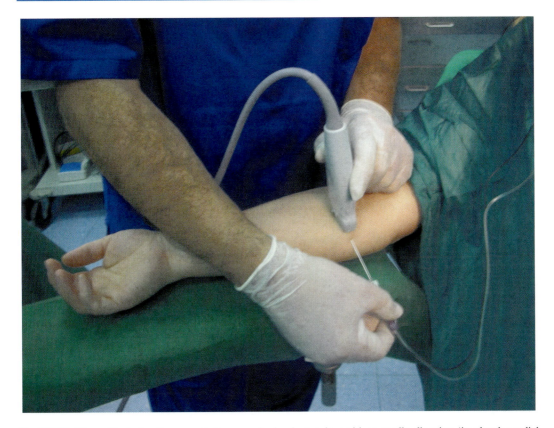

Fig. 11.10 Elbow block (median nerve): linear probe in short axis position; needle direction 'in plane'; medial approach

Approach
- Short axis.
- 'In plane' or 'out of plane' (Fig. 11.11).

Landmarks
- Medial and lateral epicondyles of the humerus.
- Biceps brachii muscle.

Needle
50 mm, electrically insulated or neutral.

Local Anesthetic
3–5 ml.

Technique
The anesthetist takes up position alongside the limb. With the non-dominant hand, he pilots the ultrasound probe and identifies the muscle belly and the nerve trunk (the first of its division).

If the ENS technique is also used, the muscle twitches will confirm the exact position of the needle.

Complications
Only the generic ones associated with the injection of local anesthetic.

11.4.3 Ulnar Nerve Block (US)

Figure (11.12).

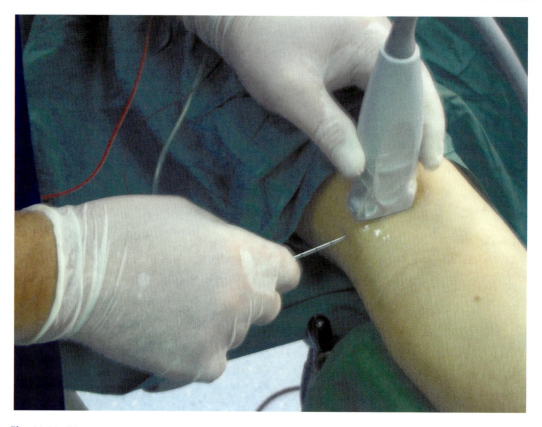

Fig. 11.11 Elbow block (radial nerve): linear probe in short axis position; needle direction 'in plane'; lateral approach

Limb Position
Limb anteriorly extended and forearm flexed (hand on the contralateral shoulder).

Probe
Linear, superficial view.

Approach
- Short axis.
- 'Out of plane' (Fig. 11.12).

Landmarks
Olecranon and medial epicondyle of the elbow.

Needle
25–50 mm, electrically insulated or neutral.

Local Anesthetic
2–3 ml.

Technique
The anesthetist takes up position alongside the limb. The landmarks are identified. With the non-dominant hand, he pilots the ultrasound probe and visualizes the nerve trunk in the cubital tunnel.

If the ENS technique is also used, the muscle twitches will confirm the exact position of the needle.

11 Truncular Blocks

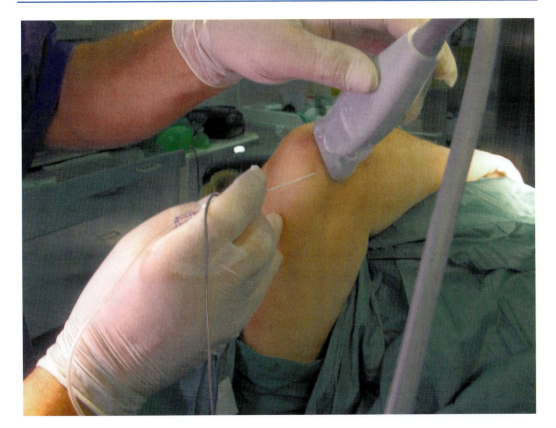

Fig. 11.12 Elbow block (ulnar nerve): linear probe in short axis position; needle direction 'out of plane'

Complications
Only the generic ones associated with the injection of local anesthetic.

11.4.4 Ulnar Nerve Block (Volar Region of the Forearm) (US)

Limb Position
Extended, supine.

Probe
Linear, superficial view.

Approach
- Short axis.
- 'In plane'.

Landmarks
- Ulnar artery.
- Flexor digitorum profundus, flexor digitorum superficialis and flexor carpi ulnaris muscles.

Needle
50 mm, electrically insulated or neutral.

Local Anesthetic
3–5 ml.

Technique
The anesthetist takes up position alongside the limb. With the non-dominant hand, he pilots the ultrasound probe and identifies the vessels and muscle bellies; he visualizes the nerve trunk and chooses the most appropriate approach.

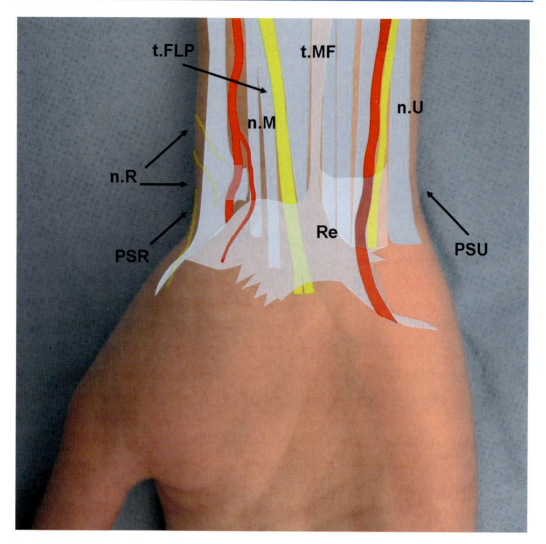

Fig. 11.13 Wrist block: *n.M* = median nerve; *n.U.* = ulnar nerve; *n.R* = radial nerve; *PSR* = styloid process of the radius; *PSU* = styloid process of the ulna

If the ENS technique is also used, the muscle twitches will confirm the exact position of the needle.

Complications

Only the generic ones associated with the injection of local anesthetic.

11.5 Wrist Region Blocks (ENS)

Figure (11.13).

11.5.1 Median Nerve Block

Limb Position

Extended, supine.

Landmarks

- Medial and lateral epicondyles of the wrist.
- Tendons of the flexor muscles of the fingers and the flexor longus pollicis muscle (Fig. 11.13).

Needle

25–35 mm, electrically insulated.

11 Truncular Blocks

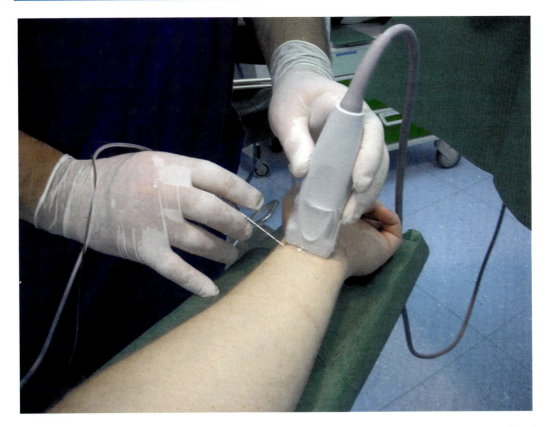

Fig. 11.14 Wrist block (median nerve). Linear probe in short axis position; needle direction 'in plane'; lateral approach

Local Anesthetic
3–5 ml.

Technique
The anesthetist takes up position alongside the limb. With the non-dominant hand, he locates the bony landmarks. Laterally to the group of tendons of the flexor muscles, he inserts the needle perpendicularly to the skin and directs it downwards advancing slowly. If the needle makes contact with bone without eliciting twitches, the needle tip must be withdrawn into the subcutaneous tissue and redirected more medially. On obtaining twitching of the flexor muscles of the fingers, the anesthetist injects the local anesthetic.

Complications
Only the generic ones associated with the injection of local anesthetic.

11.5.2 Ulnar Nerve Block

Limb Position
Extended, supine.

Landmarks
- Medial epicondyle of the wrist.
- Pulsation of the ulnar artery.

Needle
25 mm, electrically insulated.

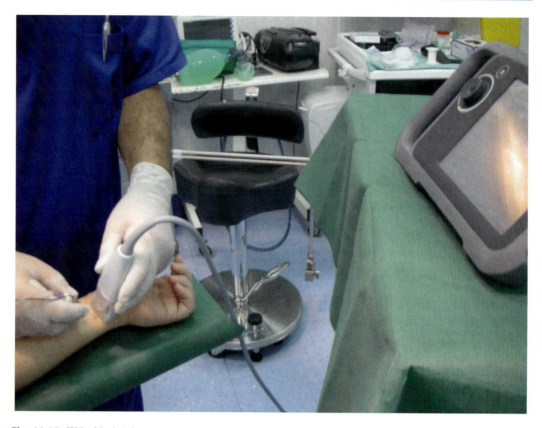

Fig. 11.15 Wrist block (ulnar nerve). Linear probe in short axis position; needle direction 'out of plane'

Local Anesthetic
2–3 ml.

Technique
The anesthetist takes up position alongside the patient. With the non-dominant hand, he locates the bony landmarks and identifies the pulsation of the artery. The needle is inserted medially to the artery and perpendicularly to the skin. On obtaining the desired twitches, the local anesthetic is injected.

NB A fan-pattern injection of local anesthetic in the region is also sufficient to achieve a complete block.

Complications
Only the generic ones associated with the injection of local anesthetic.

11.5.3 Radial Nerve Block

Limb Position
Extended, supine.

Landmarks
Lateral epicondyle of the radius.

Needle
50 mm.

Local Anesthetic
3–5 ml.

Technique
The anesthetist takes up position alongside the limb. With the non-dominant hand, he locates

the bony landmark and infiltrates the subcutaneous tissue of the dorsal and lateral volar region of the wrist.

Complications
Only the generic ones associated with the injection of local anesthetic.

11.6 Wrist Region Blocks (US)

11.6.1 Median Nerve Block

Figure (11.14).

Limb Position
Extended, supine.

Probe
Linear, superficial view.

Approach
- Short axis.
- In plane (Fig. 11.14) or out of plane.

Landmarks
- Radial and ulnar styloid processes.
- Tendons of the flexor muscles of the fingers and the flexor pollicis longus muscle.

Needle
35–50 mm, electrically insulated or neutral.

Local anesthetic
3–5 ml.

Technique
The anesthetist takes up position alongside the limb. With the non-dominant hand, he pilots the ultrasound probe and identifies the muscle tendons; he visualizes the nerve trunk and chooses the most appropriate approach.

If the ENS technique is also used, the muscle twitches will confirm the exact position of the needle.

Complications
Only the generic ones associated with the injection of local anesthetic.

11.6.2 Ulnar nerve block

Figure (11.15).

Limb Position
Limb extended, supine.

Probe
Linear, superficial view.

Approach
- Short axis.
- 'In plane' or 'out of plane' (Fig. 11.15).

Landmarks
- Ulnar styloid process.
- Ulnar artery.
- Tendons of the flexor carpi ulnaris and flexor digitorum superficialis muscles.

Needle
35–50 mm, electrically insulated or neutral.

Local anesthetic
2–3 ml.

Technique
The anesthetist takes up position alongside the patient. He identifies the ulnar artery and the muscle tendons, visualizes the nerve trunk and

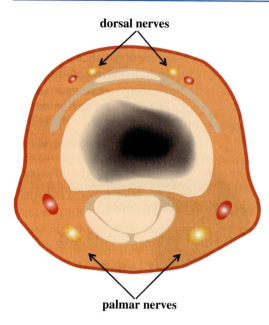

Fig. 11.16 Cross section of finger

chooses the most appropriate approach. If the ENS technique is also used, the muscle twitches will confirm the exact positioning of the needle.

NB: A fan-pattern injection of local anesthetic in the region is also sufficient to achieve a complete block.

Complications

Only the generic ones associated with the injection of local anesthetic.

11.6.3 Blocks of the Fingers

Figure (11.16).

Limb Position

Limb extended and hand prone.

Landmarks

Base of the finger.

Needle

35 mm, neutral.

Local Anesthetic

2–3 ml per side.

Technique

The anesthetist identifies the base of the finger and, starting from the dorsal region, infiltrates the entire side as far as the palmar portion. He then performs the same manoeuvre for the other side of the finger.

Complications

Only the generic ones associated with the injection of local anesthetic.

Bibliography

Aliaga L, Castro MA (2001) Anestesia regional hoy. Publicaciones Permanyer, Barcelona (Espana)

Barbati A, D'ambrosio A (2006) Blocchi periferici: Manuale di ALR: Mediprint s.r.l., Roma

Bouaziz H, Narchi P, Mercier FJ, Labaille T, Zerrouk N, Girod J, Benhamou D (1997) Comparison between conventional axillary block and a new approach at the midhumeral level. Anesth Analg 84:1058–1062

Cuvillon P, Dion N, Deleuze M, Nouvellon E et al (2009) Comparison of 3 intensities of stimulation threshold for brachial plexus blocks at the midhumeral level: a prospective, double-blind, randomized study. Reg Anesth Pain Med 34(4):296–300

De Windt AC, Asehnoune K, Roquilly A, Guillaud C, Le Roux C, Pinaud M, Lejus C (2010) An opioid-free anesthetic using nerve blocks enhances rapid recovery after minor hand surgery in children. Eur J Anaesthesiol 27(6):521–525

Grossi P, Barbati A, et al (2006) I blocchi anestetici dell'arto superiore. guida multimediale di anestesia loco regionale. Fidenza, Mattioli 1885 spa

Hadzic A, Vloka JD (2004) Blocchi nervosi periferici. Torino, UTET S.p.A

Pippa P, Busoni P (2010) Anestesia Locoregionale. Verduci Editore, Roma

Urmey WF, Grossi P (2006) Use of sequential electrical nerve stimuli (sens) for location of the sciatic nerve and lumbar plexus. Reg Anesth Pain Med 31(5):463–469

Intravenous Retrograde Anesthesia

M. Raffa, M. Greco and A. Barbati

Intravenous retrograde anesthesia (IVRA) of the limbs is an anesthesiological technique performed for the first time by Bier in 1908, who enjoyed a certain measure of success only after 1946, which was the year when new, less toxic local anesthetics became available on the market.

It is a technique that is easy to perform with failure rates below 1 % and is used in surgical operations on the forearm, hand, leg and foot lasting not more than 90 min. It is particularly indicated in allergic patients or in patients with COPD, in patients with a full stomach and in outpatient surgery.

The technique is based on the injection of an anesthetic solution into the vein of the limb to be submitted to surgery and rendered ischaemic at the root. It has a short onset time and affords good muscle relaxation.

M. Raffa
Complex Operative Unit, Anesthesia and Resuscitation, Avellino Local Health Authority, Ariano Irpino, AV, Italy

M. Greco
Simple Operative Unit, Resuscitation and Intensive Care, Avellino Local Health Authority, Ariano Irpino, AV, Italy

A. Barbati (✉)
Pain Therapy Service, Padre Pio Hospital, Mondragone, CE, Italy
e-mail: aldobarbati@hotmail.com

The mechanism whereby the anesthesia sets in with this technique is still controversial. There are two different theories:
- peripheral: penetration of the local anesthetic injected, via the vasa nervorum and the capillaries, into the nerve trunks with distal block and subsequent penetration of the peripheral fibres with retarded proximal blockade;
- truncular: distribution of the anesthetic mainly at the level of the joint of the limb.

The most likely hypothesis is the peripheral theory inasmuch as the local anesthetic reaches both the main nervous system and the peripheral nerve endings via the vascular route. A number of authors, on the other hand, have proposed nerve ischaemia as the mechanism of action of IVRA, but this is only suggestive in that the onset varies in relation to variations in the local anesthetic used.

To shorten the latency of the block, an adjuvant such as sodium bicarbonate (alkalinization) can be used in conjunction with the local anesthetic as well as an analgesic agent for prolonging the analgesia (local peripheral action).

12.1 Indications and Contraindications

The characteristics and advantages of IVRA indicate it, if properly executed, as the technique to be preferred in outpatient surgery and in urgent operations on the distal segments of the limbs.

IVRA is contraindicated when it is impossible to obtain satisfactory arterial occlusion in the presence of:
- major obesity (BMI >35);
- severe hypertension;
- major arterial calcifications;
- intolerance or allergy to local anesthetics.

It is not indicated in patients with:
- drepanocytosis;
- acute ischaemia of the limb;
- BAV grades II–III, not conducted;
- infectious cellulitis;
- arteritis;
- ischaemic cardiopathy; and
- severe liver failure.

12.2 Advantages and Disadvantages

The advantages of this technique are mainly related to its ease of execution, and the minimal complication rates and side effects, together with good stability of the vital functions, rapid onset of anesthesia, rapid reversibility, muscle relaxation and low cost.

Patient bed rest, fasting and postoperative somnolence are to be avoided. After a few hours, the patient can return home in a state of perfect well-being.

The disadvantages, on the other hand, are due to the potentially severe systemic toxic effects, the patient's poor tolerance of the tourniquet cuff (sometimes even painful), the short-lasting surgical time and the impossibility of controlling the surgical haemostasis before removing the cuff.

12.3 Technique

The preparation of the patient, as in the case of all anesthesiological procedures, entails the performance of laboratory examinations with coagulation screening, ECG and the preoperative anesthesiological visit, with the signing of informed consent. Chest X-rays can be omitted.

The technique must be performed after first monitoring the patient's vital parameters (ECG, blood pressure, SpO_2) to be maintained throughout the entire intervention.

A vein of the upper limb not involved in the intervention is cannulated for the fluid therapy and the administration of drugs; we then proceed with the premedication.

The vein is then sought for the execution of the technique as close as possible to the surgical site and a small-calibre (e.g. 22 G) needle cannula is positioned—equipped with an occlusion system—which is fixed to the skin (Fig. 12.1).

In order to avoid the entry of local anesthetic into the systemic circulation, also via the interosseous vessels, before it is completely absorbed, a double-cuff tourniquet with independent inflation control is applied above the main joint of the limb (elbow or knee) (Figs. 12.2, 12.3), or, failing that, two pneumatic cuffs at a distance of approximately 10 cm from one another and connected up to an inflation system capable of maintaining constant pressure of the cuffs throughout the entire procedure (e.g. the Tourniquet System produced by Officine Rizzoli in Bologna).

12.4 Drugs

The most commonly used local anesthetics are, in order of frequency of use, lidocaine (2–3 mg/kg bw), levobupivacaine or ropivacaine (0.25 mg/kg bw) and mepivacaine (1 mg/kg bw).

Bicarbonate solution is used for alkalinization, and opioids, NSAIDs or clonidine for prolonging the analgesia.

12.5 Procedure

First of all, the limb is rendered ischaemic either with the Esmarch bandage or by keeping the extremity of the arm raised for 10–15 min (Fig. 12.4). The proximal cuff is then inflated up to a pressure of at least 100 mm Hg above the patient's systolic pressure.

12 Intravenous Retrograde Anesthesia

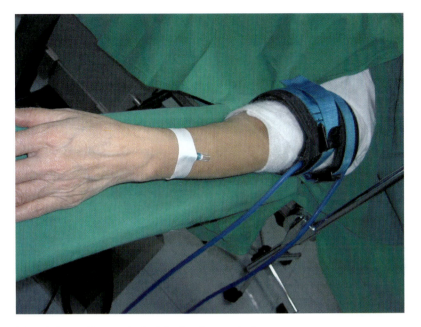

Fig. 12.1 Position of the needle cannula for injecting the anesthetic

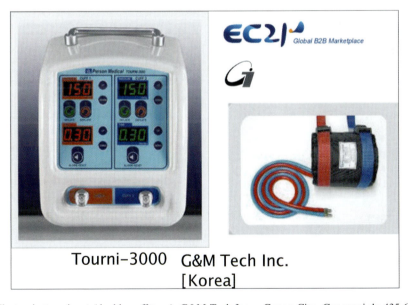

Fig. 12.2 Electronic tourniquet (double-cuff type). G&M Tech Inc.—Gunpo City, Gyeonggi-do 435-632 Korea

After verifying the perfect sealing of the cuff, the limb is brought back to the resting position and the previously prepared anesthetic solution is injected via the predisposed needle cannula (Fig. 12.5).

The local anesthetic solution plus any adjuvants or synergistic agents is diluted with saline to a volume of 30–40 ml for the upper limb or 50–70 ml for the lower limb and injected slowly in at least 4–5 min.

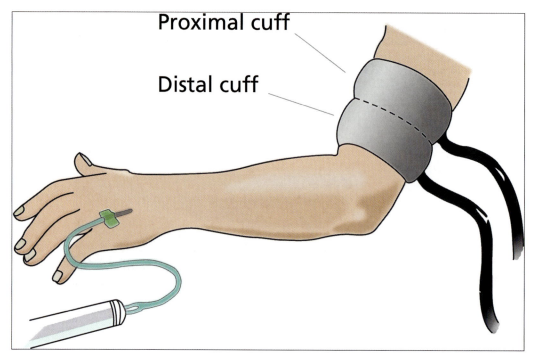

Fig. 12.3 Double-cuff tourniquet for IVRA

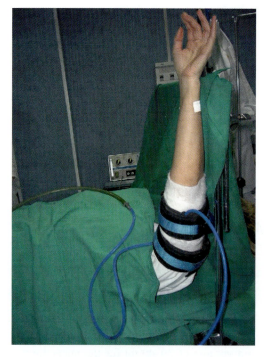

Fig. 12.4 Induction of ischaemia of the limb. The limb is raised for 10–15 min before inflating the tourniquet

The anesthesia sets in the space of approximately 15 min.

After checking that the anesthesia has set in also in the region immediately proximal to the distal cuff, the anesthetist proceeds to inflate the second (distal) cuff to the same pressure as the first and, only after ascertaining that the cuff is sealed, is the proximal cuff deflated.

In the anesthesia induction phase, the patient may manifest distress or pain due to the pressure exerted by the proximal cuff. To avoid this discomfort, anesthetic infiltration of the medial cutaneous nerve of the arm at the level of the axilla can be performed.

The duration of the intervention is limited by the ischaemia time of the limb concerned, which is normally set at 90 min. However, also in the case of very brief surgical interventions, the distal cuff should never be deflated at less than 40 min in order to avoid the massive entry of as yet unabsorbed or non-metabolized local anesthetic into the bloodstream. For the same reason, at the end of the intervention the cuff should be deflated

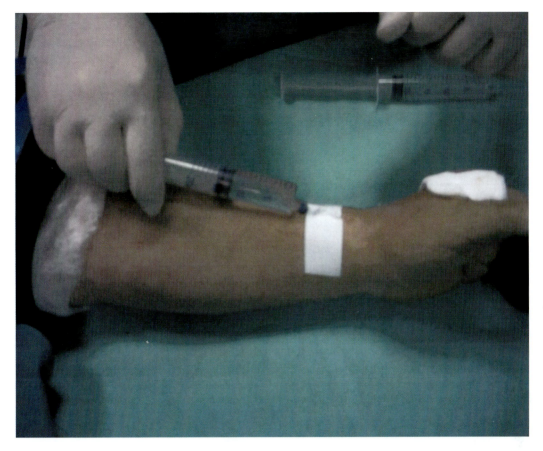

Fig. 12.5 Injection of local anesthetic

slowly. Also, the reappearance of the circulation in the ischaemic limb may cause disagreeable sensations, as may the entry into the bloodstream of free radicals accumulated in the segments of the ischaemic limb.

The anesthesia persists for about 10 min after completely deflating the cuff, and the analgesia persists for a period of 60–90 min. The addition of an analgesic agent to the anesthetic solution enables a postoperative analgesia of approximately 6 h to be obtained. In the postoperative period early walking and feeding are advisable so as to avoid the need for infusion therapy.

12.6　Side Effects

These include the following:

- The massive entry of local anesthetic into the bloodstream with numbness, tinnitus, palpitations or eye accommodation disorders;
- At revascularization of the limb, intense heat and numbness;
- Entry of free radicals into the bloodstream with consequent hypotension and transient skin rash.

12.7　Complications

The complications are caused by the prolonged ischaemia of nerve structures that may give rise to transitory or permanent lesions, and by the sudden, massive entry of local anesthetic into the bloodstream by direct injection due to a lack of or inadequate inflation of the cuff, or to accidental or premature deflation of the latter. The sudden entry of local anesthetic into the bloodstream may cause disorders ranging from simple paresthesias of the tongue and lips to bradycardia and/or severe arrhythmia, agitation, tachypnea, nausea, vomiting and dizziness. In extremely severe cases, the patient may suffer convulsions, respiratory failure and even heart failure.

12.8 Conclusions

IVRA of the limbs does not require expensive equipment for its execution and has a very rapid learning curve. The cost of the materials used is very modest, and the frequency of accidents, complications and side effects is very low. Patient satisfaction, after an initial period of perplexity, is very good, as is that of the surgeons.

Bibliography

Atanassoff PG, Hartmannsgruber MW (2002) Central nervous system side effects are less important after iv regional anesthesia with ropivacaine 0.2 % compared to lidocaine 0.5 % in volunteers. Can J Anaesth 49(2):169–172

Bier A (1908) New method for local anaesthesia in extremities. Ann Surg 48:780

Guay J (2009) Adverse events associated with intravenous regional anesthesia (Bier block): a systematic review of complications. J Clin Anesth Guay J 21(8):585–594

Hartmannsgruber MW, Silverman DG, Halaszynski TM, Bobart V, Brull SJ, Wilkerson C, Loepke AW, Atanassoff PG (1999) Comparison of ropivacaine 0.2 % and lidocaine 0.5 % for intravenous regional anesthesia in volunteers. Anesth Analg 89(3):727–731

Johnson CN (2000) Intravenous regional anesthesia: new approaches to an old technique. CRNA 11(2):57–61

Sen S, Ugur B, Aydin ON, Ogurlu M, Gezer E, Savk O (2006) The analgesic effect of lornoxicam when added to lidocaine for intravenous regional anaesthesia. Br J Anaesth 97(3):408–413

Sethi D, Wason R (2010) Intravenous regional anesthesia using lidocaine and neostigmine for upper limb surgery. J Clin Anesth 22(5):324–328

Simon MA, Gielen MJ, Alberink N, Vree TB, van Egmond J (1997) Intravenous regional anesthesia with 0.5 % articaine, 0.5 % lidocaine, or 0.5 % prilocaine. A double-blind randomized clinical study. Reg Anesth 22(1):29–34

Singh R, Bhagwat A, Bhadoria P, Kohli A (2010) Forearm IVRA, Using 0.5 % lidocaine in a dose of 1.5 mg/kg with ketorolac 0.15 mg/kg for hand and wrist surgeries. Minerva Anestesiol 76(2):109–114 IVRA

Sedation in Regional Anesthesia

13

F. Alemanno and F. Auricchio

Not all patients are suitable candidates for brachial plexus anesthesia.
Brendan T. Finucane

13.1 Sedation with Neuroleptoanalgesia

F. Alemanno

Whereas regional anesthesia, from the pharmacological point of view, is less invasive than general anesthesia, on the other hand, it involves the patient more from the emotional standpoint, inasmuch as he or she participates as a spectator, and not just as an object, both in the execution of the anesthesia technique and in the actual surgery. Moreover, since only a part of the body is anesthetized, the rest of the body may be subject to discomfort for various reasons such as a position on the operating table that might initially have seemed just a little uncomfortable but which rapidly becomes intolerable. Sometimes it may happen that the patient is unable to put up with his or her state of immobility for more than a certain amount of time and will have an impelling desire to change position. A successful regional anesthesia and a patient who, with a reasonable degree of detachment, is able to cope with the stress first of the anesthesiological procedure and then of the surgical intervention will be a source of substantial satisfaction both for the patient and for the surgeon. The anesthetist has always two 'customers' to serve, the patient and the surgeon.

It may also happen that a block may prove incomplete or patchy with distress on the part of the patient, irritation on the part of the surgeon and embarrassment on the part of the anesthetist. In this case, the anesthetist must not hesitate to go over to a general anesthesia, albeit of a lighter nature, with orotracheal intubation or with a laryngeal mask.

If the patient is particularly anxious, or worse still, psychologically unstable in the sense that, for example, after giving his consent to regional anesthesia, he goes back on his decision and changes his mind, one should not try insistently to convince him at all costs of the advantages that regional anesthesia may have to offer him.

It is clear, in this context, how important a proper preoperative talk with the patient may be. I say 'may be' because, in actual fact, very often this is done through some third party. It often happens that a single anesthetist has to examine and obtain consent from a number of patients in a crowded anesthesiological outpatient consulting room, who after an unspecified number of days will be anesthetized by another anesthetist.

A widely consulted German pocket manual of anesthesia, in the chapter entitled 'The Preoperative Visit', began with the statement 'Any patient to be submitted to a surgical operation should be visited by his anesthetist on the day

F. Alemanno (✉)
Institute of Anesthesiology, Resuscitation and Pain Therapy, University of Verona, Verona, Italy
e-mail: fernando@alemannobpb.it

F. Auricchio
Anesthesia and Resuscitation Service, Bolzano Regional Hospital, Bolzano, Italy

before the operation is scheduled'. In daily practice, however, this is simply wishful thinking.

After the history-taking and initial assessment talk, the anesthetist may realize that regional anesthesia is not indicated for a given patient for objective (organic disease) or subjective reasons (mental illness). In these cases, one should not hesitate to propose a blended anesthesia or exclusively general anesthesia.

In a surgical operation, the purpose of the anesthetist is that the patient should experience no pain, whether as a nociceptive signal if the patient is awake, or as a thalamic signal if the patient is under general anesthesia. Anxiety amplifies the pain, and therefore, it is important that it should be eliminated before the operation is performed.

The pain phenomenon is composed of the sum of two factors: the actual nociceptive signal and its amplification as a result of the state of anxiety of the patient.

It is well known that some people respond with an exaggerated reaction of defence or flight to even the slightest noxious stimulus, whereas others react in a manner more proportionate to the nature of the stimulus.

The ancient Roman soldier Mucius Scaevola, who was asked by the shocked and amazed bystanders if he felt any pain on plunging his fist into a blazing charcoal burner, replied stoically *Non dolet*—'It doesn't hurt'.

Anxiety is caused in the human body by an incorrect production and/or presence at the synaptic level of catecholamines, whose effects have repercussions also on the periphery with the manifestation of various neurovegetative reactions which, if they last for any length of time, may give rise to psychosomatic diseases.

Effective drugs for combating anxiety are the neuroleptic agents (phenothiazine, butyrophenones) and the benzodiazepines, that is, all drugs that are catecholamine antagonists.

Obviously, pain not sufficiently blocked by an imperfect regional anesthesia technique produces anxiety and, if experienced at the subconscious level in the case of too superficial a general anesthesia, brings about an increase in sympathetic activity and the entry of catecholamines into the bloodstream, hence the importance of the use of analgesics concomitantly with the neuroleptic agents.

As we can see, anxiety and pain are closely intertwined: anxiety amplifies pain, and pain produces anxiety. It is on the conflict between these two—anxiety and/or pain—that proper general anesthesia is based, even in its lightest form, 'vigilant or subvigilant anesthesia' which is called conscious analgosedation with neuroleptoanalgesia.

We have made this reference to general anesthesia, and for this reason, it may be a good idea to bear in mind what parameters general anesthesia is based on. These are well known, that is, analgesia, neurovegetative protection, sleep (for patient comfort), and muscle relaxation (for the comfort of the surgeon).

Up until the 1940s, these concepts were not so clear and general anesthesia, in clinical practice (despite Guedel's classification), tended to be more superficial than deep and therefore not protecting the patient adequately against the surgical aggression, among other things because of the inadequacy of the drugs available at the time.

In the postoperative period, the surgeon feared the onset of the ill-famed postoperative disease. This was a syndrome characterized by parasympathetic inhibition and by a relative sympathetic prevalence with hypotension, a weak, frequent pulse, hyperthermia, intestinal constipation, and oliguria to the point of anuria, which was not resolved despite the administration of hypodermoclysis or an occasional phleboclysis, heroic at the time. All things considered, this syndrome was a kind of creeping shock that sometimes resolved after one or two days, but sometimes precipitated into a state of irreversible shock leading to the death of the patient. This syndrome of the early postoperative period, together with pulmonary embolism, was defined as 'the surgeon's big disappointment,' summed up by the well-known expression 'the operation was a success, but the patient died.'

13.2 The Origins: Henri Laborit

You may say that I am approaching the subject from quite some distance, but without the observations of this young French surgeon, the basic foundations of modern anesthesia, of neuroleptoanalgesia and thus also of conscious analgosedation would not have been laid.

Henri Laborit was a medical officer in the French Navy who, immediately after the Second World War, was stationed overseas as a surgeon in a military hospital at Sidi-Abdallah near Bizerta in Tunisia. In that area, studded with landmines, there were many injuries, either accidental or incurred during mine-clearing operations in the territory, with the casualties reaching the military hospital in a state of shock. The injured population was homogeneous: the patients, all males aged from 20 to 50, had blown themselves up on antipersonnel mines with a constant payload. Every type of shock—due to pain, haemorrhage, fear and sepsis—contributed to their condition. Laborit (a surgeon!) guessed that the problem consisted in the vasoconstriction of large portions of the body, such as the splanchnic area as well as the skin, liver and kidneys. This meant hypoxia and therefore acidosis with consequent desensitization of the peripheral receptors to the action of catecholamines and transition from the reversible to the irreversible phase of shock. In this situation, little benefit could be obtained by continuous infusions of fluids or blood and even less by administering sympathicomimetic drugs.

'At the time it was believed that, even when hemostasis and surgical treatment of the injuries were performed correctly, death was caused by exhaustion of the defense systems. For this reason, once the blood mass was restored by transfusion and if the blood pressure remained low, an attempt was made to raise it by resorting to the use of pharmacological agents that caused vasoconstriction, thus reducing the capacity of the circulatory system. The results appeared to be poor…' This therapy was certainly effective in certain cases of cardiocirculatory collapse, but not in shock syndrome. This semantic confusion between collapse and shock was by no means devoid of negative therapeutic consequences! In the case of shock, once the blood mass had been restored, it was important to resolve the peripheral spasm of the arterioles and meta-arterioles in order to set in motion again the mass of blood sequestered in the vasoconstricted areas and thus restore adequate oxygenation of the tissues and organs such as the liver, kidneys and bowels, that is to say of the entire splanchnic area. With the oxygenation of the tissues and organs, there would have been a buffering of the ingravescent acidosis which, otherwise, would have led fatally not so much to exhaustion of the body's defence systems as to desensitization of the peripheral adrenergic receptors to the action of circulatory catecholamines, with consequent transition from the reversible to the irreversible phase of shock. In fact, when shock is left to its own devices, the process that sets in is what is defined—to use a term which can hardly be called scientific, but which is easy to remember as the 'cycle of death' (Fig. 13.1).

For the purposes of interrupting this vicious circle, Laborit devised a 'lytic cocktail' consisting of chlorpromazine (Largactil) with an antiadrenergic action, promethazine (Fargan) with an antiexudative action and meperidine (Dolantin) with an analgesic action.

It was only a short step, then, from the application of this cocktail in shock to its use in the operating room to perform so-called potentiated anesthesia. The French anesthetists were quick to grasp the concept and thus Huguenard, Boissier, Viars and other distinguished exponents of French anesthesiology made it their own and developed the concept, immediately followed in this by the Italian anesthetists, Carlon, Ciocatto, Gasparetto and Giron. Potentiated anesthesia made it possible to perform anesthesia procedures at a deeper level, thus preventing the postoperative disease, which, as we have already said, was a creeping shock syndrome that devastated the postoperative period of many technically well-performed surgical operations. With the use of the lytic cocktail, inhaled anesthesia (with N_2O, ether or

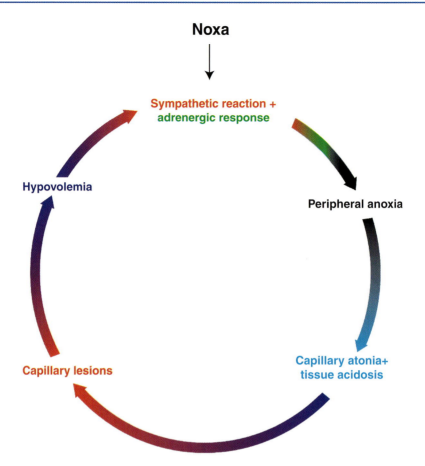

Fig. 13.1 The schematic diagram represents what is defined—to use a term which can hardly be called scientific, but which is easy to remember—as the 'cycle of death'

trichloroethylene vapour) guaranteed sleep, but also boosted the analgesia and organ protection against surgical aggression.

At the end of the 1950s, the two phenothiazines (chlorpromazine and promethazine) were replaced with a butyrophenone, haloperidol (Serenase) was replaced by De Castro and Mundeleer, and meperidine was replaced by the more potent phenoperidine. Neuroleptoanalgesia had arrived on the scene and is now known worldwide, but not many people know that the procedure originated in a French naval hospital in Tunisia.

This first form of neuroleptoanalgesia (type 1 NLA) originated in 1959 and was primarily neuroleptic. The patient was mainly left to breathe spontaneously or received assisted ventilation. Sleep was guaranteed by the use of nitrous oxide (in view of the potency of the haloperidol + phenoperidine combination, it was not always necessary to administer, albeit at low concentrations, halothane, which in those days was beginning to appear on the scene). Phenoperidine, however, soon showed a certain amount of liver toxicity and within the space of a couple of years was replaced by fentanyl, with very low toxicity at the level of the emunctories and with much more potent analgesic activity. Precisely for this reason, it induced strong respiratory depression, making it necessary to resort to controlled breathing. The plasma half-life of 20 min meant that fentanyl was a very manageable drug. Haloperidol was also replaced by dehydrobenzperidol (DBP), which with its 90 min plasma half-life was also more manageable than its predecessor. Type 2 NLA, with a prevalently analgesic action, had made its appearance.

Good analgosedation can be obtained with the type 2 NLA drugs, but applied with a prevalently neuroleptic dosage (like the type 1 NLAs). The procedure we have adopted is based on a very modest single initial administration of dehydrobenzperidol and fentanyl (5 + 0.05 or 7.5 + 0.075 mg or 10 + 0.1 mg, the last dosage should be divided in two equal administrations, at five-minute interval) depending upon the patient's weight and condition or on whether one wishes to obtain deeper sedation. After 5 min (because fentanyl crosses the blood–brain barrier rapidly, but dehydrobenzperidol takes 5 min), we inject low doses of midazolam (1 mg followed, if necessary, by 0.5 mg after 10 min).

With this method, we have always obtained:
- good analgesia (if necessary), not obtainable with benzodiazepines;
- cardiocirculatory stability with a slight tendency to hypotension;
- optimal peripheral perfusion;
- pharyngolaryngeal protective reflexes preserved.

With this technique, it is possible to produce indefinitely long sedation if the surgical operation should last for an unpredictably long time, adding as necessary, after 1 or 2 h, half doses, of neuroleptic agent or of analgesic, compared to the initial doses. It is also possible to go over, in the simplest manner, to general anesthesia with a laryngeal mask or with orotracheal intubation, after first injecting even only a modest dose of a hypnotic agent (sodium thiopental or propofol) and a muscle relaxant.

Recently, since dehydrobenzperidol disappeared from the market in Italy for a certain period, we used modest doses of haloperidol (2 mg) in its place, bearing in mind its longer duration of action and therefore using the procedure in the hospital or one-day-surgery setting.

We have often resorted to the use of tramadol as an analgesic. In this case, its tendency to induce nausea is effectively offset by the presence of dehydrobenzperidol.

The anesthetist, however, has various techniques and drugs at his disposal capable of being used in combination according to the patient's condition and the various concomitant diseases he/she may present, not least old age (*senectus ipsa morbus est*, 'old age is in itself a disease'). It is a fact that in recent years, we have been witnessing an increase in the average age of our patients. Strict surveillance of vital parameters (ECG, oxygen saturation (SpO_2), blood pressure) is absolutely mandatory and admits of no distraction.

A possible tendency towards bradycardia with heart rate equal to or less than 50 must be immediately corrected with atropine (0.01 mg/kg) and immediately afterwards, if necessary, with ephedrine or ethylephrine, in order not to run the risk of the patient slipping into the long QT syndrome, torsade de pointes or the Bezold-Jarisch syndrome.

This technique is described and published in *Acta anesthesiologica Italica,* and applied by myself in more than 40 years without ever observing any kind of adverse reaction, particularly not at the cardiac level, where the drugs used tend, if anything, to regularize any erethistic cardiac rhythm.

13.3 The Strange Case of the Long QT Syndrome

Now, in the very early years of the twenty-first century, on the basis of an article published in a journal of psychiatry reporting 10 cases of prolongation of the QT interval, torsade de pointes and sudden death, the US Food and Drug Administration has rendered 12-channel serial ECG monitoring mandatory in the postoperative period in conjunction with the use of droperidol, even at low doses as an antiemetic agent, thus in effect eliminating the drug from clinical practice.

White et al. in an article published in *Anesthesiology* in 2005, entitled 'Effect of low-dose droperidol on the QT interval during and after general anesthesia: a placebo-controlled study', make the following statement: 'Interestingly, despite the use of these high doses of droperidol as part of a neuroleptic analgesia technique for more than 30 years, there has not been a single report of a serious arrhythmia during or after anesthesia in the peer-reviewed literature (excluding the questionable case report which appeared in a Japanese journal in 2002)'.

In 2006, White, in an editorial, suggests that the action of the FDA in proscribing low doses of droperidol for the treatment of postoperative nausea and vomiting is fundamentally misguided and that it does the American people a major disservice.

In the above-mentioned study published in *Anesthesiology* in 2005, White reports that he encountered a patient with sinus bradycardia and a QT interval of 419 ms on all 12 preoperative ECG channels. A QT interval is considered prolonged if it exceeds 450 ms in men and 460 ms in women. Although this patient was not entered into the study and had not received any antiemetic or antibiotic drugs, known to prolong the QT interval, a 12-channel ECG was performed during the fairly superficial surgical operation to remove a small mass from the patient's neck. The anesthesia was administered with an intravenous anesthetic technique, which comprised the use of propofol and remifentanil. A lengthening of the QT interval to 685 ms was observed. Immediately after the surgery, the 12-channel ECG was repeated every hour, registering QT values of 720, 615, 742 and 641 ms in the 4 h period following the surgery. The postoperative period was completely uneventful, and the patient was discharged despite the prolonged QT interval. If the patient had received DBP or ondansetron for antiemetic prophylaxis, this inexplicable lengthening of the QT interval would certainly have been ascribed to the antiemetic drug.

In a recent retrospective study on drugs and the QT interval, Liu and Juurlink established that 'most of what is known about the prolongation of the QT interval is the result of spontaneously induced mechanisms. Since the FDA imposed this additional ECG monitoring (postoperative and 12-channel, Editor's note) in those cases in which this convenient antiemetic agent is administered, droperidol has in practice been eliminated from the anesthesiological armamentarium in many centers in this country and abroad'.

As pointed out by Roden in his recent review article on drug-induced prolongation of the QT interval, 'since rare secondary effects occur with many, often extremely efficacious drugs, their withdrawal from the market would probably harm the patients more than it would help them'. White concludes his article on the topic by saying: 'In the opinion of many clinicians world-wide, the recent FDA obsession with drugs that induce a prolongation of the QT interval is an example of how a mountain can be made out of a mole hill'.

In October 2007, Nuttall et al. published an article in *Anesthesiology* entitled 'Does low-dose droperidol administration increase the risk of drug-induced QT prolongation and torsade de pointes in the general surgical population?'. In this research, the authors examine QT interval values 3 years before and 3 years after the FDA proscribed the drug.

In the 3 year period prior to the proscription, out of a total of 139,932 patients, 2,321 (1.66 %) presented QT prolongation, torsade de pointes or death within 48 h of the surgery. No patients were identified as having developed torsades de pointes. The exposure to droperidol was 12 % (16,791 patients).

In the 3 years after the FDA proscription, out of a total of 151,164 patients, 2,307 (1.46 %) had a documented QT prolongation, torsades de pointes (2 cases = 0.1 %) or death within 48 h of the surgery, and the exposure to droperidol was 0 %.

The authors conclude that the FDA's decision to ban low-dose droperidol is excessive and unnecessary.

In the editorial accompanying this article, Charbit and Funck-Brentano, though admitting that effectively risks of QT prolongation and torsades de pointes are known to occur at the high doses chronically and repeatedly used in psychiatry, conclude that also for peridural anesthesia, not all anesthetists regard the risk of haematoma as negligible and therefore do not agree to practise it without taking all due prior precautions. For the same reason, according to the authors, the FDA alarm is justified by the fact that the anesthetist should pay more attention to the patient's safety rather than to the efficacy of the drug.

But if we consistently abide by this principle, which is apparently crystal clear, none of the drugs we use in our everyday practice can be defined as safe, from sodium thiopental to succinylcholine, to the halogenated anesthetics capable of inducing the decoupling of oxidative phosphorylation with the consequent unleashing of malignant hyperthermia, or N_2O, which may induce immunodepression, or propofol and remifentanil, the combination which, as reported by White, in a patient without any such preoperative findings, caused a prolongation of the QT interval to 742 ms in the postoperative period.

It is obvious that just as no anesthetist would agree to perform a peridural in a patient with impaired coagulation, likewise no anesthetist would administer neuroleptoanalgesia in a patient who already presented a QT prolongation at his or her preoperative ECG.

13.4 Sedation with Inhaled N_2O

This type of sedation, practised particularly in North America in the field of dentistry, is based on the administration of nitrous oxide at various concentrations.

This gas was introduced in clinical practice by a dentist, Horace Wells, in 1844. Endowed with a keen sense of observation and capacity for intuition, Dr. Wells, during a conference on laughing gas, followed by a practical demonstration presented by an itinerant chemist, Gardner Quincy Colton, noticed that the spectators who, at the request of the self-styled chemist, had voluntarily inhaled the laughing gas contained in a large rubber flask, became euphoric, and one of them, rolling around on the floor and splitting his sides with uncontrollable laughter, collided violently and repeatedly with the sharp corners of the front row of seats of the audience, without showing any signs of pain.

When the man had regained control of himself, Dr. Wells asked him to roll up his trouser legs, which he did, revealing his bruised and bleeding legs, much to the amazement of the injured man himself.

The next day, Dr. Wells asked the itinerant chemist to come and see him in his study, bringing with him the flask containing the laughing gas, and after inhaling the contents, he had a bad tooth extracted by a colleague, Dr. Riggs, who described the event as follows: 'Dr. Wells seated himself in the dentist's chair. I examined the tooth to be extracted with a speculum, as I usually do. Wells took a rubber bag from Mr. Colton, and sat there with the bag in his lap, while I remained standing at his side. Wells breathed in the gas until it began to have a profound effect upon him. His head fell back all of a sudden and I put my hand on his chin. He opened his mouth and I extracted the tooth. His mouth remained open for a short while. Dr. Wells, who swiftly came to his senses again, stated: 'I felt no more than a pinprick. A new era has dawned in the field of tooth extraction. This is the greatest discovery there has ever been!'.

In clinical practice, for the purposes of administering analgosedation, nitrous oxide (in addition to being a sedative, it is also quite an effective analgesic agent) is obviously combined with oxygen in concentrations ranging from 30 to 50 %.

The individual response is extremely variable. It is advisable to start the administration of the gas a few minutes before surgery, progressively increasing the concentration and stopping at the lowest effective concentration. It is then a matter of establishing the baseline, namely the optimal dose of N_2O for the patient in question. The patient is asked whether he or she feels relaxed and if he or she perceives a pleasurable heat sensation in the extremities. Generally speaking, the baseline is thought to have been reached when the patient begins to respond to our questions slowly and with difficulty, when his or her hands are warm and relaxed and the eyes tend to close. The percentage of N_2O to obtain the baseline ranges from 25 to 40 %. Signs of overdose, on the other hand, are uncontrollable laughter (nitrous oxide is called *laughing gas* in English, *Lachgas* in German and *gas esilarante* in Italian), diffuse perspiration and signs of agitation with uncoordinated and unintentional movements such as those observed by Wells during Mr. Colton's demonstration. In this case, it will be enough to raise the O_2 percentage to 100 % to obtain regression of the side effects in the space of one minute. Sedation will obviously be resumed at a lower percentage of N_2O than the one responsible for the signs of overdose. In USA, a preconstituted, ready-to-use mixture of 50 % nitrous oxide and 50 % oxygen is available on the market (ENTONOX).

N2O administration with a face mask or nose mask may present a problem due to the risk of environmental pollution.

We shall see now, in the following section, that it is possible, in the third millennium, to perform conscious analgosedation, based on the availability of extremely potent drugs, the administration of which can be programmed with the aid of new computerized procedures.

13.5 Conscious Sedation in the Third Millennium

F. Auricchio

13.5.1 General Considerations

Regional anesthesia offers indisputable advantages both from the point of view of the anesthetist (rapid postoperative recovery, cardiocirculatory stability and, above all, maintenance of spontaneous respiratory activity) and from the point of view of the patient, who sometimes wishes to remain awake during the procedure and may quickly resume ingesting food. On the other hand, numerous patients refuse regional anesthesia for fear of needles, or because staying awake during surgery may be the source of great anxiety, or for fear of not being able to keep still during the procedure. In addition, one should consider that the execution of a block is, in any event, a manoeuver that may give rise to uncomfortable or even painful sensations. Moreover, during surgery, the patient is sometimes obliged to maintain uncomfortable positions even for fairly lengthy periods. For these reasons, it may be advisable to combine the regional anesthesia with the administration of drugs acting on the central nervous system taking the form of the clinical condition called sedation. In actual fact, the term sedation comprises several meanings and is not always used in an unequivocal sense. For the American Society of anesthesiologists (ASA), sedation is a continuum of conditions ranging from anxiolysis to general anesthesia. In this classification, four main conditions are recognized. Anxiolysis, or minimal sedation, is defined as a condition in which the patient responds normally to spoken commands. Cognitive functions and coordination may be impaired, but respiratory and cardiocirculatory functions are normal. The patient is relaxed, the eyes may be closed, and responses may be lethargic, but appropriate. Moderate sedation, also called conscious sedation, is a condition of depression of the state of consciousness characterized by targeted responses to verbal commands, alone or accompanied by mild tactile stimulation. In this case, too, spontaneous ventilation is adequate and cardiocirculatory function is maintained. The patient is drowsy but can be easily awakened if called by name in a loud voice or, at least, when touched. Further depression of the state of consciousness leads to deep sedation, in which the patient responds only if stimulated repeatedly or intensely (pain stimulus). At this level, maintenance of respiratory function is no longer guaranteed: manoeuvers may be necessary to maintain the patency of the airways, and spontaneous ventilation may be inadequate. Lastly, we have general anesthesia, a condition in which the patient cannot be reawakened even by painful stimulation, requires manoeuvers for airways control and may need positive pressure ventilation to treat respiratory depression. The level of sedation that it is recommended during regional anesthesia is conscious sedation. This not only enables the anesthetist to have a collaborative patient during execution of the block, but, above all, drastically reduces the incidence of respiratory and cardiocirculatory complications. Furthermore, in the conscious sedation condition, it is much less likely that the patient will make uncontrolled movements, which may be dangerous during the intervention. Of course, these considerations do not apply to paediatric patients or to non-collaborative patients. Such patients present particular problems that will not be addressed here.

It is important to emphasize the fact that passing from a more superficial to a deeper sedation plane may occur suddenly and unexpectedly, given that even only small changes in concentration of the drug at the site of action are enough to cause important changes in the state of consciousness. Moreover, the inter-individual pharmacokinetic and pharmacodynamic variability of patients means that any therapeutic advice is purely indicative. For these reasons, the sedated patient must be continuously monitored, the level of sedation must be continuously evaluated, and the drugs must be administered in a manner that enables a constant concentration to be maintained. In addition, preference should be accorded to those drugs which, on account of their pharmacokinetic characteristics, permit a rapid onset and a rapid reduction in the concentration at the site of action.

Alongside the depression of the state of consciousness, as a corollary of the sedation, two other related pharmacological effects should be considered, that is, amnesia and analgesia. Amnesia, which is caused to different extents by the various drugs, may be a desired effect, but we should not forget that some patients by contrast wish to remember what they have said and experienced during the operation. The surgeon, too, may be interested in the fact that the patient remembers the information he or she is given during or immediately after the procedure. The anesthetist, on the other hand, may regard the amnesia as advantageous, especially if the patient has suffered some unpleasant experience during the operation. The benzodiazepines are endowed with a substantial amnesic effect, as is propofol, whereas the opioids have no such effect.

More complex, however, is the relationship between analgesia and sedation. Not infrequently, during a regional anesthesia procedure, the patient will experience pain and discomfort. One need only consider the manipulation and insertion of needles that takes place during the execution of the block, as well as the need to maintain uncomfortable positions for lengthy time periods. Often, during the execution of the block, a greater level of analgesia is required than during the subsequent maintenance phase. The extent of the painful stimulation also depends on the type of procedure, whereas the pain threshold is a subjective factor. Hypnotic sedatives such as propofol or the benzodiazepines have no analgesic effect, but act mainly on the affective component of the pain. The α_2-agonists, on the other hand, act both as sedatives and as painkillers, but, if analgesia is the primary objective, the drugs of choice are the opioids. Approximately 5–10 % of regional blocks are inadequate. It would not appear to be correct, in these cases, to expect that sedation will afford sufficient analgesia to complete the procedure, whereas, in the presence of an inadequate block, a safer and more correct policy would be to convert the sedation to general anesthesia.

All in all, anxiolysis, amnesia, hypnosis and analgesia are all components of sedation that can be obtained selectively with the drugs available to us and with appropriate dosages. What aspects of these drugs should make their use preferable depends both on the patient's needs and on the nature of the procedure opted for.

13.6 Patient Preparation

The success and safety of the sedation during a regional anesthesia procedure depend to an appreciable extent on proper preparation of the patient. The purposes of the preoperative visit are several. A thorough history-taking and physical examination must enable the anesthetist to identify any diseases of the main apparatuses, problems with previous anesthesias or sedations, current therapies, allergies and abuses. Particular

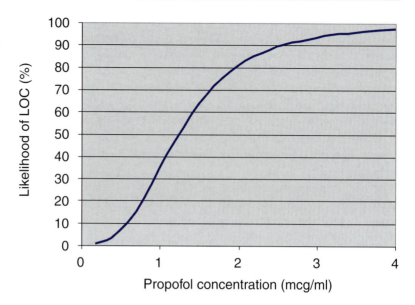

Fig. 13.2 Propofol concentration–effect curve. The effect is represented by the likelihood of suffering loss of consciousness (*LOC*)

attention must be paid to evaluating the state of the airways in order to identify possible causes of hypoventilation during the sedation (obesity, sleep apnoea, rigidity of the cervical column, hypertrophy of the tonsils, etc.). But the preoperative visit above all should represent an opportunity for properly informing the patient about what will happen in the operating room, what he or she may expect from the sedation and the methods that will be employed to assess the patient's state of consciousness. The patient, though sedated, must be collaborative, and for this reason, it is advisable that he or she be well informed. This is the time when the anesthetist can understand the patient's needs and identify those patients who, on account of their mental make-up (claustrophobics, particularly anxious subjects, etc.), may not be ideal candidates for conscious sedation. Moreover, adequate information is the best way of reducing preoperative anxiety.

As regards preoperative fasting, the same rules apply as for general anesthesia. In emergency cases, in an unfasted patient, the options to consider include delaying the procedure or, if this is not possible, choosing to protect the airways by intubation.

13.7 Modes of Administration

Particularly important in intravenous sedation is the mode of administration of the drugs. The effect of intravenous drugs depends not so much upon the dosage, as upon the concentration at the site of action. The relationship between the intensity of the effect and the concentration of the drug is the subject matter of that branch of science called pharmacodynamics. For most sedative and analgesic drugs, this relationship is described satisfactorily by the Emax model. According to this model, at very low concentrations, the effect of the drug is irrelevant. On increasing the concentration, a point is reached at which the concentration–effect curve suddenly rises steeply, that is, small increases in concentration give rise to appreciable increases in effect. This tendency is maintained up to a second critical concentration, beyond which further increases give rise only to small increments in the effect (ceiling effect). Figure 13.2 shows the concentration–effect curve for propofol. The effect is represented by the probability that the patient will suffer loss of consciousness (LOC). It may be noted that the

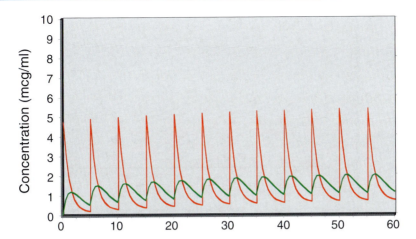

Fig. 13.3 The graph represents the trend of the plasma concentration (*red*) and the concentration at the site of action (*green*) of propofol administered in 30 mg boluses repeated every 5 min (concentrations calculated for a 40-year-old subject weighing 70 kg using Schneider's set of parameters). It may be noted that each bolus induces a peak concentration superior to that of the preceding one

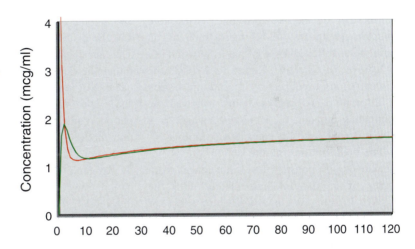

Fig. 13.4 Oscillation of propofol concentrations after a bolus of 0.4 mg/kg followed by continuous infusion at a rate of 3 mg/kg/h

steep portion of the curve identifies the therapeutic range of the drug for that particular endpoint. The steeper the curve is in this range of concentrations, the smaller will be the changes in concentration capable of inducing major variations in effect. In the case of propofol, on increasing the concentration from 1 to 2 mcg/ml, the likelihood of LOC increases from 30 to 80 %.

As we have already stressed, the ideal mode of administration must allow easy titration, enable the desired effect to be reached rapidly and maintain this effect constant for as long as is desired. In other words, it must enable the anesthetist to control the drug concentration at the action site. Intravenous drugs can be administered manually or in a computerized manner. No manual administration mode—be it a bolus, continuous infusion or a combination of the two techniques—is capable of meeting the requirement we have mentioned. Repeated boluses cause a 'saw-teeth' concentration trend, with continuous oscillations of the sedation plane (Fig. 13.3). What is more, if boluses are repeated at constant intervals in the same amounts, the effect of each successive bolus will

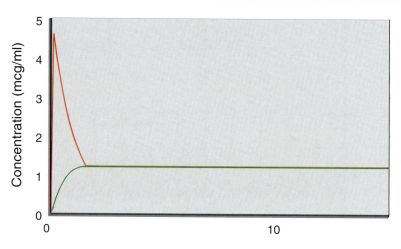

Fig. 13.5 Propofol concentrations administered using the target-controlled infusion (*TCI*) 'at the effect site' method. It may be seen that the concentration desired (1.2 mcg/ml) is reached in less than 2 min at the site of action (*green*). The algorithm for targeting the effect site gives rise to a plasma peak (overshoot), which is of very brief duration and causes no side effects

exceed that of the previous one. Also more complex administration regimens such as an initial bolus followed by continuous infusion fail to achieve the objective. Figure 13.4 shows the concentrations produced by the administration of a propofol 0.4 mg/kg bolus followed by continuous infusion of 3 mg/kg/h, which is a typical dosage used for conscious sedation.

The concentration at the action site is not maintained at a constant level, but ranges from values of 1.9 mcg/ml immediately after the bolus to 1.2 after 10 s, finally reaching a level of 1.6 after less than 2 h of infusion. These oscillations are compatible with different levels of sedation, and the patient's clinical condition will hardly remain constant. The titration process thus proves practically impossible, because even if one manages to find an optimal dosage, the concentration will change after a certain amount of time, making it necessary to repeat the evaluation of the clinical signs at brief intervals.

The problem was solved with the advent of target-controlled infusion (TCI), which is an administration method whereby a microprocessor and an appropriate computer program control the infusion pump. The program must be configured with the specific pharmacokinetic parameters for the drug to be infused, parameters that include information as to the number and amount of the different distribution volumes and the distribution and elimination clearances. The anesthetist does not set the dosage, but rather the desired concentration. The system is capable of reaching that concentration in a short space of time and of maintaining it for the entire period required. The simplest TCI administration mode is one that controls the plasma concentration. It is based on the principle described by Kruger-Thiemer, that is, on the bolus elimination transfer technique (BET). According to this model, the infusion that has to control the plasma concentration requires three components. The first of these, the initial bolus (priming dose), must enable the drug to reach the desired concentration in the central compartment of which the plasma is a part. Immediately after the bolus, two continuous infusions must start up, one at a constant rate, which must compensate for the elimination, and the other, at a progressively decreasing rate, that compensates for the distribution phenomena to the peripheral compartments. In fact, the distribution is a phenomenon that subtracts a large amount of the drug in the initial phases of the infusion, but with the progressive saturation of the peripheral compartments, it increasingly diminishes in intensity, ultimately reaching the steady state. The amount of the initial bolus and the two continuous infusions is determined on the basis of the patient's pharmacokinetic parameters.

Given that plasma is not the site of action of the drug, this mode of control is rather slow at determining the desired changes in concentration at the action site. For this reason, the effect-site TCI method has recently been developed (Fig. 13.5), which affords better control of the pharmacological effect. The 'at the effect site' algorithm comes into operation only in a disequilibrium phase, typically in the induction phase and when the target is changed during maintenance, and considers as an additional parameter the equilibration rate between plasma and effector compartment. Despite the administration of boluses of amounts greater than those used with the plasma modality, effect-site TCI is not associated with an increased incidence of side effects, but permits better titration.

The literature reports the concentration values necessary for reaching a given endpoint, in terms of a 50 or 95 % effective concentration (C_{50} or C_{95}), but the method advised is the one based on titration. In this way, one succeeds in controlling the errors that may be due to pharmacokinetic and pharmacodynamic variability. Incremental concentrations are administered until the desired effect is obtained. The TCI system maintains a constant concentration of the drug (plasma concentration or concentration at the site of action), modifying the infusion rate of the pump at regular intervals (typically every 10 s) and thus compensating for the distribution and elimination phenomena. Currently available on the market are infusion devices that enable a number of drugs to be infused according to the TCI method. The drugs currently utilizable with the system are propofol, remifentanil and sufentanil. For each of these drugs, one can choose between a plasma target and an effect target at the site of action.

13.8 Assessing the Level of Sedation

The main cause of morbidity and mortality associated with sedation and/or analgesia is

Table 13.1 Observer's assessment of alertness/sedation (OAA/S)—modified

Score	Response
5	Responds promptly to name
4	Responds lethargically to name
3	Responds only if the name is pronounced in a loud voice
2	Responds only after moderate stimulation or shaking
1	Does not respond

respiratory depression induced by the drugs and obstruction of the airways. This complication occurs with greater frequency in the course of deep sedation. For this reason, it is important to monitor the level of sedation regularly. A patient who responds to commands is a patient who, on request, can take a deep breath and who is in control of his airways. In contrast, the patient who responds only to a painful stimulus is a deeply sedated patient who may drift into a condition of general anesthesia and must be treated accordingly.

The level of sedation must be assessed by the patient himself using a visual analogue scale or by an observer. In the former case, the method can be applied only in the anxiolysis and mild sedation settings. In the latter case, different rating scales are used, such as the VAS itself, the Ramsay scale or a modified Wilson sedation scale, or the observer's assessment of alertness/sedation (OAA/S). This latter scale, unlike the others, involves the assessment of a large number of items (responsiveness, language, facial expression, eyes), but is especially indicated when particular accuracy in defining the level of sedation is required. Therefore, a modified and simplified version of this scale is widely used, which examines only the patient's responsiveness (Table 13.1). All these scales are reasonably accurate and are suitable for clinical use.

The introduction of tools for monitoring the depth of anesthesia such as the bispectral index (BIS), acoustic evoked potentials (AEPs) and entropy has suggested the possibility of using them also for monitoring the level of sedation. In actual fact, these instruments, though capable of distinguishing between extreme degrees of sedation, do not enable the anesthetist to distinguish with adequate sensitivity between minimal and moderate sedation, or between moderate and deep sedation, and it is acknowledged that these conditions can be discriminated between only by clinical evaluation.

13.9 Other Types of Monitoring

During sedation, continuous monitoring of the ECG and blood pressure is recommended at regular intervals for the early diagnosis of the unwanted effects not only of the sedative drugs but also of the local anesthetics. As regards respiratory function, it should be noted that ventilation and oxygenation must be regarded as separate processes. This means that the monitoring of pulse oximetry, albeit indispensable, is not indicated for the purposes of a timely diagnosis of a condition of hypoventilation or apnoea. When the pulse oximeter shows a drop in saturation values (SpO$_2$), due to hypoventilation or apnoea, this is diagnostic for a respiratory disorder that has occurred several seconds earlier (generally 30–90 s). The delay depends on various circumstances. In the first place, the information displayed by the pulse oximeter is 'old news'. In the case of most monitoring systems, the detection and processing of the signal take 20–30 s. Secondly, in the case of hypoventilation, the peripheral oxygenation rate depends above all on the extent of the oxygen reserve in the residual functional capacity (RFC). This oxygen reserve, in turn, depends on the volume of the RFC and on the oxygen concentration present within it. Patients with a reduced RFC, such as children, obese subjects and pregnant women, in case of hypoventilation, tend to develop hypoxia earlier, whereas in other patients, several seconds may elapse from the onset of the apnoea and the occurrence of desaturation as a result of the oxygen reserve contained in the RFC. One should consider, moreover, that it is precisely in patients with reduced RFC and thus at greater risk of apnoea that the habit of administering supplementary oxygen is advisable. This measure contributes further to delaying the diagnosis of hypoventilation when the patient is monitored with pulse oximetry alone, so much so, indeed, that the advantages afforded by administering oxygen may be completely nullified.

There are various ways of monitoring the patient's ventilation. The simplest and most effective method is auscultation, but this requires the continuous presence of a doctor alongside the patient. Many ECG monitors record the respiratory rate using the thoracic impedance meter method. The operating principle is based on the recording of variations in impedance that occur among the ECG electrodes as a result of respiratory movements of the thorax. This technique does not measure the effective passage of the flow of a gas through the airways, but rather the movement of the thorax. Therefore, it is not capable of effectively recognizing obstruction-induced apnoea, in which the respiratory effort may be conserved, even if not effective. The method of choice is the monitoring of expired CO$_2$ with the use of sidestream capnometers, which provide both numerical data (end-tidal CO$_2$) and a curve (capnograph). The interpretation of these data affords a means of continuously monitoring the patient's state. Appropriate cannulas enable gas to be sampled at both the nasal and oral levels and are not subject to any noteworthy interference as a result of the simultaneous administration of oxygen. Although the monitoring of expired CO$_2$ does not as yet represent a standard form of monitoring of spontaneously breathing patients (whereas it is mandatory in mechanically ventilated patients), various scientific societies recommend its use, particularly in the case of patients at risk of airway obstruction, in cases receiving deep sedation and in cases of supplementary oxygen administration.

13.10 Drugs

13.10.1 Propofol

Propofol is a hypnotic agent widely used as a sedative in regional anesthesia. Its action is exerted at least in part by binding with subunit β of the GABA receptor, although we cannot rule out its interaction with other receptors at the level of the CNS. It induces a dose-dependent depression of the CNS, with effects ranging from anxiolysis to sedation, and even general anesthesia. It does not possess any major analgesic effect and produces amnesia, though to a lesser extent than midazolam. Among its desirable effects, one should mention its antiemetic action. Its unwanted effects are also dose-dependent and consist in cardiocirculatory depression, defined as arterial hypotension and an increase in bradycardia, and respiratory depression. Among the adverse effects, there is also pain at the injection site, the frequency and intensity of which can be relieved by the preventive administration of a bolus of lidocaine.

The main advantages of propofol are due to its pharmacokinetic characteristics. Both the onset and the decline of its desired effects are very rapid. An intravenous bolus induces a peak hypnotic effect in less than 2 min, while the peak of the unwanted cardiocirculatory effects is present after 5–10 min. Propofol is distributed according to a three-compartment model. The main pharmacokinetic characteristics are its high elimination clearance, its reduced distribution clearances towards the peripheral compartments and its high distribution volumes. The elimination is mainly via the liver and occurs with a substantial clearance flow of around 2 l/min. This is defined as flow-dependent elimination because it is little affected by deficits of the metabolic capacity of the liver, so much so that its duration of action is not prolonged in cases of moderate hepatic insufficiency, whereas it is adversely affected by reductions in cardiac output and liver perfusion. Its short duration of action is not due solely to its high elimination clearance, but, above all, to the fact that in the postinfusional phase, the peripheral compartments continue to accumulate the drug, subtracting it from the central volume and rendering it non-bioavailable. For this reason, the context-sensitive half-life of propofol remains around 5–7 min even after a 3 h infusion. Age has a major influence on the pharmacokinetics of propofol. In paediatric subjects, the volumes are greater, which explains the need for proportionally higher dosages. With increasing age, the volumes and clearances diminish progressively, and the dosages need to be adequately reduced.

The pharmacodynamics of propofol also presents a substantial inter-individual variability. In this case, too, age is an important covariate: the C_{50} for the LOC ranges from concentrations of 2.35–1.8 and 1.25 mcg/ml at the site of action for subjects aged 25, 50 and 75 years of age. It should be noted that the concomitant administration of benzodiazepines and, albeit to a lesser extent, of opioids, synergistically potentiates both the desired effects (sedation) and the unwanted effects (respiratory and cardiocirculatory) of propofol.

Propofol can be administered manually. In this case, it is advisable to administer a priming dose (0.2–0.7 mg/kg) followed by a continuous infusion (0.5–4 mg/kg/h). But, as we explained previously, this mode of administration is not as efficacious and safe as the TCI method. The modern OpenTCI pumps enable the anesthetist not only to infuse the drug using the TCI plasma technique or TCI at the site of action, but also to choose among various sets of pharmacokinetic parameters. The possibility of choosing the most suitable parameter set reduces the errors due to the inter-individual pharmacokinetic variability, particularly with regard to the component related to the age of the subject.

In conclusion, in view of its easy titration, its lack of serious side effects at the doses inducing conscious sedation and the possibility of computerized administration, propofol may be regarded as the sedative of choice for use in conjunction with regional anesthesia procedures.

13.10.2 Benzodiazepines

The effects of the benzodiazepines are the result of its occupation of specific binding sites, the benzodiazepine receptors, extensively present in the CNS. At this level, they favour the inhibitory action of GABA on neuronal transmission. The effects are anxiolysis, sedation, hypnosis, anticonvulsant effects, amnesia and muscle relaxation. These are drugs that are preferred above all for their elevated safety margin from both the respiratory and cardiocirculatory points of view. Other advantages are the raising of the convulsive threshold of local anesthetics, which may be useful in the course of regional anesthesia, and the availability of an antagonist, flumazenil. Unfortunately, they possess unfavourable pharmacokinetic characteristics. What is more, when combined with opioids, they considerably potentiate the respiratory depression effects of the latter. Among these adverse effects, there is also the possibility of paradoxical reactions, especially in elderly patients.

Among the benzodiazepines available, only midazolam possesses pharmacokinetic characteristics that permit its use in the operating room. Despite this, the peak effect of a bolus of midazolam occurs after 13 min and the recovery phase is also prolonged as compared to that of propofol, with an elimination half-life of 2–6 h. The main weakness of midazolam's pharmacokinetics is the elimination phase. The main metabolite, which is formed as a result of the action of cytochrome P450 3A4, is $1'1$-hydroxymidazolam, which is subsequently conjugated and excreted with the urine. Cytochrome activity presents great inter-individual variability both on account of differences of constitution and for acquired reasons. Among the latter, one factor studied with particular attention has been the role of substances with an inhibiting or an inducing action. The substances that reduce the activity of cytochrome P450 3A4 include erythromycin, calcium antagonists, antacids such as ranitidine, antimycotics such as fluconazole and even grapefruit juice. Carbamazepine and phenobarbital, on the other hand, exert an inducing activity. Furthermore, it should be noted that $1'1$-hydroxymidazolam possesses an activity comparable to that of midazolam itself. The glucuronated compound also possesses pharmacological activity which is approximately one-tenth that of midazolam. All things considered, the slow onset, great inter-individual variability of the elimination clearance, the presence of active metabolites and the pharmacodynamic variability of midazolam make it an unpredictable drug as regards its effects and duration of action, and one which is not very suitable for titration. Among other things, currently there are no infusion devices available for the computerized administration of midazolam. Therefore, any therapeutic recommendations are only of indicative value. Midazolam is generally administered in manual boluses in dosages of 0.03–0.05 mg/kg, bearing in mind that its peak action occurs after more than 10 min and that elderly patients may be very sensitive to the action of this drug. Moreover, particular caution is essential when monitoring the patient's ventilation when midazolam is used in conjunction with opioids.

13.10.3 α_2-Agonists

In the past, the α2-agonists were used as antihypertensive agents and in the treatment of alcohol or drug addiction. Recently, by virtue of their analgesic and sedative effects, their use has been extended to intensive care and the operating room. Their effects are exerted through binding to the α_2-receptors, of which there exist sundry subtypes (α_{2A}, α_{2B}, α_{2C}). The various receptor subtypes are distributed ubiquitously and are responsible for the various effects of these drugs. Thus, the hypotensive effect would appear to be mediated by the α_{2A} subtype at the level of the arterial smooth muscle cells, whereas for the analgesic, sedative and sympathicolytic effects, the α_{2B} subtype is involved at the central level. The mechanism whereby this category of drugs induces a state of sedation consists in the hyperpolarization of noradrenergic neurons in the locus coeruleus, with consequent suppression of the ascending noradrenergic pathway. In this way, the inhibitory action on the ventrolateral preoptic nucleus is suppressed, with the release of gamma-aminobutyric acid and a reduction in the release of histamine. This response is similar to that which occurs during physiological sleep. The result is a very particular type of sedation, not associated with respiratory depression or with a reduced ventilatory response to CO_2. The analgesic effects are attributable to an inhibitory action both on the locus coeruleus and at the spinal level. The α_2-agonists interfere with the thermoregulation processes and antagonize postoperative shivering. Unfortunately, the sympatholytic and vagomimetic effects may give rise to side effects at the cardiocirculatory level, characterized by hypotension and bradycardia, especially in hypovolemic and vasoconstricted patients or in patients with cardiac conduction disorders. In addition, the effects of other sedatives and opioids are potentiated.

The two representative drugs of this category are clonidine and dexmedetomidine. Clonidine is a drug mainly used as an antihypertensive agent, but it is also indicated in the treatment of opioid drug addiction, attention deficit hyperactivity disorder (ADHD) and Gilles de la Tourette syndrome. It has proved to be an effective sedative at the dose of 1.5 mcg/kg/h, without any side effects worthy of note. Unfortunately, it is characterized by a slow onset and, above all, by a long offset, with a distribution half-life of 1.2 h and an elimination half-life of 8–14 h. Dexmedetomidine presents numerous advantages. In the first place, it has a seven times greater affinity than clonidine for α_2-receptors over α_1-receptors, which reduces the side effects and makes it mainly a sedative and anxiolytic drug. In addition, it presents more advantageous pharmacodynamic properties, with an elimination half-life of 2 h, which makes it an ideal drug for intravenous titration. It has been used as a sedative in intensive care, in fibrobronchoscopy intubation, and for paediatric sedation, but there are few studies describing its characteristics as a sedative in the course of regional anesthesia. It is commonly used at the dosage of 1 mcg/kg, possibly followed by continuous infusion at the rate of 0.1–0.7 mcg/kg/h. As compared to midazolam, it produces similar sedation but with less amnesia, greater analgesia and a greater incidence of bradycardia and hypotension.

In conclusion, dexmedetomidine, though as yet not sufficiently studied, is an interesting drug, above all because it induces sedation without respiratory depression, a state very similar to physiological sleep, from which the patient can be easily awakened. This is combined with an analgesic effect and with a potentiation of analgesic agents that is much greater than that induced by the other sedatives. On the other hand, however, we should not underestimate the cardiocirculatory depressive effects of the drug, especially in patients at risk.

13.10.4 Opioids

There is an increasingly widespread use of opioids, either alone or in combination with sedatives, in pharmacological support strategies in regional blocks. We have already emphasized that in the course of these procedures, it is a by no means rare occurrence for patients to have distressing or painful sensations both during performance of the block and during surgery (position, use of tourniquets, etc.). By definition, a patient under conscious sedation is reawakened and reacts in the eventuality of painful stimulation, and if one seeks to control this situation with sedatives alone, there will sometimes be a risk of slipping towards a deep sedation plane, with the consequent repercussions as regards the safety of the procedure. Opioids offer a potent analgesic effect associated with a modest sedative effect, and for this reason may constitute an efficacious tool in the anesthetist's armamentarium, provided they are used properly.

The effects of opioids are mediated by their interaction with the receptors both at the spinal and the supraspinal levels. Their main effect then is analgesia. They do not possess an anxiolytic effect, and indeed, in some patients, when they are not combined with benzodiazepines or propofol, they give rise to an unpleasant anxiety sensation. Nor do they possess any evident amnesic effect, but they do exert a dose-dependent sedative effect, which, however, is manifested at dosages that cause respiratory depression. In fact, in comparison with propofol or midazolam, when the patient reaches a level of sedation corresponding to level 3 on the modified OAA/S scale (the patient responds only if his or her name is pronounced in a loud voice), an unacceptable respiratory depression occurs with the use of opioids. The other side effects are nausea and vomiting, itching and cardiocirculatory depression, along with hypotension and bradycardia. They can be used alone or in combination with sedatives. In the latter case, it is advisable to be thoroughly familiar with the interactions between these two categories of drugs. In the first place, the opioids, although they do not induce a marked sedative effect, potentiate the sedation produced by other drugs to a considerable extent. For this reason, if in a patient who finds himself in a condition of conscious sedation obtained with a benzodiazepine or with propofol, this is combined with a modest dose of opioids, for example 1 mcg/kg of fentanyl, he may suddenly become deeply sedated, unresponsive, apnoic and hard to ventilate with a face mask. On the other hand, sedatives potentiate the analgesic effects of opioids: 2 mg of midazolam enables the anesthetist to halve the dose of remifentanil, maintaining the patient's level of comfort unaltered in the course of conscious sedation. Unfortunately, the respiratory depression is also potentiated, even if the combination eliminates the sensation of anxiety that sometimes manifests itself with the opioid alone and induces an amnesic effect. When, however, the opioids are used alone, the aim must not be to sedate the patient, but rather to enhance his comfort and relieve the pain.

The various opioids available to the anesthetist differ only in their pharmacokinetic properties. Both remifentanil and alfentanil have a rapid onset: the peak effect of an intravenous

Table 13.2 Plasma half-life (minutes) of opioids after different continuous infusion durations. The half-life of remifentanil is insensitive to the infusion duration

	1 h	2 h	3 h
Remifentanil	5	5	5
Alfentanil	33	39	42
Sufentanil	23	32	32
Fentanyl	30	45	75

bolus for these drugs occurs after approximately 1.5 min, whereas for sufentanil and fentanyl, it occurs at around 4–6 min. As regards the offset, remifentanil offers advantages in absolute terms as compared to all the other drugs in this category. In particular, its half-life is independent of the duration of the infusion and holds steady at around 5 min, whereas for the other opioids, it depends to a major extent on the duration of the infusion (Table 13.2). The main pharmacokinetic characteristics of remifentanil are its small distribution volumes, its limited liposolubility effect and its rapid elimination clearance due to its particular esterase-dependent metabolism, which is not subject to the functionality of the emunctories, but occurs in all the tissues of the body as a result of the effect of a ubiquitous enzyme. These characteristics make the drug ideal for intravenous titration and safer than the other opioids, because, in the case of adverse events, it is enough to suspend the infusion for 2–3 min to put a stop to these unwanted effects. The pharmacokinetic profile of remifentanil, described by Minto, depends on the subject's lean body mass (LBM) and age. For example, a continuous infusion of 0.1 mcg/kg/min in a 20-year-old young man for 10 min produces a concentration of 1.8 ng/ml at the action site, whereas in an 80-year-old subject receiving the same dosage, a concentration of 2.6 ng/ml is reached at the action site. Consequently, when the drug is administered manually, the dosage must be adequately reduced. This problem does not arise with the TCI modality, where the target concentration desired is set on the infusion pump. The computer incorporated in the pump calculates the dosage necessary to reach and maintain this concentration in relation to the patient's characteristics according to the pharmacokinetic model described by Minto.

Bolus administration is not advisable because it is associated with an increased incidence of side effects. Continuous infusion at the rate of 0.05–0.1 mcg/kg/min with 0.025 mcg/kg/min adjustments according to the clinical responses guarantees the execution of the block and the subsequent maintenance of patient comfort and analgesia. At higher doses, the incidence of respiratory depression and other side effects increases. The concomitant administration of 2 mg of midazolam reduces the need for remifentanil by 50 %. With the TCI technique, the concentration value recommended is 1 ng/ml with 0.2 ng/ml adjustments, taking care not to exceed the concentration of 2 ng/ml, beyond which respiratory depression occurs. In the effect-site TCI modality, the desired target is reached in only 90 s. In this way, a rapid titration can be achieved. Despite the fact that remifentanil is a drug with a rapid onset and a rapid offset, it has been demonstrated that its use in the TCI modality constitutes an advantage in terms of safety compared to the manual administration methods.

13.11 Future Developments: Patient-Controlled and Patient-Maintained Sedation

In the treatment of postoperative pain, we have recently been witnessing the widespread successful use of techniques involving the self-administration of drugs by patients (patient-controlled analgesia, PCA). For several years, now sedation procedures based on the principle of drug management by the patient have been studied, although they have yet to become standard clinical practice. The rationale is the same: the very possibility of modifying the perception of pain simply by pressing a button may be a potent analgesic in its own right comparable to the drug itself. The purpose is to obtain patient satisfaction with a minimum of side effects, lower drug consumption and a faster recovery. Two main methods have been studied. Patient-controlled sedation (PCS) consists in the administration of the drug completely controlled by the patient, who self-administers manual boluses of the drug as necessary. Given that an excessively sedated patient will be unable to activate the pump, he or she is protected against overdosing, and this guarantees the intrinsic safety of the procedure. The drug most studied with this technique is propofol, which has proved more efficacious than midazolam. PCS pumps are modified syringe pumps capable of administering a predetermined drug bolus in a predetermined time, with or without a lockout interval. An initial bolus to speed up the induction can be programmed, but like all procedures based on the administration of manual boluses, unwanted peaks are possible as well as a fluctuating sedation trend. On the whole, PCS is associated with greater patient satisfaction compared to anesthetist-based techniques, with a lower consumption of propofol and a comparable incidence of side effects.

In patient-maintained sedation (PMS), a TCI pump is set by the anesthetist with an appropriate target, generally 1 mcg/ml for propofol, and the patient can increase the drug concentration by pressing the button (0.2 mcg/ml increments) with a variable lockout period. The system will reduce the target concentration if the patient does not press the button in a determined time period. PMS avoids the problem of the fluctuation of the sedation plane and, generally speaking, patients prefer it to PCS. Initially, PMS was used with plasma-target TCI, but one of the main problems was the slow onset of sedation. More recently, PMS targeting the site of action has been proposed, presenting equal efficacy and greater rapidity in achieving the desired sedation plane. PCS and PMS have been studied, for example, for sedation in the course of dental extraction, for gastrointestinal tract endoscopic procedures, during arthroprosthesis surgery or during awake craniotomy. Despite the fact that these are still experimental techniques, the substantial measure of patient satisfaction and the possibility of involving him or her directly in the sedation titration process are the premises for predicting their widespread use in the near future.

Bibliography

American Society for Gastrointestinal Endoscopy (2008) Standards of practice committee. Sedation and anesthesia in GI endoscopy. Gastrointest Endosc 68:205–216

American Society of Anesthesiologists Task Force on Sedation and Analgesia by Non-Anesthesiologists (2002) Practice guidelines for sedation and analgesia by non-anesthesiologists. Anesthesiology 96:1004–1017

Bailey JM, Shafer SL (1991) A simple analytical solution to the three-compartment pharmacokinetic model suitable for computer-controlled infusion pump. IEEE Trans Biomed Eng 38:522–525

Bellucci G (1982) Storia della anestesiologia. Piccin Editore, Padova

Busato G, Alemanno F (1974) Praticità dell'Associazione Propanidide-NLA nelle Anestesie di Breve Durata. Acta Anaesth It 3:335–338

Carlon CA, Cavalloni L (1953) Importanza e significato dei riflessi neurovegetativi durante narcosi e nella genesi della malattia postoperaroria. Acta Anaesth Italica 4:1

Carollo DS, Nossaman BD, Ramadhyani U (2008) Dexmedetomidine: a review of clinical applications. Curr Opin Anaesthesiol 21:457–461

Charbit B, Funk-Brentano C (2007) Droperidol-induced proarrhythmia. The beginning of an answer? Anesthesiology 107:524–526

Collins VJ (1976) Principles of anesthesiology. Lea & Febiger, Philadelphia

Damia G (1987) La sedazione cosciente con N2O nelle cure odontoiatriche dell'adulto in L. Dall'Oppio, GF Di Nino: L'intervento odontostomatologico in sedazione e narcosi. MASSON, Milano, Parigi, Barcellona, Messico, San Paolo

De Castro J, Mundeleer P (1959) Anesthésie sans barbituriques: la neuroleptoanalgésie (R1406, R1625, Hydergine, Procaine). Anesth Analg Réan 16:1022

De Castro J, Mundeleer P (1962) Deidrobenzoperidolo e fentanyl. Due nuovi farmaci d'interesse anestesiologico che danno nuove possibilità alla neuroleptoanalgesia. Symposium sulla Neuroleptoanalgesia al Primo Congresso Europeo d'Anestesiologia. Vienna 5 settembre

Du Bouchet N, Le Brigand J (1957) Anesthesie reanimation. Editions Medicales Flammarion, Paris

Du Bouchet N, Passelecq J (1982) Anestesia. Marrapese Editore—D.E.M.I. Roma1982

Finucane BT (1999) Complications of regional anesthesia. Churchil Livingstone, Philadelphia

Giardina B, Tempo B, Azzolini CV, Ciocatto E (1976) Libro di anestesia. In: Libreria (ed) Scientifiche Cortina, Torino

Glassman A, Bigger JJ (2001) Antipsychotic drugs: prolonged QT interval, torsade de pointes, and sudden death. Am J Psychiatry 158:1774–1782

Herrick IA, Craen RA, Gelb AW, Miller LA, Kubu CS, Girvin JP, Parrent AG, Eliasziw M, Kirkby J (1997) Propofol sedation during awake craniotomy for seizures: patient-controlled administration versus neuroleptanalgesia. Anesth Analg 84:1285–1291

Höhener D, Blumenthal S, Borgeat A (2008) Sedation and regional anaesthesia in the adult patient. Br J Anaesth 100(1):8–16

Huguenard P (1950) Association diparcol-dolosal: anesthésie locale. Anesth Analg 7:569

Huguenard P (1951) Essais d'anesthésie générale sans anesthésique. Anesth Analg 8:5

Huguenard P (1966) Neuroleptoanalgesie: aspect doctrinal. Ann Anesth Franc 7(Special 1):1

Janssen P, Niemegeers CJ, Schellekens KH, Verbruggen FJ, Van NuetenJM (1963) The pharmacology of dehydrobenzperidol. A new potent and short acting neuroleptic agent chemically correlated to Haloperidol. Arzneimittel-Forsch 13:205–211

Kamibayashi T, Maze M (2000) Clinical uses of a2-Adrenergic agonists. Anesthesiology 93:1345–1349

Kazama T, Ikeda K, Morita K, Kikura M, Doi M, Ikeda T, Kurita T, Nakajima Y (1999) Comparison of the effect-site k(eO)s of propofol for blood pressure and EEG bispectral index in elderly and younger patients. Anesthesiology 90:1517–1527

Kruger-Thiemer E (1968) Continuous intravenous infusion and multicompartmental accumulation. Eur J Pharmacol 4:317–324

Laborit H (1965) Les regulations métaboliques. Masson & Cie, Paris

Laborit H, Huguenard P, Alluaume R (1952) Un nouveau stabilisateur végétatif, le 4560 R.P. (Largactil). Presse Méd 60:206

Laborit H, Leger L (1950) Utilisation d'un antihistaminique de syntése en thérapeutique pré et post-opératoire. Presse Méd 58:492

Laborit H (1951) L'anesthésie facilitée par les synergies médicamenteuses, vol I. Masson et Cie, Paris

Liu B, Juurlink DN (2004) Drugs and QT interval: caveat doctor. N Engl J Med 351:1053–1096

Malamed SF (1985) Sedation: a guide to patient management. The C.V. Mosby Company, St. Louis Missouri

Minto CF, Schnider TW, Schafer SL (1997) Pharmacokinetics and pharmacodynamics of remifentanil: II. Model Application. Anesthesiology 86:24–33

Nuttall GA, Eckerman KM, Jacob KA, Pawlaski EM et al (2007) Does low-dose droperidol administration increase the risk of drug-induced QT prolongation and torsade de pointes in the general surgical population? Anesthesiology 4(107):531–536

Powers KS, Nazarian EB, Tapyrik SA, Kohli SM, Yin H, van der Jagt EW, Sullivan SJ, Rubenstein JS (2005) Bispectral index as a guide for titration of propofol during procedural sedation among children. Pediatrics 115:1666–1674

Raeder J (2009) Opioid or propofol: what kind of drug for what kind of sedation? Manual dosing or target-controlled infusion? Anesth Analg 108(3):704–706

Roden DM (2004) Drug-induced prolongation of the QT interval. N Engl J Med 350:1013–1022

Rodrigo MR, Irwin MG, Tong CK, Yan SY (2003) A randomised crossover comparison of patient-controlled sedation and patient-maintained sedation using propofol. Anaesthesia 58:333–338

Rosenberg MB, Campbell RL (1991) Guidelines for intraoperative monitoring of dental patients undergoing conscious sedation, deep sedation, and general anesthesia. Oral Surg Oral Med Oral Pathol 71:2–8

Schnider TW, Minto CF, Shafer SL, Gambus PL, Andresen C, Goodale DB, Youngs BJ (1999) The influence of age on propofol pharmacodynamics. Anesthesiology 90(5):1502–1516

Servin F, Watkins W (1999) Remifentanil as analgesic adjunct in local/regional anesthesia and in monitored anesthesia care. Anesth Analg 89(45)S:28

Shafer SL, Gregg KM (1992) Algorithms to rapidly achieve and maintain stable drug concentrations at site of drug effect with a computer-controlled infusion pump. J Pharmacokinet Biopharm 20:147–169

Shafer SL, Varvel JR (1991) Pharmacokinetics, pharmacodynamics, and rational opioid selection. Anesthesiology 74(1):53–63

Stöcker L (1976) Narkose. Georg Thieme Verlag, Stuttgart

White PF, Song D, Abrao J, Klein KW, Navarette B (2005) Effect of low-dose droperidol on the QT interval during and after general anesthesia: a placebo controlled study. Anesthesiology 102:1101–1105

Perineural Adjuvants for Postoperative Analgesia

14

F. Alemanno

The story began in the late 1990s with a visit I paid to the Pain Therapy Center of the University of Würzburg in Germany, directed by Professor Sprotte, who is familiar to everyone on account of the spinal needle he devised. He was treating cases of cervicobrachialgia, performing a stellate ganglion block with one tenth of an ampoule of buprenorphine, further diluted with 7 ml of saline. The results were astonishing.

On returning to Bolzano Hospital, I successfully treated several cases of cervicobrachialgia, which my orthopaedic and neurosurgery colleagues were only too happy to refer to me.

At the time, I thought I might be able to use the same molecule to prolong the postoperative analgesia of the brachial plexus block technique I myself had devised. Proportionally, using on average 30–40 ml of anesthetic to block the plexus, I found I had to use not one tenth of an ampoule of buprenorphine, but half an ampoule.

The articles by Candido in 2001 and 2002 published in *Regional Anesthesia and Pain Medicine* further confirmed the soundness of my thinking. Particularly interesting was the 2002 article because the procedure was applied at the axillary level and therefore gave no reason to suspect a transdural spread of the buprenorphine.

14.1 Rationale

The article by Scott Young published in *Science* in 1980 provides the basis for the rationale. The opioid receptors produced in the unipolar neurons of the ganglion of the posterior root are subject to the flow of axonal liquid. To be able to trace these, two molecules with high receptor affinity, enkephalin and naloxone, were labelled, the former with tritium (H3) or with iodine-125, and the latter with iodine-125.

The same year, HL Fields published in *Nature* the article entitled 'Multiple opiate receptor sites on primary afferent fibres', claiming that '… there is evidence that both the exogenous opioids and the enkephalins act both at the presynaptic level blocking the release of neurotransmitters (nociceptive, editor's note) from the primary afferent nerve endings and at the level of the postsynaptic receptors'.

Christoff Stein of Berlin, in a review article entitled 'The control of pain in peripheral tissues by opioids', published in *The New England Journal of Medicine* in 1995, reported that opioids bind to the receptors in the ganglia, on the spinal and peripheral nerve endings and reduce the excitability of the primary afferent neurons by inhibiting adenyl cyclase (Fig. 14.1). In a previous article, published in *Anesthesia and Analgesia* in 1993 entitled 'Peripheral mechanism of opioid analgesia', the same author states: 'both exogenous and endogenous opioids are capable of producing specific effects on the

F. Alemanno (✉)
Institute of Anesthesiology, Resuscitation and Pain Therapy, University of Verona, Verona, Italy
e-mail: fernando@alemannobpb.it

opioid receptors in areas outside the central nervous system'. He concludes, however, by complaining that '... the evidence from the clinical studies is inconclusive so far'.

Other review articles have also demonstrated that the application of perineural opioids has yielded ambiguous results. Putzu and Casati agree that, in actual fact, when using the main morphine-based drugs (morphine, fentanyl, sufentanil), the results are often contradictory and disappointing.

Only two opioids, as reported by McCartney, have shown promising and lasting efficacy if administered at the perineural level. These are buprenorphine and tramadol.

Adenyl cyclase

3'5' cyclic AMP

Phosphodiesterase

Fig. 14.1 All the signals, whether hormonal or due to neuromediators, that reach the membrane receptors or the synaptic receptors in the case of the central nervous system, would in themselves be very weak, if it were not for the fact that there is a signal amplifier in the membrane receptor at the postsynaptic level. This neuromediator consists in the molecule 3'5'-cyclic AMP. The metabolism of this molecule is in constant equilibrium and is regulated by two enzymes with antithetical actions, namely adenyl cyclase that activates its synthesis and phosphodiesterase that activates its hydrolysis. Obviously, any drug that depresses adenyl cyclase, as in our case the opioids, gives rise to a reduction in the signal as a result of the diminished presence of 3'5'-cyclic AMP molecules, and thus also to a reduction in the nociceptive signal. On the other hand, any drug that depresses phosphodiesterase gives rise to an increase in the number of 3'5'-cyclic AMP molecules and thus to an increase in the signal. Thus, for example, the xanthines (caffeine, teine and theobromine) bring about an amplification of various signals, among which the adrenergic signal is the one we may note subjectively

14.2 Clonidine

Before addressing these two abnormal and to some extent curious molecules, we feel we should first mention a classic adjuvant in regional anesthesiological practice, namely clonidine.

14.2.1 Mechanism of Action

This classic α_2-agonist, normally used in general medicine as an antihypertensive drug, acts in this sense by interfering with the cells of the central nervous system whose receptors are responsible for blood pressure regulation. They normally activate a diastaltic arc, which uses the paravertebral sympathetic chain to regulate the production of circulatory catecholamines by the adrenal medulla. Clonidine deceives the brain cells regarding the level of circulatory catecholamines, inducing the cells to estimate them at a higher level than they actually are, thus causing a reduction in the signal arriving at the adrenal gland.

The posterior horn of the spinal cord is endowed with α_2-receptors that perform an analgesic function by inhibiting the presynaptic release of excitatory neurotransmitters such as glutamate (an NMDA agonist) and substance P.

If administered at the subarachnoid level, clonidine induces an increase in acetylcholine. This neuromediator presents itself mainly, in the closed chain state, in what are called the nicotinic synapses (it also resembles nicotine in shape), located in the muscles and peripheral ganglia, or mainly, in the open-chain state, at the level of the muscarinic receptors located in the peripheral endings of the vegetative nervous system and in the synapses of the central nervous system. The central stimulation of the muscarinic receptors induces and gives rise to an increase in GABA at the level of the primary afferent fibres, which results in suppression of the release of glutamate and substance P, two neuromediators with an excitatory action, and in hyperpolarization due to the opening of chloride channels.

Many studies have been conducted in which clonidine has been used as a perineural adjuvant. The most interesting of these is the study by Singelyn et al. who, by adding a 150 mcg dose of clonidine to 40 ml of 1 % mepivacaine for axillary brachial plexus block, obtained an analgesia lasting twice as long as that achieved with the local anesthetic alone. With the long-lasting local anesthetics (levobupivacaine and ropivacaine), the addition of clonidine would not appear to be particularly useful because the duration of the analgesia induced does not exceed that of the typical analgesic after-effect of the local anesthetic. In the opinion of Culebras et al. it is also believed to cause problems of haemodynamic instability. According to Hutschhala et al. and Casati et al. however, the drug will in any case prolong the analgesia induced by the local anesthetic.

14.3 Buprenorphine

Buprenorphine, a thebaine derivative, has a rather complicated mechanism of action. It is a mu receptor agonist and its receptor affinity is 24 times that of fentanyl and 50 times that of morphine. It also binds to delta and kappa receptors, but the affinity for the delta receptors is ten times less.

At the level of the posterior horn, most of the receptors are of the mu type. Mu and delta agonists inhibit pain, but the role of the kappa receptors is controversial. Activation of the mu and delta receptors inhibits adenyl cyclase, opens the K^+ channels and closes the Ca^{++} channels. These actions lead to a reduced release of the pain transmitters, substance P and glutamate. After the discovery of the mu, delta and kappa receptors, a fourth receptor has been identified which has been called the opioid receptor-like 1 (ORL1). It has nociceptin as a neuromediator, with a hyperalgesic effect which differs from the other antalgic neuromediators due to the lack of tyrosine in its constituent amino acid sequence (hence the name orphanin as it is called by some authors). Buprenorphine at high doses, unlike the other opioids, despite its potency, does not yield a maximal response; its dose-effect curve is not hyperbolical but submaximal, plateau like or even bell shaped, probably because, on account of its potency, it also manages to activate the opioid receptors-like 1 which have an antagonist effect on the drug, curbing its own potent pain-killing properties. Lutfy and Cowan assert that the potency of buprenorphine is related to its lipophilia, which determines a high receptor affinity and which, together with its low molecular weight, facilitates its axonal penetration.

Its receptor affinity is so strong that it cannot be antagonized by naloxone. Barbara Pleuvry has even postulated that naloxone may reinforce its agonist action in the presence of high doses of the drug, succeeding in detaching buprenorphine only from the opioid receptors-like 1.

To complicate matters, there is also norbuprenorphine, an active metabolite of buprenorphine, which has an agonist action on the mu receptors and a fairly weak action on the OPRL1.

14.3.1 Perineural Application

Among the clinical studies conducted with buprenorphine, the most interesting are those published in *Regional Anesthesia and Pain Medicine*, by Candido, Franco et al., regarding the interscalene block by Candido et al. in 2001 and by Candido, Winnie et al. regarding the axillary block in 2002. Unfortunately, the study population was not homogeneous.

In their study of the supraclavicular block, Candido, Franco et al. examined two groups each comprising 40 patients, anesthetized with a mixture of 1 % mepivacaine and 0.2 % tetracaine. In one of the two groups, 1 ampoule of buprenorphine (0.3 mg) was added to the local anesthetic mixture. The result was an analgesia time of 17.4 ($\pm$ 1.26) h in the buprenorphine group as against 5.3 ($\pm$ 0.15) h in the control group.

For our part, we have recently conducted a study in 150 patients, all with the same pathology, consisting in a rotator cuff injury, scheduled to be operated on by shoulder arthroplasty performed by the same surgical team.

The patients were subdivided into three groups and anesthetized with a middle interscalene block with a dose of 40 ml of 0.75 % levobupivacaine and receiving half an ampoule of buprenorphine (0.15 mg) combined with an anesthetic mixture in one of the three groups. In the second group, the half ampoule of buprenorphine was injected intramuscularly into the contralateral deltoid muscle. In the second and third group the anesthetic was added with half a ml of saline.

In the first group, the analgesia duration was 17 h and 29 min, calculated from the time the anesthesia was induced; in the second group, it was 13 h and 40 min; and in the third group, it was 10 h and 37 min.

At this point, we wondered how it was that Candido et al. with an entire ampoule of buprenorphine (0.3 mg) obtained more or less the same analgesia time as we did with only half an ampoule (0.15 mg). The cause of this incongruity, I believe, is due not only to the use of different local anesthetics, but also to the dose—response curve of buprenorphine, which, unlike the other opioids, beyond a certain dose, presents a submaximal plateau-like or even a bell-shaped curve due to activation of the opioid receptors-like 1. It might be objected that such low doses of buprenorphine are incapable of activating the opioid-like receptors, but here we are not operating via a systemic route, but on the posterior horn of the spinal cord by an axonal route. At the subarachnoid level, a dose of 0.1 mg of morphine is sufficient to guarantee good analgesia.

14.4 Tramadol

As early as 1980, Stoffregen used a tramadol infusion to boost the effect of general anesthesia, and even earlier in 1978, Flohe et al. had established that the drug was associated with few signs of development of tolerance after repeated administrations and lent itself poorly to being used as a substitute for morphine in morphine-dependent patients. According to Arend, it also gave rise to no euphoria-inducing effects or psychological dependence. The drug therefore proved to be paradoxically different from morphine with regard to its subjective effects, despite its substantial analgesic efficacy.

This apparent contradiction was solved by the studies conducted by Kaiser et al. (1991); Reimann et al. (1992); Raffa et al. (1992) who identified two distinct mechanisms (opioid and non-opioid) in the antalgic action of the molecule.

Tramadol is a synthetic molecule structurally similar to morphine and codeine. The formulation is racemic, and therefore, the drug is composed of two enantiomers present in equal parts—one clockwise rotated (+)-tramadol (1R,2R-2-[(dimethylaminomethyl)methyl]-1-3-(methoxyphenyl) cyclohexanol hydrochloride); the other counterclockwise rotated (−)-tramadol (1L,2L-2-[(dimethyaminomethyl)methyl]-1-3-(methoxyphenyl) cyclohexanol hydrochloride).

(+)-Tramadol has a weak affinity for mu receptors (6,000 times less than morphine and 10 times less than codeine). Even weaker is its affinity for delta and kappa receptors; in addition, it inhibits serotonin reuptake. (−)-Tramadol inhibits the reuptake of noradrenaline. The analgesia induced by tramadol depends on the synergistic action of the two enantiomers. There is no particular advantage to be gained from using one or the other of the enantiomers; for example, the (+)-enantiomer, compared to the racemic mixture, is associated with a greater incidence of nausea.

Tramadol is only 30 % antagonized by naloxone. Evidently, the non-antagonizable analgesic effect is independent of the opioid-related antalgic system. On the other hand, according to Desmeules et al. yohimbine, a classic synaptic antagonist of noradrenaline, only partially blocks (67 %) the antalgic activity of the racemic formulation; ondansetron, too, according to Arcioni et al. has a similar effect.

The α_2-adrenoreceptors are present not only in the periventricular diencephalon and in the periaqueductal grey matter, but also in the spinal cord. Noradrenaline exerts an inhibitory action on the cells of the posterior horn, inhibiting their activation by the arrival of nociceptive stimuli with an effect similar to that of clonidine, which like noradrenaline is antagonized by yohimbine. In actual fact, it has never been proved that tramadol binds to the α_2-receptors. In the opinion of Desmeules et al. it is very likely that tramadol acts via the indirect activation of postsynaptic α_2-receptors. Norepinephrine and serotonin are potent inhibitors of the pain stimulus which the spinal descending pathway avails itself of in order to modulate the pain at the level of the posterior horn of the spinal cord.

Tramadol, therefore, is believed to act: with its (+)-enantiomer, as an opioid on the mu receptors (effect antagonized by naloxone), inhibiting the reuptake of serotonin; with its (−)-enantiomer, on the reuptake of noradrenaline, like clonidine, increasing the presence of noradrenaline in the synaptic space, with an effect antagonized by yohimbine and ondansetron.

14.4.1 Perineural Application

Among the first to use tramadol at the perineural level were Kapral and co-workers in 1999. They added one ampoule of tramadol (100 mg) to 1 % mepivacaine in order to perform a brachial plexus block via the axillary route with significant differences compared to a second group who were treated with intravenous administration of the drug, and a third group in whom the 2 ml of tramadol were replaced by 2 ml of saline.

In 2001, Antonucci published a paper in *Minerva Anestesiol* comparing the addition of tramadol to the local anesthetic in the axillary block to the addition of clonidine and sufentanil.

In 2004, Robaux et al. conducted a dose-ranging study with progressive doses of tramadol added to a standard dose of 1.5 % mepivacaine. The most effective dose was 200 mg at which level the incidence of side effects is still acceptable.

In a recent study, by Alemanno et al. in 120 patients scheduled to undergo arthroscopic surgery for rotatory cuff injuries performed by the same surgical team, the middle interscalene block with 0.5 % levobupivacaine (0.4 ml/kg) was applied. The patients were subdivided into three groups; in the first group, a dose of 1.5 mg/kg of tramadol (maximum limit 100 mg) was added to the anesthetic mixture and an equivalent volume of saline was injected intramuscularly into the ipsilateral deltoid muscle. In the second group, the tramadol dose was injected intramuscularly into the ipsilateral deltoid muscle and an equivalent volume of saline was added to the anesthetic mixture. In the third group, saline solution was added both to the anesthetic mixture and was injected in an equal volume intramuscularly.

The duration of the analgesia was calculated as the time elapsing between the injection of the anesthetic mixture and the patient's first request for analgesia in the postoperative period.

The first request for analgesia was made on average after 14.5 h for the patients in the first group (perineural tramadol), after 10.1 h in the second group (intramuscular tramadol) and after 7.6 h in the control group.

In the two studies (both with buprenorphine and with tramadol), the side effects were modest, basically amounting to a few additional cases of nausea and vomiting (easily resolved with 25 mg of levosulpiride i.v.) compared to the group not treated with the respective analgesics.

We can therefore confirm that buprenorphine and tramadol administered into the perineural space of the brachial plexus, in addition to the local anesthetic, produce longer-lasting postoperative analgesia compared to that obtained with local anesthetic alone without any significant increase in side effects.

Full of enthusiasm at these results, we attempted to extend the experience to other types of block. Thus, tramadol and buprenorphine were added in the same proportions to the 'single-shot' femoral nerve block, but with such disappointing results that we were obliged to desist from continuing with a study that had failed to yield any positive results.

On the other hand, Candido et al. in a recent article published in *Anesthesiology* in 2010, report that buprenorphine, when used as an adjuvant in sciatic nerve blocks, failed to achieve the same longer-lasting analgesia as in the brachial plexus blocks.

In our experience, we have noticed no difference between patients receiving the two drugs at the perineural level compared to those to whom they were administered intramuscularly into the ipsilateral buttock.

The fact is that the topographical situation of the brachial plexus is unique in the human body. The brachial plexus is, in fact, surrounded by an extroflection of the deep cervical fascia, which fuses with the vertebral prolongation of the superficial cervical fascia. The two fascias together constitute the sheath that envelops the entire neurovascular bundle (this is the anatomical situation that Winnie had the merit of evidentiating). In the first place, this space is made up of loose cellular tissue, and therefore with a poor absorption capacity, like the caliber vessels themselves, both arterial and venous, that pass through it. The adjuvant molecules thus remain in contact with the nerve elements for a lengthy period of time and therefore have time to penetrate into the axon. This is quite different from injections in other more vascularized districts where the vascular absorption is faster and comparable to the intramuscular absorption, and consequently where the adjuvant molecules do not have time to overcome, in efficacious amounts, the difficult barrier posed by the axonal sheath.

Bibliography

Alemanno F, Danelli G, Fanelli A, Ghisi D, Bizzarri F, Fanelli G (2012) Tramadol and 0.5 levobupivacaine for brachial interscalene block: effects on postoperative analgesia in patients undergoing shoulder arthroplasty. Minerva Anestesiol 78(3):291–296

Antonucci S (2001) Adiuvanti nel blocco del plesso brachiale per via ascellare: confronto tra clonidina, sufentanil e tramadolo. Minerva Anestesiol 67:23–27

Arcioni R et al (2002) Ondansetron inhibits the analgesic effects of tramadol: a possible 5-HT3 spinal receptor involvement in acute pain in humans. Anesth Analg 94:1553–1557

Arend I, von Arnim B, Nijssen J, Scheele J, Flohé L (1978) Tramadol und Pentazocin im Klinischen-Doppelblind-Crossover Vergleich. Arzneim Forsch 28:199–208

Baba H, Kohno T, Okamoto M, Goldstein PA, Shimoji K, Yoshimura M (1998) Muscarinic facilitation of GABA release in substantia gelatinosa of the rat spinal dorsal horn. J Physiol 508:83–93

Behr A, Freo U, Ori C, Westermann B, Alemanno F (2012) Buprenorphine added to levobupivacaine enhances postoperative analgesia of middle interscalene brachial plexus block. J Anesth, 26(5):746–751

Candido KD, Franco CD, Kahn MA, Winnie AP, Raja DS (2001) Buprenorphine added to the local anesthetic for brachial plexus block to provide postoperative analgesia in outpatients. Reg Anesth Pain Med 26:352–356

Candido KD, Hennes J, Gonzalez S, Mikat-Stevens M, Pinzur M, Vasic V, Knezevic NN (2010) Buprenorphine enhances and prolongs the postoperative analgesic effect of bupivacaine in patients receiving infragluteal sciatic nerve block. Anesthesiology 113:1419–1426

Candido KD, Winnie AP, Ghaleb AH, Fattouh MW, Franco CD (2002) Buprenorphine added to the local anesthetic for axillary brachial plexus block prolongs postoperative analgesia. Reg Anesth Pain Med 27:162–167

Culebras X, Van Gessel E, Hoffmeyer P, Gamulin Z (2001) Clonidine combined with a long acting local anesthetic does not prolong postoperative analgesia after brachial plexus block but does induce hemodynamic changes. Anesth Analg 92:199–204

Dayer P, Desmeules J, Collart L (1997) Pharmacologie du tramadol. Drugs 53(Suppl. 2):18–24

Desmeules JA, Piguet V, Collart L, Dayer P (1996) Contribution of monoaminergic modulation to the analgesic effect of Tramadol. Br J Clin Pharmacol 41:7–12

Driessen B, Reimann W (1992) Interaction of the central analgesic tramadol, with the uptake and release of 5-hydroxytryptamine in the rat brain in vitro. Br J Pharmacol 105:147–151

Fields HL, Emson PC, Leigh BK, Gilbert RF, Iversen LL (1980) Multiple opiate receptor sites on primary afferent fibers. Nature 284:351–353

Fleetwood-Walker SM, Mitchell R, Hope PJ, Molony V, Iggo A (1985) An alpha 2 receptor mediates the selective inhibition by noradrenaline of nociceptive responses of identified dorsal horn neurones. Brain Res 334:243–254

Flohe L, Arend I et al (1978) Klinische Prüfung der Abhängigkeitsentwicklung nach Langzeitapplikation von Tramadol. Arzneim Forschung 28:213–217

Ian Carrol et al (2007) The role of adrenergic receptors and pain: the good, the bad, and the unknown. Semin Anesth Perioper Med Pain, 26:17–21

Kaiser V, Besson JM, Guilbaud G (1991) Effects of analgesic agent Tramadol in normal and arthritic rats: comparison with effects of different opioids, including tolerance and cross-tolerance to morphine. Eur J Pharmacol 195:37–45

Kapral S, Gollmann G, Waltl B et al (1999) Tramadol added to mepivacaine prolongs the duration of an axillary brachial plexus blockade. Anesth Analg 88:853–856

Kuraishi Y, Hirota N, Sato Y, Kaneko S, Satoh M, Takagi H (1985) Noradrenergic inhibition of the release of substance P from the primary afferents in the rabbit spinal dorsal horn. Brain Res 359:177–182

Lutfy K, Cowan A (2004) Buprenorphine: a unique drug with complex pharmacology. Curr Neuropharmacol 2(4):395–402

McCartney CJL (2007) Analgesic adjuvants in the peripheral nervous system. In: Hadzic A (ed) Textbook of regional anesthesia. Mc Graw Hill, New York, p 149

Pertovaara A (2006) Noradrenergic pain modulation. Progr Neurobiol 80:53–83

Pleuvry B (2005) Opioid mechanisms and opioid drugs. Anaesth Intens Care Med 6:1

Putzu M, Casati A (2007) Local anesthetic solutions for continuous nerve blocks. In: Hadzic A (ed) Textbook of regional anesthesia. Mc Graw Hill, New York, p 163

Raffa RB, Friderichs E, Reimann W et al (1993) Complementary and synergistic antinociceptive interaction between the enantiomers of tramadol. J Pharmacol Exp Ther 267(1):331–340

Reimann W et al (1990) Does a non-opioid component contribute to the efficacy of the central analgesic tramadol? 10th european winter conference on brain research, March 3–10

Robaux S, Blunt C, Viel E, Cuvillon P et al (2004) Tramadol added to 1.5 % mepivacaine for axillary brachial plexus block improves postoperative analgesia dose-dependently. Anesth Analg 98:1172–1177

Sawinor J (2003) Topical and peripherally acting analgesics. Pharmacol Rev, 55:1–20. http://en.wikipedia.org/wiki/clonidine

Scott LJ, Perry CM (2000) Tramadol: a review of its use in perioperative pain. Drugs, 60(1):139–176

Singelyn FJ, Dangoisse M, Bartholomée S, Gouverneur JM (1992) Adding clonidine to mepivacaine prolongs the duration of anesthesia and analgesia after axillary brachial plexus block. Reg Anesth 17:148–150

Stein C (1993) Peripheral mechanism of opioid analgesia. Anesth Analg 76:182–191

Stein C (1995) The control of pain in peripheral tissues by opioids. New Engl J Med 332(25):1685–1690

Stoffregen J (1980) Kombinationnarkose mit Tramadol-Infusion. Anaesthesiol Intensivmed 29:673–674

Viel EJ, Eledjam JJ, de la Coussaye J, D'Athis F (1989) Brachial plexus block with opioids for postoperative pain relief: comparison between buprenorphine and morphine. Reg Anesth 14:274–278

Young WS 3rd, Wamsley JK, Zarbin MA, Kuhar MJ (1980) Opioid receptors undergo axonal flow. Science 210:76–78

Postoperative Analgesia

15

F. Coluzzi

15.1 Physiopathology of Postoperative Pain

Pain is defined by the International Association for the Study of Pain (IASP) as 'an unpleasant sensory and emotional experience primarily associated with actual or potential tissue damage or described in terms of such damage'.

Postoperative pain is a form of acute pain, closely related to the surgical procedure and may set in after the operation or may occur on top of an already existing chronic pain related to the disease responsible for the surgical indication.

Postoperative pain is mainly of the nociceptive type, even though, in certain particular conditions, it may present a chronic course and take the form of neuropathic pain.

Nociceptive pain or nociception is a complex mechanism whereby a nociceptive stimulus is capable of generating a pain sensation in the person on the receiving end. Four neuronal processes defining nociception can be distinguished: transduction, transmission, perception and modulation.

The first step in the nociception process consists in the transduction of a nociceptive stimulus to an electrical stimulus, which can be transmitted to higher central nervous system structures. The primary afferents specialized in this function, called nociceptors or pain receptors, are neurons whose cell bodies reside in the ganglia of the dorsal sensory roots (dorsal root ganglia, DRG) and whose axons divide early into T-shaped branch points (T-junctions) thence giving rise to a peripheral (centrifugal) extension that runs through the peripheral nerve and a central (centripetal) extension that runs through the posterior root of the spinal cord. The nociceptive stimuli capable of causing tissue damage may be of a thermal, chemical or mechanical type. There is a certain degree of specificity between the type of nociceptive stimulus and the type of sensory fibre activated.

The primary sensory afferents are classified on the basis of their anatomical and electrophysiological characteristics. The A-beta fibres (Aβ) are fast-conducting large-calibre myelinated fibres that are not involved in the nociceptive process. Pain transmission occurs, in fact, via amyelinic fibres (C-fibres) or poorly myelinated fibres (A-delta fibres, Aδ). Type-I A-delta fibres respond to mechanical and chemical stimuli but also to high temperatures (>50 °C). Type-II A-delta fibres respond to thermal and mechanical stimuli. C-fibres are defined as polymodal because they comprise a heterogeneous population of neurons that respond to hot, cold and mechanical stimuli. Some of these fibres are so-called silent fibres in that they are activated only in the presence of tissue damage or inflammation. The C-fibres that innervate the viscera are known to respond to

F. Coluzzi (✉)
Department of Medico-Surgical Sciences and Biotechnologies, Faculty of Pharmacy and Medicine, Sapienza University, Rome, Italy
e-mail: flaminia.coluzzi@uniroma1.it

over distension of the hollow organs and are often responsible for the so-called referred pain.

The A-delta fibres, thanks to their myelin sheath, are capable of conducting the nociceptive stimulus faster than the C-fibres and are, therefore, responsible for the so-called first pain, which is acute and of brief duration. The C-fibres, by contrast, being slower, transmit the so-called second pain, which is diffuse, dull and longer lasting.

An explanation as to what the mechanism is whereby a nociceptive stimulus is 'transducer' to a biological signal proved possible after the discovery of the family of ion channels defined as transient receptor potentials (TRPs) which permit the flow of sodium and calcium ions, thus giving rise to depolarization and generating an action potential. The TRPV1 channel (initially identified as the vanilloid type 1 receptor—VR1) is characterized by being activated by capsaicin and produces a burning sensation as a result of contact with temperatures >43 °C. This receptor is present on most of the nociceptive fibres activated by high temperatures. Other TRPV receptors have subsequently been identified and are responsible for the response to different temperatures: TRPV2 is activated by temperatures >52 °C; TRPV3 and TRPV4, on the other hand, are responsible for heat sensations at temperatures ranging from 25 °C to 35 °C. Similarly, there are receptors that respond to low temperatures: the TRPM8 receptor (where M stands for menthol) is activated by temperatures <25 °C, whereas TRPA1 is activated by temperatures <17 °C and also by a number of inflammation mediators. Other receptors, identified as mechanoreceptors, respond to membrane stretching and osmotic swelling, namely MDEG (mammalian degenerin) receptors and the TREK-1 (TWIC-related) potassium channel. In conditions of tissue damage and inflammation, the purinergic P2X receptors respond to changes in adenosine triphosphate (ATP) (Fig. 15.1).

Sodium and calcium channels thus play a fundamental role in the transmission of pain.

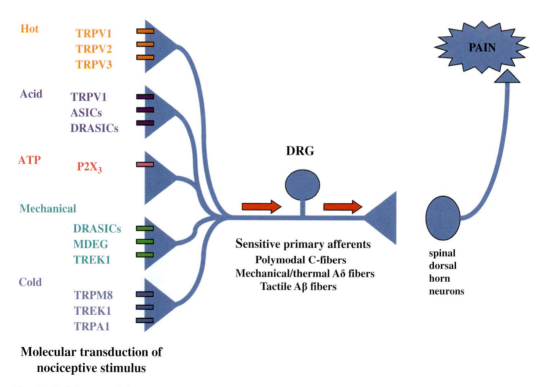

Fig. 15.1 Pain transmission

The voltage-gated sodium channels (VGSCs) most expressed on nociceptors are of three types: NaV 1.7 (sensitive to tetrodotoxin—TTX), NaV 1.8 and NaV 1.9 (resistant to TTX). Subjects suffering from erythromelalgia (paroxysmal burning pain and vasodilation of the extremities) present a mutation of the gene coding for the ion channel NaV 1.7 in such a way as to increase its activity. Conversely, the mutations that render this channel inactive are responsible for the congenital insensitivity to pain (CIP). Experimental studies in animal models have demonstrated that nerve lesions result in a redistribution of the NaV 1.8 sodium channels which are reduced on the damaged neurons and tend to increase in concentration in the healthy neurons surrounding the lesions. The concentration of NaV 1.9 channels is also significantly reduced in animal models of neuropathic pain.

The voltage-gated calcium channels (VGCCs) are the other critical element that modulates the neuronal excitability and the transmission of the nociceptive stimulus. These channels are basically of two types. N-type VGCCs are present mainly on the terminal portion of the sensory neurons and play a key role in the release of neurotransmitters such as substance P, glutamate and calcitonin gene-related peptide (CGRP) by the primary afferents. T-type VGCCs are present both on the primary afferents and on the spinal cord postsynaptic neurons and are activated by low voltages. The activation of these channels acts in synergy with neurokinin 1 (NK1) at the level of the spinal dorsal horn via activation of the complex N-methyl-D-aspartate (NMDA) calcium/receptor channel responsible for the central sensitization process.

Once the electrical stimulus has been generated, for it to be perceived, it has to be transmitted via an intact conduction system from the periphery to the central nervous system. The primary afferents described above enter the central nervous system via the dorsal horns of the spinal cord, which are functionally subdivided into laminae that receive inputs from various types of fibres. The A-delta fibres and part of the C-fibres terminate in the external part of lamina I and lamina II, thus forming the substantia gelatinosa. Other C-fibres terminate in the internal part of lamina II, whereas the deeper laminae from III to V mainly receive fibres that do not conduct nociceptive stimuli, such as the A-beta fibres. Lamina V also receives part of the A-delta fibres. Supraspinal projections depart from laminae I and V leading to the thalamus, amygdala and basal nuclei which, in turn, transmit information to the cerebral cortex.

The transmission then occurs in three steps: (1) from the periphery to the spinal cord; (2) from the spinal cord to the thalamus; and (3) from the thalamus to the cerebral cortex. The first-order sensory neuron transmits the electrical impulse from the periphery to the spinal cord, entering via the posterior horn. It then synapses with the second-order neuron, and the impulse travels up via the spinal pathways towards the thalamus, where, together with a third order neuron, the information is transmitted to the sensory cortex where it generates the pain sensation.

The transmission of the pain impulse at the spinal level occurs via two ascending pathways to the brain, namely the neospinothalamic and paleospinothalamic tracts.

The second-order neurons of the neospinothalamic bundle are endowed with long axons that rapidly crossover to the opposite side of the spinal cord and terminate at the thalamic level in the ventrobasal complex and partly in areas of the reticular formation. The paleospinothalamic tract, on the other hand, as the name suggests, is phylogenetically a much more ancient structure, that mainly transmits information coming from the C-fibres and part of the information coming from the A-delta fibres. At the level of the brain, we distinguish between the areas where this pain pathway terminates: the reticular nuclei, the tectal area and the periaqueductal grey area.

The information is transmitted from the thalamic nuclei to the sensitivity areas (parietal lobes), cognitive areas (temporal lobes) and emotivity areas (frontal lobes) of the brain. The fourth and last fundamental process in nociception is modulation of the nociceptive impulses which enables their intensity to be physiologically controlled. In conditions of stress or immediate danger, the human body is known to resist much more easily to pain stimuli. There exists, in fact, a so-called analgesic system consisting in three main structures: the periaqueductal grey area (PAG), the nucleus raphe magnus and the complex of inhibitory neurons situated at the level of the spinal dorsal horns. Electrical stimulation or microinjections of morphine at the level of the PAG give rise to a substantial antinociceptive reaction. The PAG sends inputs to the rostral ventromedial medulla (RVM), from which depart, in turn, descending projections that cross the dorsolateral funiculus and go on to reach the spinal cord. At the level of the medulla, these neurons synapse with primary afferents or second-order neurons, modulating their nociceptive inputs. The main neurotransmitters involved in this 'descending inhibitory system' are serotonin and noradrenaline. The other basic system involved in the nociception modulation mechanism is the system of endorphins produced by pro-opiomelanocortin which interacts with the opioidergic receptors present in the central and peripheral nervous systems.

15.2 Postoperative Pain Management

The treatment of postoperative pain is one of the indispensable aspects of any correct anesthesiological management and, to all intents and purposes, must be regarded as a patient's 'right'. It has been abundantly demonstrated that inadequate postoperative pain relief significantly increases the perioperative morbidity, the duration of the hospital stay and the costs, particularly in the case of major surgery or in patients at high anesthesiological risk (ASA > 3). Pain generates a series of alterations of the body's homoeostasis: it increases metabolic demands, tachycardia, blood pressure, respiratory effects (increased incidence of postoperative lung infections); it also causes increased fluid retention, reduced limb mobility (with a consequent increased risk of deep vein thrombosis), reduced gastrointestinal motility and immunological effects. Therefore, adequate postoperative analgesia is a priority in the postoperative management of surgical patients.

Pain, then, figures as the fifth vital parameter in the postoperative period, alongside heart rate, blood pressure, respiratory rate and diuresis.

For the purposes of accurately assessing postoperative pain, it is advisable to use an instrument that is simple, repeatable and common to all those involved in the pain evaluation process (anesthetists, surgeons, nurses and patients). The visual analogue scale (VAS) is the most commonly used rating scale in the strictly scientific setting, but in day-to-day clinical practice, it may be more practical to use an 11-score numerical rating scale (NRS), where 0 denotes no pain and ten stands for the maximum pain imaginable. In some subjects, such as the elderly, it may be necessary to adopt a verbal scale, whereas for children a visual scale is advisable, with graphic representation of facial expressions reflecting the different intensities of the pain experience. It is advisable to assess both resting pain and pain in motion.

The variety of operations performed on the upper limbs means that the approach to postoperative pain is correspondingly extremely varied. The pain intensity ranges from mild to moderate pain, as in the case of minor operations on the hand (trigger finger, carpal tunnel syndrome), to severe pain, such as that resulting from major shoulder surgery. The analgesic techniques to be used range therefore from systemic analgesia (intravenous or oral) to regional anesthesia techniques (continuous peripheral blocks). The possibilities of interacting with the nociceptive system are multiple and range from those involving the periphery to those involving the central nervous system (Fig. 15.2).

15.3 Systemic Analgesia

There are two fundamental types of approach to the receptors directly involved in the nociceptive process, namely direct administration of the

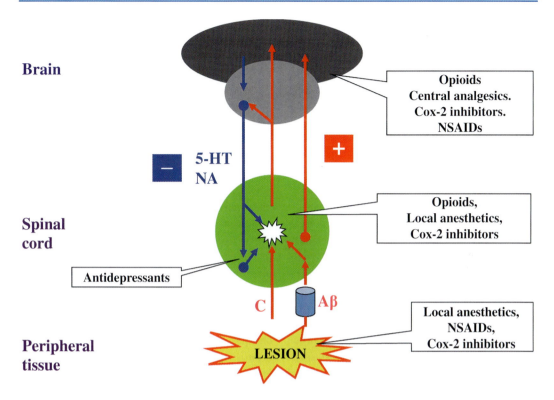

Fig. 15.2 Analgesic drugs and sites of action

drug in the immediate vicinity of the receptors (central or perineural approaches) and indirect administration systemically whereby the drugs reach their action site via the bloodstream. In systemic analgesia, the intravenous route is the one most commonly used in the postoperative setting, in that it bypasses the gastrointestinal absorption process necessarily involved in oral administration. Nevertheless, in particular circumstances, alternative administration routes may also be opted for. For example, in day surgery, the oral route is a first choice solution for pain treatment at home. In minor paediatric surgery, the rectal route (paracetamol) is a widely used therapeutic approach.

15.3.1 Non-opioid Analgesics

The management of mild-to-moderate postoperative pain is based fundamentally on the use of non-opioid analgesics, such as non-steroidal anti-inflammatory drugs (NSAIDs), selective cyclooxygenase-2 inhibitors (coxibs) and paracetamol. These drugs may also be used in the management of moderate-to-severe pain in combination with opioids in a multimodal analgesia regimen. The use of two or more analgesic drugs which act at different points along the pain transmission and modulation pathway makes it possible to reduce the dosage of the individual drugs and consequently to limit the incidence of their side effects. The interaction between the two drugs chosen or between two or more antalgic techniques may be of the additive or synergistic type. The multimodal approach improves the postoperative outcome and speeds up the discharge both of hospital inpatients (reducing the number of days' stay in hospital) and of patients operated on in the day-surgery setting. This phenomenon is part and parcel of the broader concept of fast track surgery, which assigns a new role to the anesthetist, no longer confined to the operating room, but as the main figure in perioperative medical care. As introduced by Kepler in the 1990s, a perioperative multimodal programme that guarantees reduced morbidity and early discharge capability comprises: correct preoperative patient information, a reduced response to stress, adequate pain relief, early enteral nutrition and early physiotherapy and mobilization.

15.3.2 NSAIDs and Coxibs

NSAIDs exert an anti-inflammatory and analgesic action by means of the non-selective inhibition of the central and peripheral cyclooxygenases, thus reducing the level of prostaglandins. This lack of selectivity underlies the known side effects associated with these drugs at the gastrointestinal, renal and platelet level. The prostaglandins perform a series of important physiological functions for the homoeostasis of the body: protection of the gastric mucosa and of renal tubule function, intrarenal vasodilation, bronchodilation, production of prostacyclines that induce vasodilation, and of thromboxanes that induce platelet aggregation and vasospasm. These physiological functions are controlled mainly by the so-called constitutive isoenzyme COX-1, whereas the COX-2 isoenzyme is thought to be involved mainly in inflammatory and pain processes as a result of tissue damage and which, at the level of the spinal cord, may contribute to the process of central sensitization. For these reasons, in the past decade, selective COX-2 inhibitors (coxibs) have come onto the market which guarantee good analgesic efficacy with none of the unwanted gastrointestinal side effects associated with the NSAIDs. In the postoperative period, coxibs have been used successfully in both oral and intravenous formulations. Coxibs significantly reduce postoperative pain and opioid intake and increase the measure of patient satisfaction. Despite these drugs having an opioid-sparing effect, no reduction in the opioid-related incidence of side effects has been observed. The preoperative administration of celecoxib or parecoxib (pre-emptive analgesia) offers no advantage in terms of postoperative pain and perioperative opioid intake when compared to administration at the end of surgery. At the renal level, the side effects of coxibs are similar to those of NSAIDs, since the COX-2s also participate in maintaining an adequate renal blood flow. At the platelet level, on the other hand, the coxibs do not interfere with platelet agreeability and therefore do not increase postoperative bleeding. When used chronically, some coxibs (rofecoxib) have caused cardiovascular alterations and specifically an increased incidence of myocardial infarction and for this reason have been withdrawn from the market. However, the short-term use of parecoxib and valdecoxib postoperatively after non-cardiac surgery does not increase the risk of cardiovascular side effects. At the respiratory level, it has been demonstrated that coxibs, unlike NSAIDs, do not induce bronchospasm in patients sensitive to aspirin. In arthroscopic shoulder surgery, the addition of etoricoxib 120 mg *per os* to subacromial analgesia with bupivacaine significantly reduces the level of postoperative pain for up to 7 days after the operation and reduces the patient's hospital stay.

15.3.3 Paracetamol

Paracetamol is a centrally acting drug endowed with analgesic and antipyretic activity. Unlike the NSAIDs, it does not interfere with peripheral cyclooxygenase activity and therefore does not have either the classic side effects of the NSAIDS related to COX-1 inhibition nor any of the pronounced anti-inflammatory activity related to COX-2 inhibition. Although it has been available on the market for more than a century, its actual mechanism of action is still a subject of study. Recent studies have led researchers to postulate a possible potentiation of the descending inhibitory serotoninergic system, a possible interaction with the endocannabinoid system (paracetamol being metabolized to the compound AM404, which is an inhibitor of the cellular reuptake of anandamide and therefore an indirect activator of cannabinoid CBI receptors) and the possible inhibition of substance P-mediated hyperalgesia and therefore an interaction with the nitric oxide synthase system.

The recent introduction of a ready-to-use intravenous formulation has given this molecule a new lease of life for the management of postoperative pain. The ideal dosage is 1 g every 6 h, to be administered in an approximately 15 min infusion. At this dosage, the intravenous formulation crosses the blood–brain barrier rapidly and affords a good level of rapid, predictable analgesia. A number of authors have proposed an initial priming dose of 2 g, which has proved more efficacious than the 1 g dose, but is not currently recommended in everyday clinical practice. Paracetamol has an approximately 20 % opioid-sparing effect on morphine and therefore has not been found to significantly reduce the incidence of opioid-related side effects but may significantly increase patient satisfaction.

The risk of hepatotoxicity is negligible at the doses recommended. Retrospective studies have shown that the mean dose taken by patients presenting acute paracetamol-induced hepatotoxicity is approximately 24 g, that is, far higher than the 4 g per day recommended for intravenous administration. Even in patients suffering from alcoholic liver disease, the administration of 4 g of paracetamol a day for three consecutive days does not give rise to any significant increase in transaminases. The hepatotoxic effects are therefore to be regarded as being exclusively related to accidental overdoses or to voluntary overdoses for the purposes of committing suicide.

15.3.4 Opioids

Opioids are the mainstay of postoperative systemic analgesia for surgery causing moderate-to-severe pain. They exert their analgesic efficacy by interacting with the mu opioidergic receptors present at the level of the central and peripheral nervous systems, and belonging to the G-protein-coupled receptor family.

There is no evidence of any analgesic superiority of one opioid over another, if used at the appropriate dosage. The conversion tables of equianalgesic doses used in order to identify the right dose of a drug compared with another of the same category are partly flawed by the degree of inter-individual pharmacokinetic and pharmacodynamic variability. These tables are often based on studies conducted on single administrations of a drug and fail to take proper account of repeated exposure in the course of time to the same molecule.

Nevertheless, for reasons of pharmacokinetics, metabolism and elimination, a number of opioids are to be preferred to others in certain special types of patients. For example, since morphine is a strongly hydrophilic drug, it is particularly indicated in obese subjects. Fentanyl, in turn, thanks to its prevalently hepatic metabolism, would appear to be particularly indicated in subjects with renal insufficiency. In any event, in these specific categories, such as the elderly, the obese, patients suffering from obstructive sleep apnoea (OSA), and patients with renal or hepatic insufficiency, the doses must be carefully calibrated for each subject on an individual basis.

In particular, in the immediate postoperative period, it is always advisable to perform the titration of the opioid until an adequate level of analgesia is obtained, usually estimated as a VAS value of less than 4.

The use of opioids is burdened, to various extents, with unwanted side effects unavoidably related to the pharmacological action of these substances. The most feared adverse event is unquestionably respiratory depression, but, in the postoperative setting, the most frequent unwanted side effects are nausea and vomiting, constipation, itching, sedation and possibly hemodynamic effects (bradycardia, hypotension, arrhythmias).

For surgeries that give rise to mild-to-moderate pain, the so-called weak opioids can be used, such as tramadol or codeine. These opioids are also available in combination with paracetamol, in fixed-dose oral formulations.

15.3.5 Tramadol

Tramadol is defined as an atypical opioid on account of its combined effect on opioidergic receptors and on monoaminergic transmission. Tramadol has an effect on mu receptors, which is 6,000-fold less than that of morphine and an inhibitory effect on serotonin and noradrenaline reuptake that potentiates the descending inhibitory pathway.

Tramadol is available as a racemic mixture: The (+) enantiomer mainly has an effect on serotonin, while the (−) enantiomer mainly affects noradrenaline.

Tramadol is subject to a cytochrome-dependent hepatic metabolism, related to CYP2D6, that produces tramadol's main analgesic metabolite MI, which is 200 times more potent than the molecule from which it derives. This is responsible for the profound inter-individual variability of the response to the drug. Subjects who are so-called poor metabolizers have significantly lower blood concentrations of MI compared to the so-called extensive metabolizers, whether homo- or heterozygous, who therefore fail to obtain adequate pain relief. Moreover, the perioperative use of 5-HT3 receptor inhibitors, such as ondansetron, for antiemetic treatment may reduce its efficacy.

Unlike the other opioids, tramadol presents the advantage of carrying only a minimal risk of respiratory depression and having less of an impact on gastrointestinal motility. However, its use is burdened by a certain incidence of postoperative nausea and vomiting. When compared to the NSAIDs, particularly in patients potentially at risk, it presents the advantage of having no effects on the gastric mucosa or on platelet function.

15.3.6 Codeine

Codeine, too, is subject to metabolism on the part of cytochrome CYP2D6. At the hepatic level, approximately 10 % of the drug is demethylated to morphine. In extensive metabolizers, the morphine blood concentration, as a result of the oral administration of codeine, is approximately 50 % greater than that of normal subjects. Therefore, in addition to an altered renal clearance, also a genetic modification of the metabolism may be responsible for the side effects observed after the administration of codeine. There are more than 100 allelic variants of the cytochrome CYP2D6 gene. In the Caucasian population, there are at least 10 % of poor metabolizers and 5 % of extensive metabolizers. The latter, in particular, are at high risk of side effects due to elevated blood concentrations of morphine.

In cases of major surgery of the upper extremity (fractures, shoulder prostheses) causing severe pain, in which it is decided to implement systemic analgesic therapy, the most commonly used pure opioid agonists are morphine, fentanyl and sufentanil.

15.3.7 Morphine

Morphine still remains today the most widely used drug in the postoperative period. Its metabolism is mainly via the liver which, by glucuronidation, produces two main metabolites—M3G and M6G. The M6G metabolite is also a mu opioidergic receptor agonist that crosses the blood–brain barrier more slowly than morphine, but possesses an analgesic potency superior to that of the drug from which it derives. The M3G metabolite, on the other hand, has no analgesic effect but is responsible for the neuroexcitatory effects of morphine, such as hyperalgesia, allodynia and myoclonus. The accumulation of morphine metabolites in patients with renal insufficiency is responsible for side effects such as sedation and respiratory depression.

The genetic polymorphism of the mu opioidergic receptor may be responsible for the variability of the individual responses to morphine. In particular, the nucleotide A118G that codes for the mu receptor has been identified. Whereas homozygous subjects (AA) respond well to morphine, heterozygous subjects (AG) or homozygous subjects for the G variant of the allele (GG)—particularly frequent in the Asian and Caucasian populations—show an increased intake of opioids in patient-controlled analgesia (PCA). Other polymorphisms concern genes that code for enzymes participating in the metabolism of morphine (UGT2B7) or for the glycoprotein for transporting the drug across the blood–brain barrier (MDRI).

15.3.8 Fentanyl

Fentanyl is structurally related to pethidine. It is a strongly lipophilic drug, metabolized mainly at the hepatic level. Less than 10 % is excreted via the kidneys, which makes it particularly suitable for subjects with renal insufficiency. Furthermore, the absence of active metabolites constitutes another important advantage over morphine in postoperative pain management. The polymorphism of the mu A304G opioidergic receptor may affect the analgesic response to fentanyl.

15.3.9 Sufentanil

Sufentanil is a synthetic lipophilic opioid, which is from five to ten times more potent than fentanyl. It has a pharmacological profile similar to that of fentanyl, with a mainly hepatic metabolism.

Opioid Dose Determinants

There is a great deal of inter-individual variability with regard to the amount of opioid drug necessary for adequate postoperative analgesia. A number of factors, however, have been identified as indicators of a greater or lesser opioid requirement. It is well known that age, more than body weight, contributes to a patient's postoperative analgesic needs. With advancing age, the mean dosages are reduced to a half or a quarter of those for younger subjects, the reasons for this reduced opioid requirement are changes in the pharmacokinetic parameters (metabolism) and in the percentage penetration at the cerebral level. In the immediate postoperative period, women present significantly higher pain levels than men, surgical procedures being equal, as well as a significantly greater opioid intake. Obviously, as mentioned previously, genetic factors may significantly modify the opioid requirement postoperatively.

In the light of these observations, administration modes must be used that can be modulated on the basis of the individual patient's specific requests. Titration of the opioid at the end of surgery is undoubtedly the first step for an appropriate use of opioids in the management of postoperative pain. The choice of a suitable intravenous infusion modality is equally important in order to guarantee adequate analgesia.

15.3.10 Modes of Administration: Patient-Controlled Analgesia

Patient-controlled analgesia (PCA) is a pain relief modality which permits the patient to self-administer small doses of analgesic drugs on the basis of his or her effective needs. Worldwide it constitutes one of the most commonly used postoperative pain treatment modalities. PCA fulfils two fundamental requirements for effective opioid therapy: It enables the dose to be individualized by titrating the right amount to ensure adequate pain relief and avoids the so-called 'peak and valley' phenomenon in which phases of excessive analgesic cover alternate with phases of acute pain.

For the use of intravenous PCA to be effective, it is necessary to administer a priming dose that stabilizes the intensity of the patient's pain at a predefined acceptable level, corresponding to a VAS rating of less than 4. This stabilization is obtained by titrating the intravenously administered opioid in the immediate postoperative period before discharging the patient from the surgical unit or the recovery room.

The pumps for PCA are programmed by setting a number of basic parameters: the bolus dose (how many millilitres of solution injected in the device are released per bolus delivered), the lock-out time (the time interval between two doses—the doses required are not delivered until the predetermined time interval has elapsed) and the maximum dosage that can be delivered per hour or over a 4 h period.

PCA pumps are also capable of delivering a continuous basal infusion, when programmed to do so. It has been demonstrated, however, that this mode of use (infusion + boluses) does not improve the quality of the postoperative analgesia and increases the risk of side effects. Continuous basal infusion is not recommended in that it bypasses the negative feedback mechanism on which the safety of the PCA system rests. The most feared unwanted side effect of opioids is respiratory depression. When implementing PCA, the use of appropriate doses of opioids at predetermined intervals means that, in the case of an overdose, sedation is manifested before respiratory depression. In this situation, the patient will be so sedated as not to require a subsequent dose. For this reason, it is important that the patient should be the only person managing the PCA pump, and that he or she should understand the mode of use in advance and be informed, together with the family, of the possible complications deriving from an inappropriate use of drugs such as opioids.

There is no evidence in the literature that any given type of programming is more effective than another. Morphine is certainly the opioid most commonly used, at a bolus dose of 1 mg with lock-out intervals of 6 min. The bolus dose should be sufficient to afford a certain degree of analgesia, but should not be so large as to risk generating side effects due to an acute overdose. Similarly, the lock-out interval should be long enough to allow the patient to avail himself to the full of the beneficial effects of the single dose delivered before receiving the next, but not so long as to risk gaps in the analgesic cover. On the basis of the periodic review of the PCA pump and the relationship between the doses required and those effectively received by the patient, the programming of the system can be appropriately modulated in the course of postoperative antalgic therapy.

Intravenous analgesia with PCA affords a superior level of analgesia and greater patient satisfaction when compared to the conventional use of opioids via the parenteral route. There is, however, no evidence of a reduction in the intake of opioid analgesics, nor of any reduction in the incidence of side effects related to these drugs.

The electronic pumps for PCA are available in hospital versions, to be attached to stands, and in versions for use at home which are small and portable so as not to encumber the patient's movements.

One of the problems associated with the use of these devices is the possibility of a pump programming error. An error in the concentration of the drug or in the programming of the boluses may even have very serious consequences. Available on the market today are particularly sophisticated PCA pumps, designed to comply with the strict acknowledged standards for reducing errors. The CADD Solis Smart Pump uses the CADD Solis Medication Safety Software which allows up to 500 different protocols to be programmed directly by the computer and catalogued in specific libraries. The infusion history can be called up directly on the computer with graphics both in PDF and in Excel. The infusion profiles are extremely flexible with absolute and relative limits that can be programmed by the user. Despite its very considerable potential, the structure of the work menus is extremely simple so as to simplify the work of the users (Fig. 15.3).

Another system designed to avoid programming errors is transdermal PCA by means of the fentanyl iontophoretic transdermal system (IONSYS^{TM}). The application of a small amount of energy, by means of a battery applied to a patch containing fentanyl, permits the administration of predetermined 40 mcg boluses at 10 min intervals (maximum 6 doses per h) up to a total of 80 administrations. This system has proved effective in different types of surgery—abdominal, pelvic and orthopaedic. What is more, the degree of patient satisfaction has proved distinctly superior with this transdermal system when compared to the traditional intravenous PCA system with morphine. However, the system is not yet available for clinical use.

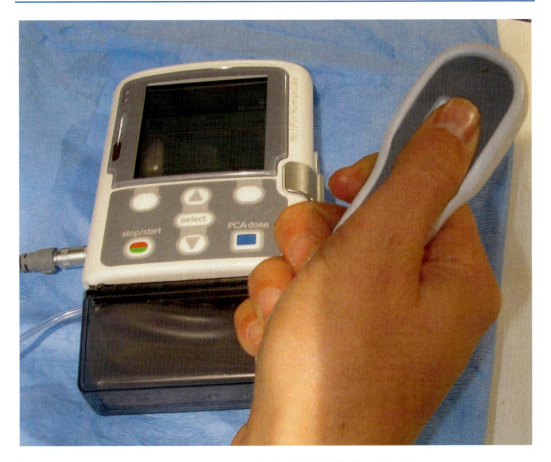

Fig. 15.3 Electronic pump for patient-controlled analgesia (CADD Solis Smart Pump)

15.3.11 Elastomeric Pumps

Elastomeric pumps consist of a PVC tubing connected up to a reservoir, the elasticity of which ensures that, once filled, it tends to empty progressively as a function of its own elastic springback characteristics (Fig. 15.4). These pumps are available with various capacities (60–300 ml) and different flow rates (0.5–12 ml/h). The reservoir is protected by an external shell, which prevents it from suffering damage with loss of the analgesic-containing solution. Obviously, this system fails to comply with any of the PCA principles, inasmuch as the infusion, once initiated, proceeds without any regard for the effective analgesic needs of the patient. The decision to use these devices is based mainly on considerations of an economic nature. Therefore, to avoid unwanted side effects, in the devices with a fixed infusion rate, there is a tendency to deliver under doses of the analgesic drug scheduled for the treatment period. To overcome this limitation, variable flow elastomeric pumps have been designed (multirate infusor systems) which, while maintaining the simplicity principle (they do not require electricity, have no alarm system, cost less than electronic pumps, and are single-use disposable, light and practical to use), they permit easier modulation of postoperative analgesic treatment. These pumps enable the flow rate of the analgesic solution to be varied from a minimum of 0.5 ml/h to a maximum of 7.5 ml/h. A further therapeutic possibility is offered by the availability of elastomeric pumps equipped with a control module for the self-administration of boluses within predetermined posological

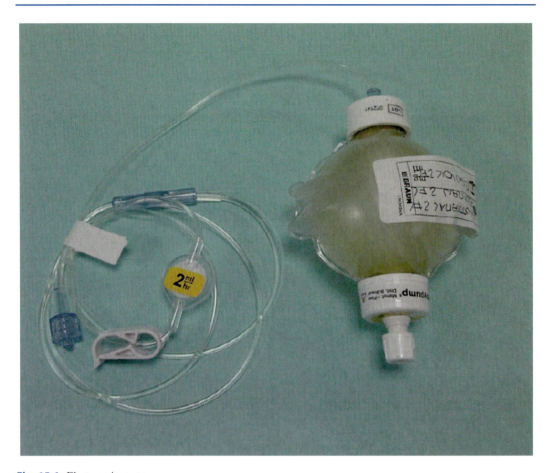

Fig. 15.4 Elastomeric pump

limits set at the patient's request. These devices permit the administration of simple, economic PCA, but with none of the complex technology associated with the latest electronic PCA pumps.

15.4 Continuous Peripheral Nerve Blocks

Continuous peripheral nerve blocks (CPNBs) prolong the duration of postoperative analgesia beyond the maximum period of analgesic cover guaranteed by peripheral blocks with single-shot injection of local anesthetic. Their use has increased over the years for the management of moderate-to-severe pain of the upper and lower limbs.

The first continuous peripheral nerve block for upper limb surgery was described in 1946 by Paul Ansbro, who infused 220 ml of 1 % procaine in repeated boluses for an operation lasting approximately 4 h, positioning a non-cutting needle laterally to the subclavian artery, with a supraclavicular approach.

Since then, continuous peripheral nerve blocks for analgesia of the upper limb have evolved and have been used both in traditional surgery and in the day-surgery setting.

It has been amply demonstrated that, when compared to systemic analgesia with opioids, CPNBs afford better analgesia and a lower

Table 15.1 Continuous peripheral nerve block versus systemic analgesia with opioids

Study	Surgery	Catheter positioning	Infusion	Opioid	Outcome
Borgeat 1997	Major shoulder surgery	Interscalene	0.15 % Bupivacaine	Nicomorphine i.v.	Reduced VAS at 12 and 18 h less vomiting and itching
Borgeat 1998	Major shoulder surgery	Interscalene	0.2 % Ropivacaine	Micomorphine i.v.	Greater patient satisfaction reduced VAS less nausea and itching
Lehtipalo 1999	Acromioplasty	Interscalene	0.25 % Bupivacaine	Morphine i.v.	Reduced VAS at 12 and 24 h no difference in side effects or opioid intake
Borgeat 2000	Major shoulder surgery	Interscalene	0.2 % Ropivacaine	Nicomorphine i.v.	Greater patient satisfaction reduced VAS at 12 and 24 h less nausea and itching
Klein 2000	Open rotator cuff repair	Interscalene	0.2 % Ropivacaine	Morphine i.v.	Reduced VAS at 12 and 24 h less morphine intake
Ilfeld 2002	Elbow day surgery	Interscalene	0.2 % Ropivacaine	Oxycodone p.o.	Reduced VAS at 24 and 48 h less nausea and sedation
Ilfeld 2003	Shoulder day surgery	Interscalene	0.2 % Ropivacaine	Oxycodone p.o.	Reduced VAS at 24 and 48 h less nausea, sedation and itching less opioid intake

incidence of nausea, vomiting itching and sedation (Table 15.1).

The ideal local anesthetic concentration to be used, however, still remains a controversial issue. Various long-acting local anesthetics have been used at different concentrations (Table 15.2). There are no significant differences between the use of 0.2 % ropivacaine and 0.125 % levobupivacaine infusions. Nevertheless, in a recent study, Borgeat et al. have demonstrated that it is possible to use 0.3 % ropivacaine at an infusion rate of 14 ml/h in interscalene CPNB, significantly reducing the intake of opioids (compared to 0.2 % ropivacaine) without increasing the intensity of the motor block or the incidence of side effects.

Shoulder arthroprosthetic surgery is one of the main indications for the placement of a catheter for interscalene continuous infusion; 0.2 % ropivacaine can be used at an infusion rate of 8 ml/h for the first 40–72 h postoperatively. The analgesia obtained with the perineural infusion can be supplemented with NSAIDs, paracetamol or PCA with morphine, if necessary. Even so-called minor shoulder arthroscopic procedures may benefit from a continuous block. The use of a 0.2 % ropivacaine infusion via the interscalene route significantly reduces pain due to movement in the first 24 h.

In traumatized patients, continuous peripheral nerve blocks are an excellent analgesic aid for limb fractures. In the case of injuries to the forearm or hand, a catheter can be placed at the axillary or infraclavicular level, whereas for shoulder, humerus or elbow injuries an interscalene or supraclavicular approach will be necessary. Obviously, the execution of an axillary block will be possible only in patients in whom the injury does not prevent the abduction of the injured limb and, in any event, maintaining a catheter in that site always presents distinct management problems.

In an attempt to enable patients operated on in the day-surgery setting to be discharged early, some authors have proposed CPNB also for the management of postoperative pain at home after shoulder or elbow surgery.

The continuous infusion can be done with an elastomeric system or with a pump for regional PCA.

Table 15.2 Continuous peripheral nerve blocks for upper limb surgery: comparison between different local anesthetic concentrations

Study	Surgery	Catheter positioning	Infusion	Outcome
Casati 2003	Open shoulder surgery	Interscalene	a 0.125 % Levobupivacaine b 0.2 % Ropivacaine	Similar analgesia. Lesser volume infused in the first 24 h (a versus b)
Eroglu 2004	Open shoulder surgery	Interscalene	a 0.15 % Bupivacaine b 0.15 % Ropivacaine	No significant difference between a and b (analgesia, opioid intake, total volume infused, side effects)
Borghi 2006	Open shoulder surgery	Interscalene	a 0.25 % Levobupivacaine b 0.25 % Ropivacaine c 0.4 % Ropivacaine	No significant difference between a and c (analgesia, opioid intake, motor block intensity)
Borgeat 2010	Rotator cuff repair	Interscalene	a 0.3 % Ropivacaine b 0.2 % Ropivacaine	Less opioid intake (a versus b). Better quality sleep (a versus b). No difference in motor block. Intensity or side effects

In continuous infusions, the anesthetist must bear in mind the toxic potential of local anesthetic agents. It has recently been demonstrated by Bleckner et al. that even prolonged infusions of 0.2 % ropivacaine at a rate of 6–14 ml/h lasting more than 120 h in traumatized patients (supraclavicular or infraclavicular block) do not give rise either to dangerous increases in blood concentrations of free ropivacaine (more than 0.6 mg/L) or to local anesthetic systemic toxicity phenomena.

15.4.1 Subacromial or Intra-Articular Infiltration

Since major shoulder surgery is associated with severe pain, there is often a need for high doses of opioids for prolonged periods. For the purposes of reducing the use of these drugs, various different analgesic techniques have been studied, in addition to CPNB. The intra-articular or subacromial approach is particularly easy to use. The surgeon himself, at the end of the surgical procedure, may inject 20–50 ml of local anesthetic in a single administration or may insert an indwelling catheter. This technique was successfully used early in this decade as an alternative to the interscalene block on account of its simplicity and reduced risks. The first studies were conducted in minor surgery (shoulder arthroscopy) and yielded positive results. More recent studies, conducted in major shoulder surgery (open surgery or rotator cuff repair), have failed to show significant advantages compared to placebo, and therefore, the technique has witnessed something of a decline in recent years. Furthermore, attention has recently been drawn to the possibility of direct toxicity of intra-articularly administered local anesthetics on chondrocytes. Fredrickson et al., in a recent meta-analysis of analgesic techniques for shoulder surgery, conclude that, in the light of the latest results, this technique can no longer be recommended.

15.5 Day Surgery: Analgesia at Home

Pain is the main cause of readmission to hospital after surgical operations in the day-surgery setting. Up to one-third of patients undergoing surgery in the day-surgery regimen complain of moderate-to-severe pain within 24 h of the operation. Orthopaedic surgery, in particular, is associated with a higher incidence of severe postoperative pain than the other surgical specialties. In recent years, we have witnessed a substantial rise in orthopaedic surgical procedures performed in the day-surgery setting, as reflected by the numerous difficulties encountered in the management of postoperative pain at home.

The therapeutic options for postoperative pain management in the orthopaedic day-surgery setting consist basically in three techniques: oral analgesics, intra-arterial analgesics or local anesthetics, or CPNBs.

The ideal analgesic treatment for the management of day-surgery postoperative pain must be not only effective but also safe and simple for patients to use autonomously at home. From this point of view, oral analgesia is certainly the most commonly used therapy, particularly NSAIDs, paracetamol and tramadol. Unfortunately, all too often there is as lack of any methodical outcome assessment. One of the main reasons for the inadequate treatment of postoperative pain in day surgery is failure to detect the pain, at rest or due to movement, at the time the patient is discharged and allowed to go home. This leads to an underestimate of the extent of the postoperative pain accompanying a given surgical procedure and, consequently, failure to provide an adequate antalgic treatment. It is therefore necessary to ensure the availability of simple assessment instruments (diary cards) to be filled in by the patient and handed into the facility delivering the medical care at the first check-up visit.

In a study conducted in 120 patients undergoing ambulatory hand surgery, Rawal et al. demonstrated that the postoperative pain lasts for up to 2–3 days after the surgery and that paracetamol (1 g every 6 h) presents an excellent analgesic and tolerability profile, whereas tramadol (100 mg every 6 h), despite being the most effective drug, is associated with a higher incidence of unwanted side effects.

Since home treatment needs to guarantee maximum compliance with the therapy prescribed, and the compliance is related to the simplicity of the dosage regimen, an easy solution may be to use fixed drug combinations to be administered orally, which, with a single administration, meet the needs of a multimodal approach. In hand surgery, the fixed combination of paracetamol + tramadol (325 + 37.5 mg) has been used successfully, with analgesic efficacy equal to tramadol 50 mg and a lower incidence of gastrointestinal and central nervous system side effects. In day surgery, even more than in hospital inpatients, the tolerability profile of an analgesic acquires greater importance, inasmuch as the drug is taken in the home setting. Postoperative nausea and vomiting (PONV) are a major problem in day surgery, where approximately one-third of patients manifest these side effects after being discharged, regardless of the anesthetic and/or antalgic treatment opted for.

In the field of upper extremity surgery, the main limitation of a number of operations in the day-surgery setting is precisely the difficulty encountered in the management of postoperative pain at home, particularly as relating to shoulder surgery. Alongside systemic analgesia, more sophisticated techniques have also been proposed, for which thorough assessment of the patient's cognitive capacities and adequate preoperative information are absolutely mandatory. Continuous peripheral nerve blocks have been proposed by some authors for the postoperative management of arthroscopic shoulder surgeries. Fredrickson, in more than one study, has demonstrated the efficacy and safety of CPNBs in ambulatory surgery, making it possible to significantly reduce home consumption of opioids.

The interscalene use of 0.2 % ropivacaine significantly reduces movement-induced pain in the first 24 h after arthroscopic shoulder surgery. A continuous interscalene block with a posterior approach using 0.2 % ropivacaine has been employed for orthopaedic day surgery on the shoulder, with an improvement in pain relief, a reduced opioid intake, better quality sleep and enhanced patient satisfaction compared to the single-shot block.

Rawal et al. have evaluated the efficacy and safety of patient-controlled regional analgesia (PCRA) at home, using the axillary block in patients undergoing hand surgery (0.125 % ropivacaine or 0.125 % bupivacaine—10 ml boluses). This self-administration approach has proved effective and safe in the domiciliary management of postoperative pain. Adequate patient selection, telephone follow-up and 24 h anesthesia availability are deemed indispensable.

The use of CPNBs in day surgery, however, still remains a controversial issue inasmuch as the postoperative pain as a result of ambulatorial surgery is usually regarded as being of a mild-to-moderate level of intensity and therefore well controlled with oral systemic analgesia in most patients. It would therefore not appear to be appropriate to use invasive and expensive techniques when not strictly necessary, given the availability of simple, low-cost alternative therapies.

Bibliography

Bleckner LL, Bina S, Kwon KH, McKnight G, Drogavich A, Buckenmaier CC (2010) Serum ropivacaine concentrations and systemic local anesthetic toxicity in trauma patients receiving long-term continuous peripheral nerve block catheters. Anesth Analg 110(2):630–634

Borgeat A, Aguirre J, Marquardt M, Mrdjen J, Blumenthal S (2010) Continuous interscalene analgesia with ropivacaine 0.2% versus ropivacaine 0.3% after open rotator cuff repair: the effects on postoperative analgesia and motor function. Anesth Analg 111(6):1543–1547

Borghi B, Facchini F, Agnoletti V, Adduci A, Lambertini A, Marini E et al (2006) Pain relief and motor function during continuous interscalene analgesia after open shoulder surgery: a prospective, randomized, double-blind comparison between levobupivacaine 0.25%, and ropivacaine 0.25 or 0.4%. Eur J Anaesthesiol 23(12):1005–1009

Casati A, Borghi B, Fanelli G, Montone N, Rotini R, Fraschini G et al (2003) Interscalene brachial plexus anesthesia and analgesia for open shoulder surgery: a randomized, double-blinded comparison between levobupivacaine and ropivacaine. Anesth Analg 96(1):253–259

Coluzzi F, Bragazzi L, Di Bussolo E, Pizza G, Mattia C (2011) Determinants of patient satisfaction in postoperative pain management following hand ambulatory day-surgery. Minerva Med 102(3):177–186

Dayer P, Desmeules J, Collart L (1997) Pharmacologie du tramadol. Drugs 53(Suppl. 2):18–24

Eroglu A, Uzunlar H, Sener M, Akinturk Y, Erciyes N (2004) A clinical comparison of equal concentration and volume of ropivacaine and bupivacaine for interscalene brachial plexus anesthesia and analgesia in shoulder surgery. Reg Anesth Pain Med 29(6):539–543

Fredrickson MJ, Ball CM, Dagleish AJ (2010) Analgesic effectiveness of a continuous versus single-injection interscalene block for minor arthroscopic shoulder surgery. Reg Anesth Pain Med 35(1):28–33

Fredrickson MJ, Ball CM, Dagleish AJ (2008) Successful continuous interscalene analgesia for ambulatory shoulder surgery in a private practice setting. Reg Anesth Pain Med 33(2):122–128

Fredrickson MJ, Krishnan S, Chen CY (2010) Postoperative analgesia for shoulder surgery: a critical appraisal and review of current techniques. Anaesthesia 65:608–624

Grass AJ (2005) Patient controlled analgesia. Anesth Analg 101:S44–S61

Ilfeld BM, Enneking FK (2005) Continuous peripheral nerve blocks at home: a review. Anesth Analg 100:1822–1833

Ilfeld BM, Morey TE, Enneking FK (2002) Continuous infraclavicular brachial plexus block for postoperative pain control at home: a randomized, double-blinded, placebo-controlled study. Anesthesiology 96:1297–1304

Mariano ER, Afra R, Loland VJ, Sandhu NS, Bellars RH, Bishop ML et al (2009) Continuous interscalene brachial plexus block via an ultrasound-guided posterior approach: a randomized, triple-masked, placebo-controlled study. Anesth Analg 108(5):1688–1694

Mattia C, Coluzzi F, Sonnino D, Anker-Møller E (2010) Efficacy and safety of fentanyl HCl iontophoretic transdermal system compared with morphine intravenous patient-controlled analgesia for post-operative pain management for patient subgroups. Eur J Anaesthesiol 27(5):433–440

Mattia C, Coluzzi F (2009) What anesthesiologists should know about paracetamol (acetaminophen). Minerva Anestesiol 75(11):644–653

Rawal N, Allvin R, Amilon A, Ohlsson T, Hallén J (2001) Postoperative analgesia at home after ambulatory hand surgery: a controlled comparison of tramadol, metamizol, and paracetamol. Anesth Analg 92(2):347–351

Rawal N, Allvin R, Axelsson K et al (2002) Patient-controlled regional analgesia (PCRA) at home: controlled comparison between bupivacaine and ropivacaine brachial plexus analgesia. Anesthesiology 96:1290–1296

Richman JM, Liu SS, Wong R et al (2006) Does continuous peripheral nerve block provide superior pain control to opioids? A meta-analysis. Anesth Analg 102:248–257

Russon K, Sardesai AM, Ridgway S, Whitear J, Sildown D, Boswell S et al (2006) Postoperative shoulder surgery initiative (POSSI): an interim report of major shoulder surgery as a day case procedure. Br J Anaesth 97(6):869–873

Scott LJ, Perry CM (2000) Tramadol, a review of its use in perioperative pain. Drugs, 60(1):139–176

Toivonen J, Pitko VM, Rosenberg PH (2007) Etoricoxib pre-medication combined with intra-operative subacromial block for pain after arthroscopic acromioplasty. Acta Anaesthesiol Scand 51(3):316–321

Trompeter A, Camilleri G, Narang K, Hauf W, Venn R (2010) Analgesia requirements after interscalene block for shoulder arthroscopy: the 5 days following surgery. Arch Orthop Trauma Surg 130(3):417–421

Stellate Ganglion Block

16

F. Alemanno and B. Westermann

As an appendix to this monographic study on the brachial plexus block techniques performed in order to obtain anesthesia of the upper extremities, we feel it is appropriate to include this chapter on the stellate ganglion (SG) block. This block has no surgical indications, but only postoperative, medical and pain therapy indications.

The most important of these indications are cervicobrachialgia, the prophylaxis of reflex sympathetic dystrophy as a consequence of trauma, Raynaud's disease, Bürger's disease, scalene syndrome, Volkmann's ischaemic contracture, lymphoedema after radical mastectomy with emptying of the axillary fossa, chronic upper limb infection, subacromial bursitis, herpes zoster, and the postoperative management of surgical reconstruction of the neck and face or of upper limb, after catheter removal.

16.1 Anatomy of the Cervical Sympathetic System

The cervical sympathetic system (CSS) is situated between the base of the skull and the seventh cervical vertebra. It continues superiorly with its endocranial part, passing via the carotid canal and continues caudally with its thoracic part.

The cervical sympathetic chain lies above the transverse processes of the cervical vertebrae, separated from the latter by the longus capitis muscle superiorly and by the longus colli muscle inferiorly. The longus capitis muscle extends from the basilar apophysis of the occipital bone and then goes on to divide en route into four small fascicles which insert progressively, with an oblique path inferiorly and laterally, on the anterior tubercles of the transverse processes of the third, fourth, fifth and sixth vertebrae. The longus colli muscle, in a position posterior to that of the longus capitis muscle, is in direct contact with the vertebral column. It divides into three parts: (1) an oblique descending part that runs from the anterior tubercle of the atlas, reaching the anterior tubercles of the transverse processes of the third, fourth, fifth, sixth and seventh cervical vertebrae; (2) an oblique ascending part that runs from the bodies of the second and third thoracic vertebrae, reaching the anterior tubercles of the fourth and fifth cervical vertebrae via an oblique path travelling upwards and laterally; and (3) a longitudinal part, in a medial position in relation to the other two, which runs from the anterior tubercle of the atlas and from the crest of the epistropheus, inserting on the bodies of the last four cervical vertebrae and the first three thoracic vertebrae. Both muscles are invested by the deep cervical fascia.

F. Alemanno (✉)
Institute of Anesthesiology, Resuscitation and Pain Therapy, University of Verona, Verona, Italy
e-mail: fernando@alemannobpb.it

B. Westermann
Consultant Anesthesiologist, Division of Anesthesiology and Pain Medicine, Jeroen Bosch Ziekenhuis, Hertogenbosch, The Netherlands

Thus, the CSS adheres to this fascia which splits and thereby endows the apparatus with a tenuous anterior investing layer.

Along the CSS are situated three ganglia named according to the position they occupy—the superior cervical ganglion, the middle cervical ganglion and the inferior cervical ganglion. The latter, if fused with the first thoracic ganglion is called the stellate ganglion (SG).

The superior cervical ganglion is by far the largest of the three, measuring 2–4 cm in length and 5–7 mm in width and even reaching half a centimetre in thickness. It is oval-shaped, oblong and cranio-caudally oriented; it adheres, at the level of the transverse processes of the second and third cervical vertebrae, to the greater rectus muscle of the head. It stems from the fusion of the first four cervical ganglia and this is sometimes shown by the presence of symmetrical notches along its longitudinal profile.

The middle cervical ganglion, sometimes absent, is the smallest of the three. It is to be found at the level of the transverse processes of C5 and C6, crossed by the thyroid artery. Its size does not exceed one quarter of that of the superior cervical ganglion.

The inferior cervical ganglion is larger than the middle cervical ganglion, but does not reach one centimetre in length and half a centimetre in thickness. It is just a little larger if fused with the first thoracic ganglion. It lies on the transverse process of C7 or, when it is fused with the first thoracic ganglion (80 % of cases), on the first costovertebral joint. In this case, it is to be found at a point corresponding to the angle, in the form of a 'V' on its side, open-ended medially, formed by the subclavian artery together with the vertebral artery, and may be star-shaped (hence the name 'stellate ganglion') or half-moon-shaped with the concave portion embracing the neck of the first rib. The ganglion is surrounded by adipose areolar tissue which facilitates the spread of the anesthetic solution.

The most important anatomical relationship (to be avoided, for our purposes) is with the neurovascular bundle of the neck (carotid artery, internal jugular vein, vagus nerve). Cranially, the internal carotid artery is antero-medial to the sympathetic chain, while the jugular vein and vagus nerve are fairly lateral. In the midportion of the neck, the common carotid artery is slightly medial in relation to the sympathetic chain, while the jugular vein and vagus nerve are anterior to it. In the lower part of the neck, the sympathetic chain shifts laterally, passing behind the subclavian artery, while remaining medial to the point of origin of the vertebral artery. The inferior cervical ganglion is in relation to the pleural dome which protrudes above the first rib, particularly on the right, by as much even as 2–2.5 cm; on the right, the pleural dome is closer to the ganglion, whereas on the left it is at a distance of one or two cm from it. It is in relation to the apex of the lung and with the pleural suspensory apparatus, composed of fibromuscular fascial bands which run from the transverse process of C7 and insert on the pleural dome (Zuckerkandl's organ).

The cervical sympathetic chain in the more superficial planes is in relation to the omohyoid muscle which crosses it lateromedially and downwards, with the middle cervical fascia and, lastly, with the muscular plane consisting in the sternocleidomastoid muscle. It is from the posterior border of this muscle that the anesthetist has the most direct access route for reaching the sympathetic chain, even though the simplest access technique for the SG block is the 'two-finger' technique applied at the level of the anterior border of the muscle.

16.2 Stellate Ganglion Block: Anterior Approach (Two-Finger Technique)

16.2.1 Patient Position

Supine without a pillow, with the arms extended alongside the body, and with the head and neck hyperextended backwards in such a way as to straighten the oesophagus which projects slightly beyond the tracheal profile on the left.

16.2.2 Landmarks

From the mid-point of the jugulum the anesthetist measures a distance of 4 cm laterally and 4 cm cranially. In practice, 4 cm corresponds to the transverse width of two fingers. If you are operating from the right-hand side, the pad of the middle finger of the right hand is placed on the jugulum with the index finger immediately alongside it. The same two fingers of the left hand are placed at right angles to the first two in such a way that the corners of the fingernails of the two index fingers are touching one another. An X is marked on the skin of the neck at the point corresponding to the corner of the nail of the left middle finger on the internal border of the sternocleidomastoid muscle.(Fig. 16.1).

After thorough disinfection with a disinfectant based on alcoholic chlorhexidine or polyvinylpyrrolidone-iodine, wait for the disinfectant to dry (the time it takes to act). A 1.6-cm-long 25-G needle is used to induce a skin wheal with 1 ml of local anesthetic, at the point marked X. The index and middle fingers of the left hand will now delimit the X above and below it, respectively, along the medial border of the sternocleidomastoid muscle. A 10-ml syringe filled with local anesthetic with a 30-mm 23-G needle is gripped in the right hand. The anesthetist exerts a certain amount of pressure with the two fingers of the left hand in an attempt to distance the sternocleidomastoid muscle from the trachea, and with it the neurovascular bundle. At the end of this manoeuvre, the anesthetist should feel the pulsation of the common carotid artery on the pads of the two fingers (but not on the fingertips!). The left hand will remain fixed in this position throughout the duration of the block. The 30-mm needle connected to the 10-ml syringe is now inserted slowly and advanced via the skin wheal, normally to the skin and perpendicularly to the plane of the bed, until it reaches the transverse process of C7 (Fig. 16.2).

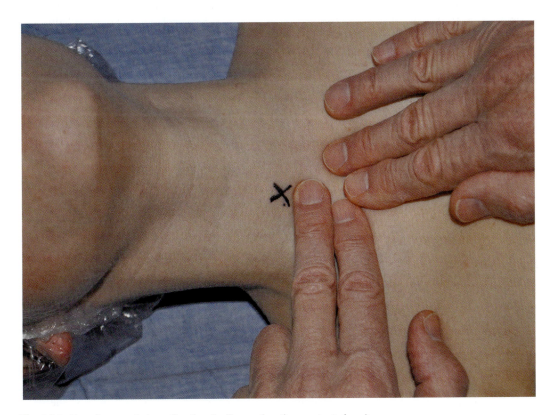

Fig. 16.1 Two-finger technique. Landmarks (for explanation see text above)

The insertion depth of the needle varies according to the patient's structure and the downward pressure that needs to be exerted with the fingers in order to feel the pulsation of the carotid artery on the finger pads. In any event, in our experience, a 30-mm needle is more than sufficient for reaching the target even in the most robust patients. If the needle should fail to make contact with the bone, it will have to be retracted and reinserted firstly more medially, then more cranially, and finally more caudally until contact is achieved. Normally, however, not all these manoeuvres will be necessary.

Once the needle has made contact with the bone of the transverse process, it is retracted 5 mm to avoid a subperiosteal injection or an injection into the longus colli muscle (Fig. 16.3).

After carefully aspirating a first time and then a second time after rotating the syringe to check on failed aspiration due to a wall-obstructed bevel, 1 ml of anesthetic solution is injected and after 30 s, if there is no adverse reaction, another 1 ml is injected, with aspiration at intervals, again waiting for 30 s before injecting the entire solution. The need for caution with the initial mini doses is due to the possibility that blood may not be aspirated into the syringe for two reasons: That is, the bevel of the needle may be up against the vessel wall, or the vertebral artery (especially in young patients) is subject to spasm as a result of puncture. The injection, albeit of small amounts of anesthetic, into the vertebral artery gives rise to dizziness, nausea and blurred vision, but also loss of consciousness with the falling back of the tongue.

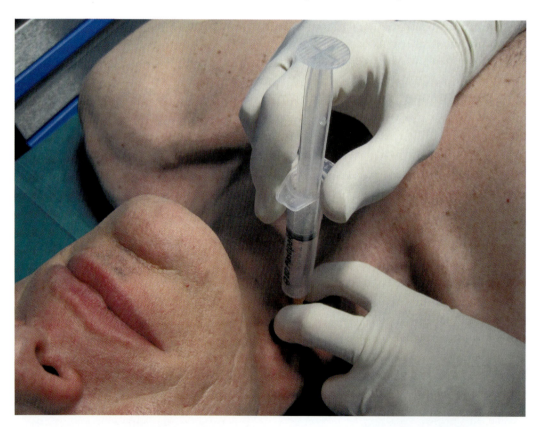

Fig. 16.2 The *index* and *middle fingers* of the left hand, situated, respectively, *above* and *below* the X marking the transverse process of C6 grip the sternocleidomastoid muscle in order to shift the carotid neurovascular bundle to the point where the pulsation of the carotid artery is felt on the finger pads. In this case, a 16-mm 25-G needle was sufficient to reach the periosteum of the transverse process, thanks to the pressure exerted by the two fingers towards the plane of the bed

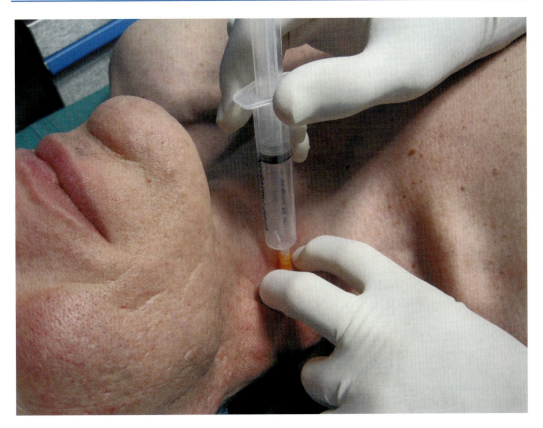

Fig. 16.3 After making contact with the bone, the needle is retracted 5 mm and after proper aspiration, 1 ml of anesthetic solution is injected, followed 30 s later by another 1 ml and after a further 30 s by the rest of the solution in small boluses at additional aspiration intervals

A second reason for caution makes it advisable to perform the block at the level of C6 in order to stay away as far as possible from the pleura. Even injecting as small an amount as 10 ml of anesthetic solution at this level is sufficient to reach the SG, particularly if, once the block has been performed, the patient is made to assume the reclining 'beach-chair' position, which favours the caudal flow of the anesthetic bolus along the cleavage plane of the deep cervical fascia.

The anesthetic agents to be used are those endowed with a long duration of action (ropivacaine or levobupivacaine) because, if the indication is of the medical or antalgic type, than what is wanted is that the effect should be as long as possible. No doubt it is advisable to choose the least concentrated formulations (0.2 % for ropivacaine and 0.25 % for levobupivacaine) in order to avoid some root of the brachial plexus being anesthetized with concern and discomfort on the part of the patient as a result. In any case, the small amyelinic C fibres of the sympathetic innervation chain will be more than amply anesthetized even by a relatively weak solution.

16.2.3 Adjuvants

As adjuvants, our limited experience confined to the therapy of cervicobrachialgia refers exclusively to two molecules, clonidine and buprenorphine. We adopted clonidine after reading the article by Singelyn et al. published in 1992 and buprenorphine as suggested by Prof. Günther

Sprotte, Director of the Pain Therapy Center of the University of Würzburg, Germany, in 1997. The doses we use are 30 mcg of clonidine (1/5 of a 150-mcg ampoule) or 0.03 mg of buprenorphine (1/10 of a 0.3-mg ampoule). The two adjuvants can also be used in combination, amongst other things because they have completely different mechanisms of action, α_2-agonist and mu-agonist, respectively. In any event, at these dosages, they have practically no effect at the systemic level, but yield spectacular results when compared to the use of the local anesthetic alone. Ketamine at the dosage of 0.5 mg/kg may be used for vascular or neuropathic pain.

16.3 Ultrasound-Guided Stellate Ganglion Block

As we have already seen, the SG block can be performed on the basis of anatomical landmark. It may be also performed with the aid of fluoroscopic guidance or computed axial tomography.

With the increasingly widespread use of ultrasonography in the field of regional anesthesia, there is now growing interest in its use and applications in pain therapy. The first ultrasound-guided SG block was performed by Kapral et al. in 1995.

16.3.1 Anatomical Considerations (repetita iuvant)

As we have already said, the cervical sympathetic chain is composed of the superior, middle and inferior ganglia. In 80 % of the population, the inferior cervical ganglion is fused with the first thoracic ganglion, thus giving rise to the cervicothoracic ganglion or SG. The SG measures approximately 2.5 cm in length and 1 cm in width, with an anteroposterior diameter of approximately 0.5 cm.

In the eventuality that the inferior cervical ganglion and the first thoracic ganglion are not fused, the inferior cervical ganglion is located anteriorly to the tubercle of C7, whereas the first thoracic ganglion rests on the neck of the first rib. Consequently, at the level of C6, it is above all the middle cervical ganglion that is blocked, and the SG is blocked if the drug extends caudad towards the level of T1.

The fasciae of the neck are important structures which affect the distribution of anesthetic agents and the complications that may arise. These sheaths are divided as follows: the superficial cervical fascia which invests the sternocleidomastoid and trapezius muscles; the middle or paratracheal cervical fascia which invests the thyroid gland and trachea; and the deep (or prevertebral) cervical fascia which invests the cervical column together with the erector spinae muscles of the neck, the scalene muscles, the longus colli muscle and the chain of the CSS. The prevertebral (or deep cervical) fascia at the level of the sympathetic chain splits to envelop it. The grey rami communicantes penetrate anteriorly into the longus colli muscle before reaching the cervical nerves. The postganglionic grey rami emerge from the SG and reach the cervical nerves 7 and 8 and the first thoracic nerve for the sympathetic innervation of the upper limb. The preganglionic fibres of the head and neck travel craniad towards the middle and superior cervical ganglia via the cervical sympathetic chain.

The SG is located medially to the scalene muscles, and laterally to the longus colli muscle, oesophagus, trachea and recurrent nerve. It is located anteriorly to the cervical vertebral transverse processes, superiorly to the subclavian artery and the surface of the pleura dome and posteriorly to the vertebral vessels at the level of C7 (an additional reason for performing the block at the level of C6).

16.3.2 Sonoanatomy

The structures that need to be visualized in an ultrasound-guided SG block are the following:
1. The vessels contained in the carotid neurovascular bundle.

The common carotid artery and the internal jugular vein are easily recognizable within the sheath during ultrasound scanning and constitute

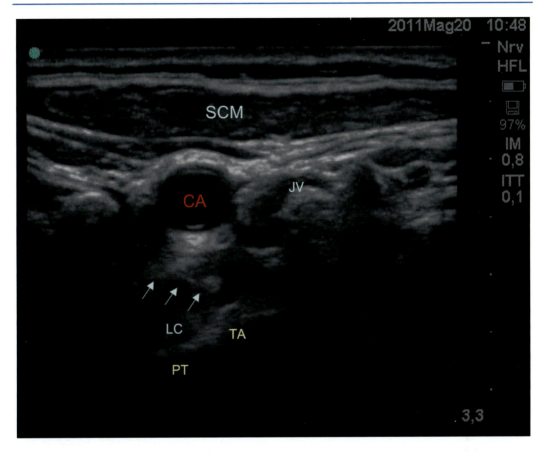

Fig. 16.4 Carotid artery (*CA*) with, on the right, the internal jugular vein (*JV*) partially crushed by pressure on the probe; *SCM* sternocleidomastoid muscle; *LC* longus colli muscle and deep cervical fascia, indicated by the *arrows*; *PT* transverse process; *TA* anterior tubercle

important landmarks. The vein is compressible (beware!) and the use of echo-colour-Doppler helps to distinguish the vessels (Fig. 16.4).

2. The vertebral artery.

This artery enters the foramen of the transverse process of C6 in 90 % of patients. In the remaining 10 % of cases, on the other hand, it is exposed to the passage of the needle because it fails to perforate C6, anatomically missing the transverse process foramen.

3. The inferior thyroid artery.

This artery can be seen more laterally than the vertebral artery where it crosses the anterior fascia of the longus colli muscle. Its course may interfere with the passage of the needle between the carotid artery and the trachea.

4. The prevertebral (or deep cervical fascia).

In the ultrasound view, a fascia is distinguished as a hyperechoic border around the muscles. In the case of the SG block, one can discern that portion of the prevertebral fascia that lies on the surface of the longus colli muscle.

5. The longus colli muscle.

6. The anterior tubercle of the transverse process of vertebra C6.

Vertebra C6 has a transverse process with an anterior and a posterior tubercle. This distinguishes it from the transverse process of vertebra C7 which lacks the anterior tubercle and which, in an axial scan, presents the so-called thumbs up appearance.

7. The thyroid gland.

The superior pole of the thyroid gland coincides with the transverse plane of C6.

8. The trachea and oesophagus.

These are important landmarks. The oesophagus may be damaged during a left SG block. Asking the patient to swallow during the procedure helps to identify the anatomical structure by watching the movement. At this level, the oesophagus frequently protrudes to the left in relation to the tracheal profile and is therefore at greater risk of injury.

The cervical sympathetic trunk is invested by the splitting of the prevertebral fascia, but the two structures prove ultrasonographically indistinguishable. In some patients, on the other hand, the ganglion and the prevertebral fascia can be distinguished at the level of the middle cervical ganglion.

In an ultrasound-guided SG block, the needle is not directed towards the SG itself; what is blocked is the cervical sympathetic chain with its grey rami communicantes at the level of C6. Effectively speaking, it would be more correct to call it a cervical sympathetic block. The cervical sympathetic chain is located within the prevertebral fascia, and the grey rami communicantes penetrate anteriorly into the longus colli muscle. For this reason, the SG block at the level of C6 can be performed by injecting the anesthetic just in front of the longus colli muscle after passing through the prevertebral fascia (subfascial approach).

16.3.3 Ultrasound-Guided Stellate Ganglion Block Technique

The patient is in the supine position with the neck slightly hyperextended in order to straighten the oesophageal profile and with the mouth half open in order to relax the muscles of the neck. Most anesthetists use the 'in-plane' approach but the 'out-of-plane' approach is also possible. Others prefer to perform the block with the patient in the lateral decubitus position, using the 'in-plane' approach.

After adequate sterile preparation of the field and probe, a high-frequency linear probe (6–13 MHz) is rested against the side of the neck at the level of C6 on the cricoid line (Fig. 16.5a, Fig. 16.6a), in order to be able to visualize the relevant anatomical structures which are the transverse process of C6, the longus colli muscle, the prevertebral fascia, the vessels and the thyroid gland.

It is advisable to perform an echo-colour-Doppler pre-scan, because it enables you to plan the direction and path of the needle. In this way, the puncturing of important structures such as the inferior thyroid artery and the oesophagus is avoided. Narouze et al. advise following the course of the inferior thyroid artery using a short-axis view with echo-colour-Doppler, then moving the transducer slightly caudad or craniad until the artery is no longer in the path of the needle on its way to the cervical sympathetic chain. If these structures should make it difficult to insert the needle between the trachea and the carotid artery, the anesthetist may choose to introduce the needle laterally in relation to the carotid artery. The needle normally used is a 35-mm 24-G Teflon-coated needle, which we ourselves prefer for reasons of ultrasound visibility.

The needle tip is directed towards the prevertebral fascia at the point where it invests the longus colli muscle and is positioned beyond the fascia (subfascial approach). The injection of the anesthetic—total amount 7 ml—is performed under ultrasound guidance, observing the spread between the longus colli muscle and the fascia, with dislocation of the latter. The absence of any such spread of the drug may indicate an intravascular injection.

If the needle is inserted laterally in relation to the probe (Fig. 16.5a), it must be directed between the carotid artery and the tip of the anterior tubercle of C6, towards the longus colli muscle in such a way as to avoid touching the C6 nerve root (Fig. 16.5b, Fig. 16.6b).

The internal jugular vein is identified by modifying the pressure of the probe. Puncturing of the vein is avoided by applying a slight amount of transverse pressure.

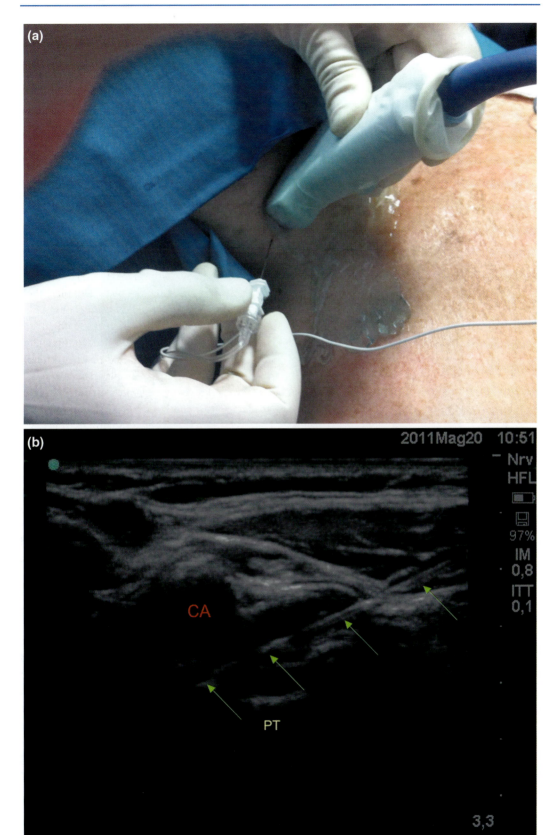

Fig. 16.5 Ultrasound-guided stellate ganglion block: in plane approach

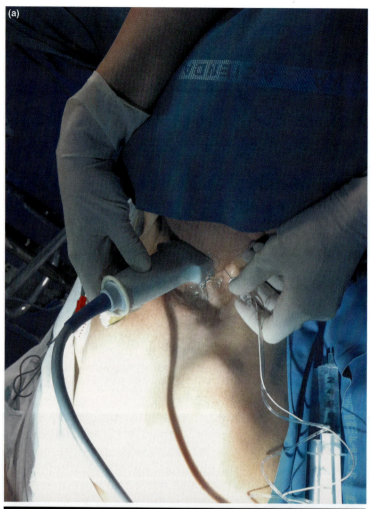
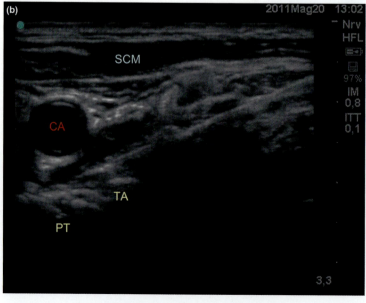

◀ **Fig. 16.6 a** Block of the right stellate ganglion. With the probe positioned on the cricoid line, the needle is inserted with an 'in-plane' lateral approach. **b** *SCM* sternocleidomastoid muscle; *CA* carotid artery; *PT* transverse process of C6; *TA* anterior tubercle. It may be noted that the insertion of the needle, between the anterior tubercle and the carotid article, is halted at the level of the longus colli muscle. Also worthy of note is the flattening in of the internal jugular vein due to the pressure of the probe

16.3.4 Complications and Other Side Effects

Claude Bernard-Horner Syndrome

This is the first thing you see; indeed, it has to be the first thing you see. Rather than a complication, it may be considered a side effect which normally regresses within 24 h and represents the most tangible sign that the block has been successful. Blockade of the CSS severs the afferences to the ciliary ganglion, which explains the miosis. The drooping of the eyelids, on the other hand, is due to blockade of the sympathetic superior tarsal nerve that innervates the smooth muscle fibres of the tarsus (the fibroelastic lamina endowed with Muller's tarsal muscles), thus giving rise not so much to ptosis as to relaxation of the eyelids and therefore narrowing of the palpebral rim. The same explanation also applies with regard to enophthalmos. Tenon's capsule, which is attached to the circumference of the orbit and envelops the eyeball in the manner of a truncated cone, is endowed with smooth muscle fibres, innervated by the sympathetic system, that confer a more or less constant tone, holding the eyeball in the right position. In the case of sympathetic blockade, the muscle fibres are relaxed, and therefore, the eyeball retracts slightly into the orbit—enophthalmos.

Intravascular Injection

The intravascular injection of local anesthetic causes an immediate cerebral toxicity with loss of consciousness, apnoea, hypotension and convulsions. The landmark for positioning the needle in the classic technique is the anterior tubercle of the transverse process of C6 (Chassaignac's tubercle). The cranio-caudal size of the tubercle is variable and may be as little as 6 mm. In this case, the needle may easily fail to make contact with the tubercle, thus increasing the risk of puncture of the vertebral artery or the C6 nerve root, or the risk of penetrating into the intervertebral foramen, or into the epidural or subarachnoid space. Even if contact with the tubercle is made, the vertebral artery may be at risk in the 10 % of cases in which the artery does not perforate the transverse process of C6 but becomes intertransverse from C5 upwards. Whereas, with the fluoroscopy-guided technique, an intravascular injection is only discovered after puncturing the artery, the ultrasound-guided technique permits visual monitoring of the needle, the adjacent structures and the spread of local anesthetic in real time.

The second structure responsible for intravascular injection is the inferior thyroid artery. Whereas, with the classic technique, there is no way of visualizing it directly, the ultrasound-guided technique enables the anesthetist to avoid approaching it too closely with the needle.

A third possible cause of intravascular injection has to do with the internal jugular vein if excessive pressure is applied to the ultrasound probe, such as to render the vein invisible. Pressure of the probe such that, impinging the needle upon the inner wall of the vessel, may make it impossible to detect the flow of blood into the syringe after aspiration, while the injection itself would than tend to shift the needle away from the vessel wall (previously sucked in) with the consequent introduction of a bolus of anesthetic into a central vein.

Oesophageal Injuries

The oesophagus is often shifted to the left in relation to the midline and rests on the middle portion of the transverse process. An oesophageal injury may occur, especially in patients with an undiagnosed Zenker diverticulum and may present clinically with a 'foreign body sensation'. The most serious outcome consists in mediastinitis. Whereas, with the classic technique, based on surface landmarks, oesophageal injury can only be prevented by making the patient hyperextend the neck, with the ultrasound-guided technique the oesophagus can be visualized.

Haematoma Formation

In the article by Kapral et al., the incidence of haematoma as a result of SG block was 25 % in the group undergoing the classic technique (based on the cutaneous landmarks), while no case of haematoma occurred in the group undergoing the ultrasound-guided technique. The formation of a retropharyngeal haematoma after a SG block manifests itself with pain in the neck, an increase in the circumference of the neck, hoarseness or alteration of the voice, and dyspnoea to the point of acute airways obstruction. This latter complication requires emergency orotracheal intubation which may be impossible due to oedema and the displacement of the trachea, requiring the use of videolaryngoscopy or, in extreme cases, an emergency tracheotomy.

Hoarseness

The cause is temporary paralysis of the recurrent nerve. With the subfascial injection of the anesthetic at the level of C6, compared to the classic paratracheal technique, it may be assumed that the drug spreads more caudad, thus obtaining a better sympathetic block of the upper limb and a lower incidence of hoarseness caused by the involvement of the recurrent nerve when the anesthetic is injected suprafascially and paratracheally, in which case the anesthetic spreads into the space between the thyroid gland and the trachea where the recurrent nerve is situated. According to Urmey, the hoarseness is not always caused by blockade of the recurrent nerve, but also by hyperemia and unilateral edema of the vocal cords (true and false) and of the hemiglottis as a whole, with consequent hoarseness and/or bitonal voice.

Cardiac Arrest

The aetiology of cardiac arrest after a SG block comprises both a toxic reaction to the local anesthetic and blockade of the sinus node, described in the classic right paratracheal SG block, whereas, on the left, it may be attributable to blockade of the sympathetic cardiac accelerator nerves (we should not forget that the embryonal position of the heart is left laterocervical and that it subsequently migrates into the thorax). The incidence of cardiac arrest during SG block complications is quite low. The block must be performed only in the presence of all the material necessary for handling an emergency, including the immediate possibility of infusing a 20 % lipid emulsion.

16.3.5 Epilogue

The use of ultrasound guidance during a block of the cervical sympathetic chain makes it possible to identify important anatomical structures such as the oesophagus and the vessels with their normal or aberrant course. The possibility of using echo-colour-Doppler enables the anesthetist to choose the safest approach for the path of the needle ('in plane' or 'out of plane', paratracheal or lateral) according to the patient's anatomical situation. Moreover, its application avoids the use of X-rays, as in fluoroscopy or CAT scans, and of contrast medium; it does not require bulky equipment or collaboration with the radiology department.

In order to achieve the maximum possible reduction in the incidence of complications (haematomas, intravascular injection), it is advisable to perform pre-scanning with echo-colour-Doppler, which makes it possible both to avoid the penetration of the needle into the vessels and to monitor the injection and spread of the local anesthetic.

As things stand at present, there is no evidence that the echo-guided SG block technique is superior to the classic technique. Above all, numerous anesthesiology services do not have adequate ultrasound equipment (but may have an ultrasonograph already stored away somewhere in the attic by the radiologists), which complicates rather than facilitating the procedure, giving the impression that one is 'entering into the misty harbour' where one is faced with the need somehow to distinguish, as Alain Borgeat has said, between 'hyper-hypoechoic holes in a foggy background'.

In the near future, we will have ultrasonographs endowed with increasingly enhanced resolution, capable of providing us with 3D images and an increasingly accurate visualization of the patient's anatomy.

Bibliography

Bonica JJ (1966) Il Dolore. Vallardi Editore, Milano

Borgeat A (2009) Axillary brachial plexus block: neurostimulation technique Pro/Con ultrasound guided technique. ASRA NEWS, pp 6–9

Charbonneau H, Marcou TA, Mazoit JX, Zetlaoui PJ, Benhamou D (2009) Early use of lipid emulsion to treat incipient mepivacaine intoxication. Reg Anesth Pain Med 34:277–278

Chiarugi G, Bucciante L (1972) Istituzioni di anatomia dell'uomo. Vallardi Editore, Mlano

Gnaho A, Erieuz S, Gentili M (2009) Cardiac arrest during an ultrasound-guided sciatic nerve block combined with nerve stimulation. Reg Anesth Pain Med 34:278

Goebel A, Lawson A, Allen S, Glynn C (2008) Buprenorphine injection to the stellate ganglion in the treatment of upper body chronic pain syndromes. Eur J Pain 12:266–74

Gofeld M, Bhatia A, Abbas S, Ganapathy S, Johnson M (2009) Development and validation of a new technique for ultrasound-guided stellate ganglion block. Reg Anesth Pain Med 34:475–479

Higa K, Hirata K, Nitahara K, Shono S (2006) Retropharyngeal hematoma after stellate ganglion block. Anaesthesiology 105:1238–1245

Ihnatsenka B, Boezaart A (2010) Applied sonoanatomy of the posterior triangle of the neck. Int J Shoulder Surg 4(3):63–74

Kapral S, Krafft P, Gosch M, Fleischmann D, Weinstabl C (1995) Ultrasound imaging for stellate ganglion block: direct visualisation of puncture site and local anesthetic spread: a pilot study. Reg Anesth 20:323–328

Kulkarni KR, Kadam AI, Namarni IJ (2010) Efficacy of stellate ganglion block with an adjuvant ketamine for peripheral vascular disease of the upper limbs. Indian J Anesth 54:546–551

Moore DC (1969) Anestesia regionale. Piccin Editore, Padova

Narouze S, Vydyanathan A, Patel N (2007) Ultrasound-guided stellate ganglion block successfully prevented esophageal puncture. Pain Phys 10:747–752

Narouze S (2009) Beware of the "serpentine" inferior thyroid artery while performing stellate ganglion block. Anaest Analg 109:289–290

Peng P, Narouze S (2010) How I Do it–Stellate ganglion block. ASRA News, pp 16–18

Peng PWH, Narouze S (2009) Ultrasound-guided interventional procedures in pain medicine: a review of anatomy, sonoanatomy, and procedures. Part 1: nonaxial structures. Reg Anesth Pain Med 34:458–474

Rastogi S, Tripathi S (2010) Cardiac arrest following stellate ganglion block performed under ultrasound guidance. Anestesia 65:1042

Shibata Y, Fujiwara Y, Komatsu T (2007) A new approach of ultrasound-guided stellate ganglion block. Anaesth Analg 105:550–551

Singelyn FJ, Dangoisse M, Bartholomée S, Gouverneur JM (1992) Adding clonidine to mepivacaine prolongs the duration of anaesthesia and analgesia after axillary brachial plexus block. Reg Anesth 17:148–150

Sonsino DH, Fischler M (2009) Immediate intravenous lipid infusion in the successful resuscitation of ropivacaine-induced cardiac arrest after infraclavicular brachial plexus block. Reg Anesth Pain Med 34:276–277

Sunder RA, Toshnival G, Dureja GP (2008) Ketamine as an adjuvant in sympathetic blocks for management of central sensitivation following peripheral nerve injury. J Brachial Plexus Peripher Nerve Inj 3:22

Testut L (1943) Anatomia umana, libro sesto, Sistema nervoso periferico. UTET, Torino

Urmey W (2000) Tecniche di anestesia loco-regionale e di terapia antalgica. Promo Leader Service Editore, Firenze, Settembre

Viel EJ, Eledjam JJ, de la Coussaye J, D'Athis F (1989) Brachial plexus block with opioids for postoperative pain relief: comparison between buprenorphine and morphine. Reg Anesth 14:274–278

Printing and Binding: Stürtz GmbH, Würzburg